The heirs of Jethro Kloss—Promise Kloss Moffett, Eden Kloss, and Doris Gardiner—authorize this as the only Kloss Family Edition of BACK TO EDEN. All have worked through the years to insure its continuation in its complete, authentic form.

JETHRO KLOSS

BACK to EDEN

by

Jethro Kloss

American herbs for pleasure and health;
natural nutrition with recipes
and instruction for living the Edenic life

Published and Distributed by

WOODBRIDGE PRESS PUBLISHING COMPANY
Post Office Box 6189
Santa Barbara, California 93111

Library of Congress Catalog Card Number: 75-585

International Standard Book Number:
Hard Cover, 0-912800-33-X
Soft Cover, 0-912800-12-7

Published simultaneously in the United States and Canada

Printed in the United States of America

Fifth Edition

FOREWORD

It is with godly fear and much humility that I undertake the task of writing this book as I am in no sense of the word a writer. I am sending forth this book for the purpose of helping humanity and giving courage to those who may have thought their cases hopeless. My prayer is that God may make this book a blessing to many.

I wish to present the truth in a practical manner, to help the human family, and to prevent my fellow men from becoming slaves to erroneous ideas, so that mothers and fathers may better care for their families.

This book contains tried, safe, and inexpensive remedies for the prevention of disease and sickness, remedies which are the result of my own practical experience of nearly forty years.

Many recipes are given herein that are not found elsewhere. They are inexpensive and can be made in any home. They contain all the elements the system requires, are very palatable when properly prepared. Millions today who have little food would be better able to keep body and soul together if they knew which foods to eat that really sustain life. There has been a growing demand for many years for a practical knowledge of non-poisonous herbs.

Actual facts and the true healing art is given in this book as handed down by physicians from Hippocrates, who was called "the father of medical literature," until 1541, when Hohemhein started the practice of using chemicals, and the idea that the human body could be purified chemically, as were the metals at Tyrol, where he worked after giving up his medical profession.

I wish to bring to the notice of the general public the untold blessings which our Heavenly Father has provided for all the world. It can be truly said, "My people are destroyed for lack of knowledge." Hosea 4:6. A lack of knowledge based on truth is accountable for much of the untold sufferings and miseries of humanity. The advice contained in this book, if heeded, will save money, suffering, and often premature death.

From practical experience, I explain how to be in health, mentally and physically. No matter how many germs get into the body, if the blood stream is clean and the blood corpuscles are in a healthy condition, you will be safe. Everyone comes in contact with many kinds of germs, but these organisms will not harm you or cause sickness and death, unless they have a place in which to propagate themselves.

Many who violate the laws of health are ignorant of the relation of the laws of living (eating, drinking, and working) to their health. Until they have some kind of sickness or illness, they do not realize that their condition is caused by violating the laws of nature and health. If then they would resort to simple means, and follow the simple laws of health that they have been neglecting— proper diet, use of pure water, fresh air, sunshine, rest, and nature's remedies, herbs, etc., nature would restore the body to its original health. Had nature been supplied with them all the time, the body would always be in good condition. When a course such as is outlined above is taken, patients will generally recover without being weakened.

There is a wonderful science in nature, in trees, herbs, roots, and flowers, which man has never yet fathomed.

All the science of ancient Egypt when it was in its glory, and the science of ancient Babylon when it was at its height, the wisdom of Solomon when he lived in obedience to God, and the science and knowledge of this enlightened age as taught in the colleges and universities, does not equal the science in nature, and yet it is little understood by the most intelligent people.

God has provided a remedy for every disease that might afflict us. Satan cannot afflict anyone with any disease for which God has not provided a remedy. Our Creator foresaw the wretched condition of mankind in these days, and made provision in Nature for all the ills of man.

If our scientists and medical colleges would put forth the same effort in finding the virtues in the "true remedies" as found in nature for the use of the human race, then poisonous drugs and chemicals would be eliminated and sickness would be rare indeed. If they would make use of only these remedies that God has given for the "service of man" it would bring an untold blessing to the world.

In these distressing days, the use of a simple natural diet would prevent much suffering and save money. The most important subject for people to study, should be: How can we live our allotted time without suffering? God has surely made this possible.

REVOLUTIONIZE THE COMMON MANNER OF LIVING, EATING, AND DRINKING, AND YOU WILL HAVE A HAPPIER AND HEALTHIER PEOPLE.

Recently a Chicago firm advertised very extensively some little tablets, claiming that they contained all the elements needed by the body, and were prepared by scientifically combining foods. The most learned scientists who ever lived on this earth cannot separate natural foods and then combine them in a better manner than nature herself has prepared them.

The fundamental principle of true healing consists of a return to natural habits of living.

Coming back to God's original plan for maintaining

health, restoring the sick, miraculous truths which have been covered up by commercial graft and tradition and neglect are being uncovered by honest men and women and brought to the front; miraculous things are in the Bible and Nature. The Creator of this universe made man in the beginning out of the ground. The different properties which are found in the earth are found in man, and the fruits, grains, nuts, and vegetables contain the same elements which are in the earth, and in man. When these fruits, grains, nuts, and vegetables are eaten in their natural state and not perverted and robbed of their life-giving properties in their preparation, health, beauty, and happiness will be the sure reward. The scripture which says, "My people are destroyed for lack of knowledge," is surely being fulfilled. But our loving heavenly Father is looking down and he, seeing the untold suffering and wretchedness, has made provision that the use of these things which He has provided will surely bring relief. Read, in this book, of the wonderful properties which are in trees, herbs, flowers and roots, and leaves of the trees, which the Holy Book says are for our medicine. Ezek. 47:12. There are also wonderful life-giving properties in fruit, if properly eaten, and not combined with other foods, the combination of which causes fermentation and other disturbances and thus destroys their life-giving properties.

If symptoms in any illness are persistent or severe, or if there is any reason whatsoever for believing that the services of a physician are essential to the patient's well-being, professional help should be sought without delay.

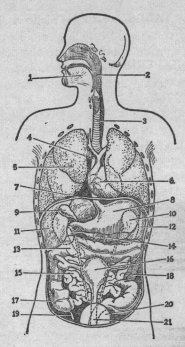

THE HUMAN BODY

1. Tongue
2. Pharynx or throat
3. Trachea or windpipe
4. Esophagus
5. Lung
6. Heart
7. Diaphragm
8. Stomach
9. Gall bladder
10. Kidney
11. Liver

12. Spleen
13. Colon
14. Pancreas
15. Small intestine
16. Uterus
17. Cecum
18. Descending colon
19. Appendix
20. Bladder — urinary
21. Sigmoid

TABLE OF CONTENTS

*An Intimate, Personal Account
by his daughter . . .*

Jethro Kloss

—the Man and the Legend

By Promise Kloss Moffett

The wisdom of Jethro Kloss on questions of health and natural living has long since made him a legendary figure among those who choose this approach to the unspoiled, good life.

Hundreds of thousands of persons have testified to their interest in his remarkable skills and insights in diet and in herbal medicine and other forms of natural healing.

A lifetime of wide-ranging experience, expressed in simple, lay terms, has been compressed in this classic work, BACK TO EDEN—cherished as a "bible" by those wishing to return to the natural principles of good health and peace of mind intended for mankind by a benevolent Creator.

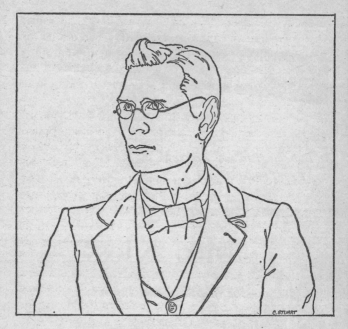

Jethro Kloss in his early years of teaching and healing.

Since it was first published more than thirty years ago, this book has become virtually the standard in its field and it is selling far faster today than ever before.

Who was Jethro Kloss? How did he acquire such wisdom in the ways of nature?

My father was born on a large farm near Manitowac, Wisconsin, on April 27, 1863. The eleven children born to his pioneering parents lived a healthy and happy life in that primitive Indian country. It was here, led by his industrious, hard-working, provident parents, that Jethro Kloss first learned the value of wild and cultivated herbs, grains, nuts, fruits and vegetables. As a child he was taught to gather from the land many kinds of leaves, barks, and berries for his parents who prepared and used them to help ailing neighbors. They experimented with these medicines of nature and developed a systematic approach to their use in both health and illness.

These early lessons Jethro Kloss never forgot as he moved on to become well educated in theology and in the principles of natural living and treating the sick. He worked closely with the then-revolutionary medical leadership of the world-renowned Battle Creek Sanitarium in Michigan. He saw clearly the disastrous results of the use of dangerous drugs then prevalent in caring for the sick. He developed further his own philosophy and understanding of the laws of nature; still remembering those things so deeply implanted in his mind from his early childhood.

This dedicated man's developing insights were based on a great faith in God and in His healing power. He believed that God had placed in the earth remedies for human ills and aids to human health. He possessed a deep thirst for knowledge on everything related to natural living and a sincere desire to share that knowledge with others.

In 1900, he was married to Miss Carrie Stilson (my mother); and for some five years they operated a branch of the Battle Creek Sanitarium in Rose Lawn, Wisconsin. In 1905, he lost his companion by death and later married Mrs. Amy Ponwith, a widow who had a small daughter, Mabel. Jethro and Amy Kloss had three children: Lucile, Eden, and Naomi.

With his second wife, my father operated an attractive sanitarium in St. Peter, Minnesota. This pleasant and efficient health center was called "The Home Sanitarium." It was conducted much as a small hospital would be today and included an operating room where local surgeons performed surgery while Kloss administered anesthetic. He and Mrs. Kloss operated men's and women's wards as well as private rooms for the care of patients. They were well equipped for electrical treatments and hydrotherapy and were unusually successful in treating cases of nervous breakdown.

This good health program was a family enterprise, with each of us children pressed into service in one way or another. At times we would be helping with some food experiment, or perhaps in typing and retyping the material that later became BACK TO EDEN, which was many years in preparation. Jethro Kloss' son Eden was for many years his right hand helper. Whatever my father did in spreading the gospel of health and natural living, he did it with all his might and trained his children in that same pattern of living.

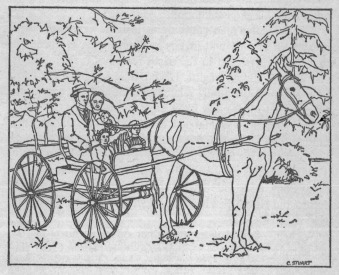

Jethro Kloss with Amy, his second wife, in Minnesota with his daughter, Promise; her daughter, Mabel; and their first child, Lucile.

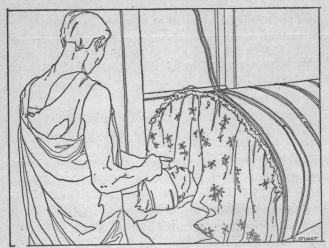

Jethro Kloss operating men's hydrotherapy treatment room at The Home Sanitarium.

We often read aloud to him from new books and magazines in the field of health—for his interests extended far beyond even his own vast experiments and studies. We read to him in order to spare his eyesight, which was not the strongest, and he could cover more ground this way. As we read along, with pencil poised, he would now and then say, "Mark!" Then a little mark in the margin would be his guide for further study as he checked author with author and compared with his own rich experience.

A later development in good health was his creation of a significant health food manufacturing operation in Amqui, Tennessee. From this center he shipped health foods throughout North America and originated many new health food recipes and herbal medicine preparations. He took a keen, almost evangelistic interest in this effort to improve the general health of the public. This health food factory was later re-established as a part of what has since become the well-known Madison Sanitarium near Nashville, Tennessee.

My father's driving energies subsequently led him into a wide variety of enterprises in the interests of healthful living, including health food cafeterias, health schools, and still other factories and stores.

A move to Washington, D.C. in the early 1930's plunged him into a career as a lecturer and teacher, including such remarkable projects as a well-publicized "Demonstration Dinner" for Washington notables; an event designed to give prominence to the principles of a healthful diet. He also lectured in Constitution Hall in promotion of the natural life.

Requests poured in for his services as a lecturer and he traveled widely throughout the country, all the while refining and perfecting the manuscript for BACK TO EDEN; and all the while continuing personally to treat the sick, often taking them into his own home where they could have a proper diet and the necessary herbs and treatments. One was continually amazed at his patience, kindness, and concern for everyone.

He was always an early riser. If some urgent work did not call him, he would be studying or writing while others were still sleeping and many times have I overheard his earnest prayers from his study corner or as he walked out of doors.

One of our favorite memories as a family is the daily hour when Father would gather his family of seven about him and we would sing hymns, read Bible verses around the circle, and pray together. He was a gentle but firm family leader--a true patriarch.

Although a strict disciplinarian, my father was warm-hearted and affectionate. When he was away from home, we invariably received a letter from "Papa" every day. We knew he loved us and was thinking of us. When he came home, there were always the little gifts--a nice piece of

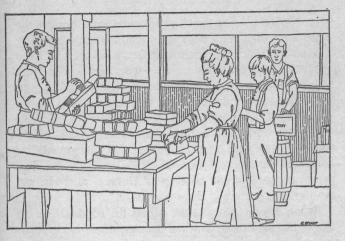

Labeling and packing cereal foods in Kloss' Tennessee manufacturing operation.

material for a dress, some choice fruit, or something else he knew we would like.

He took great pride in his children and grandchildren. I can still remember the obvious pleasure with which he presented me or his granddaughter, Doris, to lecture audiences as "evidence" of the beneficial effects of natural living.

BACK TO EDEN was at last published in 1939, the fruition of much toil and sacrifice for many years by the entire Kloss family and others who assisted in its preparation. Its wide acceptance and the appreciation expressed by so many who wrote to its author were spiritually very rewarding to my father.

After the death of Mrs. Kloss in 1944, Jethro Kloss moved to Coalmont, Tennessee, and worked together with newfound friends, Mr. and Mrs. DeLoe Robert Hiatt. There he continued treating the sick and teaching the health principles advocated in his book and in other works.

How he rejoiced in the fruit of God's green earth! After the loss of his wife he visited me and my family in northern British Columbia and delighted in the rich harvest of fruits and vegetables produced by the long summer days of that northland. I remember how he measured the length of the huge boysenberries with his pocket ruler; and how he did enjoy picking peas from the tall vines! He always relished each new and different food flavor. He loved life, and often talked of the joys and bounties of Heaven, where he was preparing to go.

When I was finally called across the continent to my father in his last illness--when the candle that for so many years had been burned at both ends was almost spent--I remember how even then his face would light up and his eyes shine at the mention of a new sanitarium he was going to build, where he could do a still greater work for "suffering humanity."

He did not know that his greatest work had already been accomplished, nor could he know then how many more thousands of lives would be benefited by his book, BACK TO EDEN.

And so, in 1946, he peacefully went to sleep--in his eighty-fourth year--and today rests in a little cemetery in Tennessee.

But the legend of Jethro Kloss, the "apostle" of natural health and healing, continues to grow. And as multiplied thousands continue to refer to this, his handbook of good health, his work goes on today--perhaps even stronger than in his lifetime.

CHAPTER I

PERSONAL EXPERIENCES

During my long years of experience along medical lines, I have worked out things that are of value to the human family. There is a crying need for an old-fashioned remedy book which people can use themselves. I have been asked many times to write out my experiences so that others may have the benefit of what I have found to be true.

When presenting the subjects on which this book treats, I have many times been asked the reason for my interest in these subjects and what my purpose is in endeavoring to interest others also. It is only fitting, that now, in putting my experience and knowledge in printed form, I should answer these questions. This I can best do by giving a brief sketch of my personal experiences during my youth and early manhood.

I was born and reared on a truck and nursery farm in the northern part of Wisconsin. We raised all kinds of vegetables, also seeds for large seed houses. My father was a practical farmer and nurseryman. We raised nearly everything that we needed, had very few things to buy. We made our own syrup and sugar from beets and carrots, and had an abundance of all kinds of fruits, such as apples, cherries, plums and the common varieties of berries, blackberries, raspberries, strawberries, also grapes and currants. We lived almost entirely upon the natural products of the earth.

After I left home, I lived in boarding houses and hotels, eating little except devitalized foods, until my health began to fail. This continued until I suffered a complete breakdown. My nerves gave way completely, and I became so weak that one time I was in bed three months, suffering with pains no tongue can describe. Death would have been a welcome release.

Finally, when I was able to be up and around again, I went to various sanitariums, and consulted with doctors and specialists. Sometimes it seemed as though I were getting a little better, and then I would get worse again. Even when I could walk around, if anyone talked to me for only five minutes, holding the most pleasant conversation, I would collapse. Some of the very best doctors said that they did not see how I lived at all, and that I certainly could not live long. My nerves were in such a condition that sometimes when I had my eyes open, I would seem to see flashes of lightning in broad daylight. In this condition I lingered for a number of years.

I had tried every remedy known to the medical profession, and none of my doctors gave me one ray of hope. I, myself, had no thought of ever getting well again, and had made my will and was lingering around, not looking for any further help from the medical profession.

It was then that I came across some books, written by a Mr. and Mrs. James White, who, though not physicians, were great medical missionaries. In those books I found statements like these: "Nine out of every ten could get well if they would use simple God-given means." And "Do not eat food robbed of its life-giving elements." "Do not eat food that makes you sick." This was an entirely new line of thought to me. At that time I had never heard such things mentioned.

Anyone desiring any of Mrs. E. G. White's writings can procure them from the Review and Herald Publishing Assn., Takoma Park, D.C., Southern Publishing Assn.,

(2)

Nashville, Tenn., or Pacific Press Publishing Assn., Mountain View, California.

These were the first things that began to open my eyes, and they gave me encouragement that there might be hope for me. This brought to my mind that in my youth, at home, we never had a doctor. For food we depended on the nuts of the forest, the fruits of the orchard, and the grains of the field. For medicine we used the herbs of the fields and gardens, teas made from the inside barks of certain trees and shrubs, and the health-giving, cooling juices of wild and tame fruits that grew all around us in abundance. Our herbs we gathered and dried in the summertime, and saved, to have on hand in case of sickness, either for ourselves or for our neighbors. Well do I remember how I gathered herbs, barks, and blossoms for the doctors. I recalled many times, when my parents were called to a neighbor's home after someone there had been given up to die, they, with their herbs, fruit juices, and vegetable broths, helped the sick one back to health again.

One time black smallpox broke out in a community a little distance from us. But we were all exposed before we knew it; and though we did not have a doctor, by means of these simple herbs, water, and simple foods, we recovered, though several children of the family had it at the same time. There were also others who used only the herbs, and not one of them died.

In those pioneer days, doctors were scarce in the northern country, and the people largely depended upon each other and the simple means of treatment, as they had a practical knowledge of their effectiveness, gained from their experiences.

All these things came vividly to my mind at this time when I was in such a hopeless physical and mental condition.

Then I began to search further in those books, and I found many useful things and it was not long until my health began to improve, and by the continued use of these simple God-given things, it improved until I was a well man.

One time there was an epidemic of typhoid fever in the locality where I was living, and most of the people were deathly afraid of it, as a great many died. Someone told me of a family, a man and wife who were afflicted, with it, and had no one to wait on them. The neighbors would come and set food on the porch, but would not go into the house, so I went to see this family. As I approached the house, I met the doctor outside the door, and asked him if he had any objections to my doing something for these folks. He said "No, no objection," and he added that the woman would recover but the man would die.

I found this man in a very critical condition. He had hemorrhage of the bowels and ulcers from his mouth through the entire digestive tract, with a severe pain in his bowels. He was very low. From all appearances, there was no hope for him. But I obtained a cot, put it in his room, and began to treat the man with the simple remedies which I found in the White books. I stopped giving poisonous drugs, and gave him plenty of water and fruit juices, and used other simple means, such as fomentations, which proved a great means of allaying his pains. These were given in the form of hot and cold applications, and I soon had his pain eased.

In about six weeks the man was up and around. When he asked me how much he owed me, I told him he owed me nothing, as I myself had been lingering for years with no hope of ever being well again, and I was glad and happy to be able to do something for him. But the man said, "No, sir. You will never do this for nothing," and he gave me a check for seventy-five dollars.

(4)

This was the beginning of my medical missionary work, as I had never before done anything for the sick. I was so pleased and happy that I had been successful in doing something for someone, that I continued nursing, having the same good results. I nursed for several doctors, who were surprised that one having had no medical training of any kind could get such results.

In a later chapter of this book, entitled, "Fevers," I will give the means I used for the treatment of these cases. I have had the same results many times since. The means are so simple that anyone can use them in his home.

I studied every case that I had, to see what I could learn further on the subject of simple methods of treating the sick. I was so aroused by this time that I began to search for and buy books on these subjects, and subscribe to medical magazines. I have continued this search for many years, writing many letters in search of things that might be a blessing to man. After I found help for myself, I kept up the search for the sole purpose of giving to the world what I might find. I studied the Bible on cooking, baking, and learned also the remedies that were used in Bible times. I found that the healing art which God gave to man to maintain and restore health was to be practiced by ministers and gospel workers. And God has never changed that plan.

I also have many bulletins from the government in which I have found valuable information, analysis of various products, etc. I had the *Journal* and many of the books which the American Medical Association publishes, from which I learned much.

Man's methods of treating disease are truly complicated and mystifying, but God's ways are so simple that anyone can understand them without a medical education. This led me to think of the simple herbs, fruits, and fruit juices, and barks which my parents used and the means which Mr. and

(5)

Mrs. White used, so simple and harmless and so inexpensive that everyone can use them for himself. This is God's plan. His remedies can be used at small expense.

Here are the simple means which Mr. and Mrs. White, with the aid of their helpers and many others, used: pure air, sunshine, properly prepared food, non-poisonous herbs, water treatments, pure water to drink, abstemiousness, foods not robbed of their life-giving properties in manufacture, cleanliness of body and premises. When we heed these things, God will do for us what we cannot do. He lets the sun shine on the just and the unjust. If any man or woman would apply these simple, God-given remedies, the results would be the same for both saint and sinner. When physical law is obeyed, by any human being, whether good or bad, he will reap the reward God has promised. When a wicked man, who does not believe in God, tills his soil properly and sows and plants properly, God gives him sunshine and rain the same as he does a righteous man, for God is no respecter of persons.

I have heard many health lectures and have read a great deal on health topics, but it was the books of Mrs. White that first opened my eyes. I have been told that Mrs. White employed as medicine the common Red Clover Blossoms, and she used them all during her life as a beverage. She lived to the age of eighty-four years.

It is going on forty years since I was given up by my doctors without hope or ever being able to do anything again in this world. Part of the time I have done the work of two or three, and many times the circumstances were such that I could not take proper care of myself, and I would work beyond my strength. Now I am getting to be an old man and have more strength and endurance than many young people. I feel grateful to my heavenly Father for all these simple God-given remedies. It was the reading of such statements as the following which led me to believe that there must be a remedy for me. "Do not eat food that makes you sick." "To eat food as far as possible in its natural state." "Foods that require cooking should be prepared in a simple, palatable way without the use of spices." God has a remedy for every ill of man. I certainly found that remedy.

A short time after I had begun to help people with these simple remedies, as I was driving along the road, a man called to me and said, "Can't you do something for my boy?" A large, strapping young fellow was sitting in the house suffering with an ingrown toenail. His toe was so sore and inflamed that he could not walk. I washed the foot with soap and water and trimmed away the toenail down to the quick. Then I took some peroxide and kept putting it on until the pus and foul matter was cleaned away. Finding there was proud flesh, I put on burnt alum powder. This killed the proud flesh. I then asked him to bathe the foot every day and soak it in hot water, as hot as he could stand, for several minutes, then plunge it into cold water. Then I had them get an old shoe, and cut the leather away at the toe, so his sore toe would not touch it. Then I put a little cotton between the toes so they would not touch each other. Three days later I came along that same road and stopped to see the boy. His father said he was out in the field working.

Along that same road, the folks were threshing. The man who was doing the feeding was cut in the palm of the hand by the bundle cutter. There was a deep cut in the flesh and the gash was nearly an inch wide. I put a little disinfectant in water and some astringent and soaked his hand in hot water for over an hour. This almost entirely closed the wound. Hot water, of course, was added at intervals to keep it hot. Then I cut some narrow strips of adhesive plaster. I pressed the wound together so it was tightly closed, and put these narrow strips across it to hold it in place. Then I put his arm in a sling. In one week his wound was entirely knit together, and in less than two weeks the man began to work again.

For a disinfectant and astringent, a tea made of white oak bark or bayberry bark is excellent. Use a heaping teaspoonful in powder form to a cup of boiling water, and steep thirty minutes, or it can be made a little stronger. Wild alum root, golden seal, and myrrh are also excellent for such purposes. Use a half teaspoonful of any of these three to a cup of boiling water.

A small teaspoonful of myrrh and one of golden seal and a half teaspoonful of red pepper to a pint of boiling water makes a very effective surgical dressing, and may be used for any kind of a wound or swelling. After the teas are steeped, there will be some sediment in the bottom of the container. The fluid or tea should be carefully poured off so that the fluid which is used will be entirely clear before it is put in the wound.

A small teaspoonful of myrrh and one teaspoonful of golden seal and a half teaspoonful of red pepper put in a pint of alcohol and allowed to stand for seven days, shaken well every day, makes an excellent liniment for sprains or bruises, and can be used anywhere as a liniment for any sore fresh wound or ulcer. Kerosene is also excellent for wounds and bruises. Look in the Table of Contents for the heading, "Kerosene."

I could multiply similar experiences with these remedies that anyone can use in his own home.

A Swollen Foot

Again I came to a home where a young man was sitting with his foot swollen. The thick part under his foot near the toes was very badly swollen and inflamed so that he was not able to walk. I had them get a large pan of hot water, and one of cold. He soaked the foot in the hot water until it was thoroughly heated, then plunged it into the cold for just a second or two, putting it immediately back into the hot water, alternating in this manner for one hour. I then took a pan with some kerosene in it, and put hit foot into this cold kerosene while the foot was hot and the pores open. We went through this process several times during this same evening and then repeated it the first thing in the morning. The young man went to work that same day. But I advised them to continue this treatment every evening for a few evenings, which entirely cured the soreness in his foot.

Treating Sore Toe With Peroxide

Many years ago I had occasion to treat a young man who had been wearing a shoe that was too tight, or at least it did not fit his foot well, and had caused his large toe to become very sore. It was swollen and had become so painful that he could not work. There was not anything available except some of that old household remedy, peroxide of hydrogen. I washed his foot in very warm water, and then applied peroxide every two or three minutes, until it was perfectly clean and did not bubble any more. This treatment alone removed the inflammation so much that the young man could resume his work. I told him that for several evenings he should soak his foot in first hot, and then cold water, and then apply the peroxide or kerosene until the soreness was entirely gone. The toe got well.

A Case of Rheumatism

One time four men came to see me and told me of a man who was crippled with rheumatism. They insisted that I go with them to see this man. We found a man about thirty-five years of age in bed with both of his legs drawn up so tightly that they could not be moved to a normal position, and his arms were the same way. His wife fed him with a spoon, as one would feed a little baby.

This man had been doctoring for years with specialists, and spent hundreds of dollars without receiving any help. What the doctors did for him at this time was to inject strychnine and morphine. Without this the man would groan night and day.

I gave him hot blanket packs to sweat in. Then later I gave him baths in the washtub. I covered him with blankets and put his feet in a pan of hot water as you would give a sitz-bath, and then rubbed him with oil. (For herbs used, see Table of Contents for herbs given for Rheumatism.) For food, I gave him zwiebach, whole wheat flakes, adding a tablespoonful of lime water to every cup of milk given, and an abundance of fresh fruits, and vegetables, and had him drink a great deal of pure water. In one week there was decided improvement, and in a comparatively short time, he was well and resumed his work again with both his arms and legs perfectly limber.

Ulcerated Stomach Causes Spasms

This case was brought to my attention by the man who had the forementioned case of rheumatism. He suggested that I might be able to do something for his aunt, who had not been able to work for a number of years. She had a bad case of ulcerated stomach and bowel trouble. When I met her I inquired about her troubles. She told me that every few days, aside from the constant pain she had, she would get a spell in the form of a spasm, with terrible pain. I said, if I could see her in one of those spells I could tell more about what was the matter. She said, "If you can do anything for me to keep me from having another spell, for God's sake do it, for I'd sooner die than have another spell."

I ordered a sitz- and sweat-bath, followed by a salt glow and a high enema. I also put her on a liquid diet, also giving her whole wheat flakes dissolved in boiling water and a little cream. She also had some whole wheat zwiebach with hot milk. A teaspoonful of lime water was added to each cup of milk. We gave her daily hot and cold applications over the stomach and liver, also the spine. I gave her herbs to heal the uclers in the stomach and to cleanse the system. (See ulcerated stomach in Table of Contents, to find what herbs to use.) In three weeks this woman was so much improved she could go home, and continue her treatment.

Fifteen years later, I received a letter from Mr. Gilson, (who was this woman's brother and had been healed of rheumatism) saying that he wished he could get a few more treatments as he was again feeling a touch of rheumatism. He added in the same letter, "It might please you to know that my aunt has been well ever since, and hat not suffered another spell, but is just now feeling a little touch of that old trouble." I had thoroughly instructed them both in the first place that the things which caused the trouble originally would do so again. I could not go to see them, but instructed them by letter what to do, and they got along all right.

Cured of Tuberculosis

About thirty-five years ago a man by the name of Stevens, in the northern part of Wisconsin, very urgently called me to see his wife. I found her sick in bed with tuberculosis. She was a young woman with one child less than a year old. Upon inquiry, we found that three in this family had already died of tuberculosis; her mother, one brother, and one sister. This lady was the fourth in the family to be afflicted with the disease. The doctors had given up her case. She was a frail woman with a small, round chest and very small lungs. A number of my friends advised me not to try to do anything for the woman, as it would be impossible for a cure to be effected. I told both the woman and her husband just what it would mean to undertake this case. I said that if they would not live up to everything I asked them to do, to the last detail that I would not undertake it, and that just as soon as I might find out that they did not live up to every requirement I would drop the case at once. Suffice it to say, it was not more than two weeks before the woman was so that she could walk around. I asked them to get her some warm felt shoes, woolen stockings, and woolen underwear extending down to her ankles, then I had her exercise outdoors every day. As her strength increased I had her exercise more and more. Nearby was a high hill which I had her walk up every day, rain or shine, unless the weather was too stormy. Walking up hill is very beneficial as it compels one to breathe deeply.

This woman got entirely well, and the last I heard of her, had reared a family of children.

There is no need for failure in such cases unless they have gone so far that there are organs of the body destroyed and you have nothing to build on. I could cite many more instances of this kind, but will only give a few more to show the results of the use of simple means that can be used in your own home.

Child Given up to Die

One time I was called to go to a home where there was a little four-year-old child. The doctor had pronounced it pneumonia. Her fever was above 104 degrees, and she had been unconscious for some time. This child was clothed in a heavy woolen undersuit, and also wore a jacket made of batting to cover her lungs, both in front and back. The house was full of people, as they expected the child to die any minute. I asked them to remove her clothes, and the grandfather, who was standing on one side of the bed, objected very seriously, saying that it would cause the child's death. But her father said to leave me alone. The doctor had said that the child would die, and unless a decided change came, they all knew that she would.

They asked me the cause of the fever. I told them I did not know the cause, but that no matter what was the cause, the fever must be reduced. We put the child, without any clothes on, between cotton blankets, gave her an enema, then sponged her with tepid water every five minutes, letting the water evaporate. I raised her head every few minutes and filled her mouth with cold water. She would take one swallow, but would not drink. We kept this treatment up all night. When she seemed to be getting a little chilly, I would stop the sponging, and put a hot water bottle to her stomach or feet. As soon as she would get warm, we would continue the sponging. At three o'clock in the morning, when she opened her eyes for the first time, and said, "Thank you." Her father, who was standing on the other side of the bed, burst into tears and said, "Now I know she is going to get better."

By this time the fever had gone down more than two degrees. We kept this treatment up until three o'clock in the afternoon, a little more than twenty-four hours from the time we started. By this time the child was quite normal, and began to talk, but would get a coughing and choking spell every little while. Upon inquiry as to what might have been the cause of this fever, I found that at suppertime three or four days before this, the child had eaten very freely of beefsteak. Shortly afterward, she became ill. I told them I thought the child was full of worms, that her choking spells were caused by the worms crawling up in her throat. I sent them to their home physician to get some worm medicine.

In three or four days the child was entirely well. The cause of this fever was the beefsteak she ate. She was unable to digest it, the worms had a feast on it, and caused a large amount of poison to accumulate. Just as soon as the poison was removed by the enema, the pores opened and the skin made active by sponging so the poisons could escape, and by constantly giving water to drink, we reduced the fever to normal.

Hemorrhage of Uterus

One time I saved the life of a person who had bled so much that she was near death. She could only whisper faintly, and could not be heard except by listening close to her mouth. I elevated the foot of the bed, and gave her hot malted nut cream, diluted with grape juice, half and half. After giving her several cups very hot, it had strengthened her so I could understand what she said while standing at the foot of the bed. (Then I followed this up with more treatment as per hemorrhages—see Table of Contents.)

Infantile Paralysis

A few years ago, a woman brought a three-year-old boy who had infantile paralysis, to me. His head was drawn clear over to his shoulder, his arm was drawn up to his chest, and his shoulder blade stuck out very much. This child had been permitted all the candy, ice cream, cakes, and cookies he wanted, and nearly all the food he had been eating was robbed of its life-giving properties. The mother said they had consulted several physicians in the city where they lived, and had taken him to another city to some of the best specialists they could find. All the physicians gave her no hope for the boy's recovery, and said that it would probably take years for him to outgrow it.

I ordered them to give the child plenty of fresh fruits and vegetables, but no candy, ice cream, cake, or cookies of any description, and no white flour products, or cane sugar products. I had them give the boy hot and cold applications to the spine, stomach, and liver, and then massage his entire body. Also hot baths, finished with short cold. I had him take lots of exercise in the open air. Anyone could notice improvement from the first few days. In six weeks this boy could throw a ball with the hand that had been drawn up to his chest. His head, which had been drawn clear down to his shoulder, was perfectly straight, and the shoulder blade was almost entirely normal. All that was done for this child anyone can do in his home. This was quite a number of years ago. The child has been well ever since, and is a normal high school student to-day. (See Table of Contents for herbs for Infantile Paralysis.)

817 DOWNING STREET, NEW SMYRNA BEACH, FLA.
September 22, 1938

DEAR MR. KLOSS:

I had a letter from my sister, Mrs. Burkhard, several days ago, telling me about the letter she had received from you. I will be glad to give the date of Harry's illness and other particulars.

Harry Peyton Cobb, Jr., became ill of infantile paralysis in April, 1925, at the age of three. It paralyzed his right side from his waist up, and his lower limbs were very weak as he could only walk a short distance without falling. He could not hold his head up and it dropped forward badly. When he would lie down, he could not sit up without being helped, nor could he stand up by himself. After three treatments from Mr. Kloss, and the proper diet, he was able to sit and stand up unassisted. After taking six-weeks treatments, he could hold his head erect, throw a ball, ride his tricycle and walk without falling. Harry is seventeen years old now and is in good health. He enters in all high school sports and no one knows he has had infantile paralysis unless we tell them. We certainly owe his strong physical condition to Mr. Kloss and enough cannot be said of his treatments.

When I see other children left so crippled from infantile paralysis, it makes me *so* thankful for Mr. Kloss's help and for God's help, that my boy has grown to be a big, fine young man. I do wish you folks could see him.

All send their best regards to you, Mrs. Kloss, Naomi, and Eden.

Yours truly,

MRS. HARRY P. COBB

Another Case of Infantile Paralysis

Not long ago my wife asked me to go and see a neighbor's child who had been stricken with infantile paralysis that day. Upon entering the home, I found the mother holding in her arms a plump baby, who was not yet a year old. The mother also was fleshy. This child was nursed exclusively by the mother and had never had any other food. Upon inquiring about the mother's diet, I found that she was practically living on white bread, and white biscuits made with soda, pork, peeled potatoes with white flour gravy. For breakfast she would have pancakes and syrup. She also used some milk, but very few vegetables. All these foods are high in calorie value and make fat, but have little life-giving properties in them. This is what caused the baby's paralysis, because the mother was not eating food that would properly nourish the nerves. We at once gave the woman oatmeal and bran water to drink, and fresh fruits. My wife cooked her a kettle of vegetable soup, carrots, onions, potatoes, and natural brown rice. We gave the baby oatmeal water and tomato juice. We then gave the baby some baths, both hot and cold, and rubbed her well, repeating this treatment several times, and in a few days every symptom of paralysis was gone, and the child got well. Of course we thoroughly instructed the mother how to eat to have a healthy baby and to avoid sickness.

Complete Paralysis

Many years ago, a man awoke me about one in the morning, saying that his wife was paralyzed all over. I went with him to his home, and began treatment at once. First, we gave her an enema, then hot and cold applications to the spine, stomach, and liver. We then gave a hot towel rub, just as hot as we could give it, following with a cold towel rub. We then gave her a thorough massage from head to foot. We kept this up practically all the rest of the night, giving hot and cold to the spine, then percussion, hacking movement, and spatting. When morning came we rested a while. We could already see marked improvement in the pulse beat, but there was as yet no sign of life or any feeling. In a short while, we repeated the treatment in full. The second day we began to see signs of life when we pricked her with a needle. We kept up this treatment for hours each day, and part of the night. The fourth day she could stand alone, without any assistance, but as yet was not able to walk. We kept up this treatment for some time, but not so vigorously or so prolonged. In less than two weeks she was up, doing her housework again. I knew this lady for years afterward, and know that she stayed well. This was nearly thirty years ago, and the last I heard she was rearing a family.

I have had many experiences with treating spinal meningitis and paralysis. I will mention just one more case, the worst that I have ever *seen or heard of*.

Two Strokes of Paralysis

This was my own wife. We had been married only a short time. One morning when I got up I noticed that my wife did not act as she usually did. Upon examination I found that she was half paralyzed from her head down to her feet. I could take a needle and stick it into one side of her face, her arm, leg or her foot and there was no sign of life. I at once called the best doctor that we knew, and in whom we had the most confidence. He gave her a thorough examination and said that nothing could be done aside from giving general good care. He said that she would be likely to die at any time, that this stroke would be followed by another stroke which would cause her death.

I started the same course of treatments which I had used with the neighbor's wife, which incident I just related. In the course of three weeks my wife was around the house in the usual way, and we could again listen to the beautiful tones which she is capable of producing on the piano.

Not long after that I arose at an early hour, as my custom was, and went about my work. When I came in for breakfast, I inquired where Mrs. Kloss was and the answer was that they had not seen her yet that morning. I went to the bedroom and found her lying in bed. When I talked to her, there was no response. When I took hold of her, it felt as if I were taking hold of a dead person, only she was not entirely cold. I tried to get her to say something, but she gave not a sound of any kind. Then I took a needle, and pricked her face and neck. But she did not flinch or wink her eye. I went down her body to her feet on both sides, but there was not a flinch or response of any description.

(18)

I called loud in her ear, and asked her if she could hear me. Then I put my finger on her eyeballs, but she did not wink. Her pulse was so weak that on the arm I could not find a pulse beat at all. There was just a very faint pulse beat on the neck.

After I saw the situation, I sent for the best doctor I knew of in that section of the country. He thoroughly examined Mrs. Kloss, and said that she was liable to drop off any minute. Then I began to work on the same line of treatments already mentioned. After one day's treatment, her pulse beat had increased materially, and in four weeks she was able to walk around. In five or six weeks she was playing the piano again and went about her work as usual. She has been well ever since, which is about twenty-six years. I wish that you could see her today. She is active, well, and cheerful.

History of My Wife's Case

I know that many would be interested to know how her health ever came to be in such bad condition. Before I met her she had had the sleeping disease. She would sleep for a week or two and no one could wake her up. The cause of all this was that she was a bookkeeper for twelve years, and instead of working six or eight hours, would work twelve to fourteen hours. Sometimes she kept two or three sets of books. That was not the worst of it. She would hurry at lunch to get a white bread sandwich, then go back to work. She did not get the proper food to nourish the nervous system. Besides auditing the books and working late into the night, she did not get enough sleep, and she lacked getting proper exercise. She kept this up until she had a complete breakdown. There was no one to advise her to do the right things.

Thank God, there is a remedy for every ill of man. The angels in heaven weep because of the dreadful suffering that is going on because of ignorance. And I have wept until I could not weep any more, when I have seen the untold amount of suffering in the world and knew that most of it might be prevented if people only knew what to do to prevent it. The only thing that I feel conscience stricken for is that I have not done more to bring to the notice of the public and show by practical experience what really can be done for suffering humanity with simple remedies which can be used in every ordinary home. I could write volumes, giving my personal experiences, but will mention only a few more for practical lessons.

Rheumatism

An elderly minister came to me, saying he was full of aches and pains, all stiffened up, and feeling very badly generally, and asked me if I would do something for him. I gave him an enema and some herbs to cleanse his system thoroughly. I put him in a tub of hot water, keeping him there several hours, rubbing his body while in the water, and at the last, gave him a vigorous salt glow, using half epsom salts and half common salt. I gave him several glasses of water to drink while in the bath, then gave him some herbs for his rheumatism. In a few days he went about his work. See Table of Contents for herbs for Rheumatism.

Pneumonia Case

Another time I was called to see a young lady who had been given up to die with a relapse of pneumonia. When I got to the house, I found the young lady in bed with a very high temperature. She had been sick for some time, and was very low. They had a graduate nurse, but she knew little about water treatments. This woman's lungs were in very bad shape. I could hardly hear a sound of air with the stethoscope on any part of the lungs.

I sent at once for one of my best graduate nurses, who understood water treatments. We started in by giving an enema. Then we placed her between cotton blankets and sponged her with tepid water, giving her frequent sips of cold water, short hot and cold applications to both the chest and back of lungs. In the course of two hours with this treatment, her lungs began to open up, and we could hear air in her lungs through the stethoscope. In four hours with this treatment, we had run the temperature down two degrees.

We kept up the treatment, sponging her body with tepid water, letting the water evaporate. Sometimes she would show signs of chilliness, and we would stop the treatment and put a hot water bag to her stomach and cover her up. We continued giving her sips of cold water, and wrapped a cold towel around her head and neck, changing it frequently. Never let a cloth on the head or neck get hot. Just as soon as IT GETS WARM, TAKE IT OFF. We gave her a liquid diet and fruit juices. In four days her temperature was normal. This woman is alive today. Her illness was nearly twenty-five years ago.

Many cases of pneumonia would get well if taken in time, and the right treatment given. I mention these cases to show what can be done in the home by using these simple treatments. There will be many times when you cannot get a doctor or nurse and it is a most blessed thing to know how to relieve suffering.

Anyone wishing the detailed particulars of this case may obtain same from the mother of this young lady, Mrs. Alma M. McGrath, 406 W. Water Street, Austin, Minnesota, or from the young lady, who is now Mrs. William Haesecke, St. Peter, Minnesota.

Pneumonia Resulting From Wrong
Habits of Living

Many years ago, before there were any automobiles, I was in the extreme northern part of Wisconsin, in a Country Club. The manager was a drinking man and a high liver. He had had frequent spells of pneumonia. The last time he had pneumonia, the doctor told him that if he got another spell there would be no means on earth to save him. He told the man not to call him, that he would not come if he were called.

There was great excitement when he came down with a high fever of 104 degrees F., and was very sick. They were fifteen miles away from a doctor. They had a fine driving team which he ordered hitched up at once. He did not know about any of my medical experience, but his wife had heard something about it. She called me in to see him, and asked the driver to wait a few minutes. The man was very much excited and urged them to hurry on for a doctor. The wife made the plea that he knew what the doctor had said. She said I had had splendid results with these cases, and urged him to give me a trial. When he got over his excitement a little, he consented for me to go ahead. The team was unhitched. I gave him an enema, removed all his clothing, had him lie between cotton blankets, and began sponging him with tepid water all over, giving him cold water to drink. The room should be 75 degrees F. and well ventilated. I kept on sponging him every five minutes. Sometimes he would get a little chilly and we would stop for a little while and cover him up. I kept up the cold water drinking and tepid sponging. Tepid sponging feels very agreeable to a patient with high fever.

The next day at three o'clock, just twenty-four hours from the time the fever began, it was almost entirely gone.

His temperature was below 100 degrees F. The man said he felt just as well as he ever did in his life, and wanted to get up. I advised him not to get up for a day or two at least. I knew this man for years afterward, and he never had another attack of pneumonia while I knew him.

In all these cases, and I might say in all cases, I constantly hold before them and remind them of the things that put them in that condition, and how to avoid sickness. (Look in the Table of Contents under heading of "Fever" and "Pneumonia" to find what herbs to use and how to feed the patient.) Never forget that water puts out fire, and that it is one of the best known remedies to cure fevers, to be used both internally and externally.

Post Mortems Reveal Secrets

I connected with an emergency hospital just to get the experience. It was a wonderful help to me in many ways. I witnessed scores of post mortems, under competent surgeons. It was very interesting to see the organs of people whose lives we had previously known, and knew just what they had been in the habit of eating and drinking.

We opened up one man who had been a great eater of meats, rich pastries, pies, cakes, puddings, white bread, and peeled potatoes, etc. We found his liver about three times its normal size. There were tumors all around the liver, and some in the liver, ranging in size from a small marble to a small-sized potato. The heart was also very much enlarged, more than once again its normal size, and the walls of the heart were very thin and flabby and of a dark color as if bloodshot. The spleen and pancreas were both enlarged and diseased, and he had gallstones and gravel in the bladder. His stomach was also very much prolapsed and diseased.

He was a middle-aged man, quite fleshy, who had died of heart-failure. One evening at about six o'clock as he prepared to take a bath, he reached up to get a drinking glass standing on a shelf about as high as his head. As he reached for it, he fell dead.

Another man, past middle age, was cancerous. He always complained of a pain right around his navel, but there was no outward sign. The only indication that could be seen on the outside of his body was a little lump under his jaw. After he had died and we opened him up, we found his bowels full of cancerous growths and where he had complained of his pain, it had eaten right into the bowels and opened them up. This, of course, seemed to cause his death. He was all full of cancerous growth from his head clear down to his feet. You could not cut him anywhere without finding cancer. All his organs were in bad shape.

I could mention many cases but it is not necessary. We have many unfailing evidences and proof of what effect a wrong diet will have upon the system.

Experience in a Small Sanitarium

Several years ago, much was said about the wonderful cures effected through operations. Many cures were said to have been obtained through the use of electricity and much expensive electrical apparatus was manufactured. The manufacturers of these instruments spent a great deal of money in advertising what their apparatus would do. I, like thousands of others, thought there might be something in it. So I equipped a small sanitarium in a beautiful little town, in the best spot in that city. It was located near a park.

I equipped it with bathrooms for both men and women, so that we could give Turkish and Russian baths, electric baths, showers, tub baths, etc. It was also equipped with a very fine operating room and a room with electrical apparatus. I bought one of the best X-ray, static and high frequency current, galvanic, and sinusoidal current. German ultra-violet rays, sun-rays, and several other rays.

I took a medical electrical course in one of the best medical electrical schools. I hired by the year one of the best medical doctors I could find. He had been graduated as a nurse, and had learned the water cure, then had taken the regular medical course, being graduated from that. He had also studied in Europe, taking several post-graduate courses. I hired graduate nurses from recognized institutions. I extended invitations to the doctors in that city to bring their cases to this institution, which they did. I gave the anesthetic for many years, prepared the patients for their operations, and took care of them after the operations, assisted by my corps of workers.

Here I had an opportunity to learn all I wanted to know about the use of electricity, also operations.

There is a remedy among herbs, correct food, sunlight, fresh air, and pure water for most cases of tonsilitis, appendicitis, gallstones, stones in the kidneys, stones in the bladder, piles, and hemorrhoids.

Health Food Factory at Nashville, Tennessee

Many years ago I purchased a large food factory near Nashville, Tennessee. Here I gained a most wonderful experience along food lines, as we were making a large variety of foods in larger quantities than I had ever made before. Here we had a large reel oven and an up-to-date cracker machine. We made a very fine line of crackers, five different kinds. Our capacity was from twelve to twenty hundred pounds per day. Besides this, we made a very fine cereal coffee and various breakfast foods, whole-wheat flour and quite a line of gluten and nut food preparations to take the place of meat, also malt honey and malt extract.

I had an experienced baker and health food maker. I subscribed for various journals on cracker making, bread making, etc., and bought the best books obtainable on bread making, canning, and cooking. I had a regular experimental outfit, which I have till this day. I have been experimenting with foods all the time, for the sole purpose of giving to the public the best.

My purpose in this was not to establish some commercial business, but to get before the public healthful things which are to take the place of the harmful articles of foods which are filling the world with chronic invalids. While I was operating this food factory, I took in people at different times who were interested and wanted to learn the business. I gave them my recipes, and helped them to find where they could get things needed to make health foods, also proper machinery. I gave them much other necessary information.

Since then I have helped others to start a food business in different parts of the United States. They are doing a successful business. I will not be satisfied until I have so many of these factories in operation—to make the foods of various sorts in the baking line as well as others—that the people who want to live right and avoid sickness, can get these wholesome products everywhere.

I am now spending my time conducting public food demonstrations, cooking schools, and health lectures. My main object is to have everyone learn in his own home how to make these things. I have spent a good deal of money and simplified these things so that everyone can make the foods in an ordinary home.

I tell the people where they can get the various products that are wholesome at a reasonable price, and condemn the hurtful articles. I help manufacturers everywhere to make wholesome articles which will take the place of many injurious articles. Anyone wishing to manufacture any of these health foods in the baking line or in canning, etc., may obtain from me my best information where to get machinery and needed articles.

I am especially interested in having people everywhere start health restaurants with a health food store in connection with them so that these products can be sold and served at the same time.

After I had run this large factory at Nashville for a number of years, I sold it to an industrial school. It was moved to their school campus and is still operating in connection with their school. A few years later I opened another factory at Brooke, Virginia, and equipped it with machinery for a large capacity. After operating this factory for a number of years, I sold it. At the same time I was teaching others how to make health foods, and they are now operating factories in different parts of the United States.

There should be a large number of factories so that these healthful articles could be obtained in every grocery store. I have a number of new articles which have not as yet been put on the market, and I am still experimenting, for the sole purpose of giving it to those who will make use of it.

[Extract from "The Sawdust Trail," by Rev. William (Billy) Sunday, in the *Ladies Home Journal,* September, 1932.]

"During the first three years of my life, I was sickly and could scarcely walk. Mother used to carry me on a pillow which she made for that purpose. There were no resident physicians in those pioneer days, and itinerant doctors would drive up to our cabin and ask, 'Anybody sick here?'

The Country Doctor

"One day, Doctor Avery, a Frenchman, called at our

(27)

cabin and mother told him, 'I have a little boy three years old who has been sick ever since he was born.'

"The old doctor said, 'Let me see him.' He gave me the once over while I yelled and screamed like a Comanche Indian. Then he said to mother, 'I can cure that boy.'

"She asked him how much he would charge, and he replied, 'Oh, if you will feed me and my old mare, that will pay the bill.'

"Mother said, 'All right, but you will have to sleep up in the garret. We have no stairs and you'll have to climb the ladder.' "He replied, 'That suits me.' He then went into the woods and picked leaves from various shrubs, including mulberry leaves and elderberries, dug up roots, and from them made a syrup and gave it to me. In a short time I was going like the wind and have been hitting on all eight ever since. From that day to this, elderberries and mulberries have been my favorite wild fruits, and I like sassafras tea.

"I do not believe that there is a disease to which human flesh is heir but that somewhere there is growing a weed or an herb or plant that will cure it. Somewhere there is a remedy for the dread plagues of the human race, consumption and cancer. God has made the cure and is waiting for man to discover it.

"The greatest doctor this world ever knew is an old Christian mother, and my mother was the greatest of all. I regret that I did not write down the names of all the herbs and roots she knew, and the diseases they would cure. When she put on her 'specks' to look at the sore and spread salve on it, that made it almost well.

"You may name this suggestive therapeutics or the power of mind over matter. All these designations are as useless as the name of the horse that Paul Revere rode. The fact remains."

CHAPTER II

SOIL

Back to the farm is my message.

It is really very interesting to take a poor piece of soil and make it productive in a short time by plowing deep and plowing under soybeans, green crops, etc., for fertilizer.

To make some interesting experiments, plow your soil eight or ten inches deep in the fall with a turn-plow. Plant corn on a piece of poor ground the first year. You will have to fertilize it so you will get big cornstalks. When you lay the corn by, plant soybeans between the rows. These beans will get big enough so you can have green shelled beans, which is an excellent food. Just as soon as the corn is glazed, pull the corn and haul it from the field, and spread it out to dry. Mow or cut down the cornstalks and soybean vines close to the ground, then plow the ground with a 12-or 14-inch plow with a rolling cutter on it. This will bring soil which has not been worn out to the surface. The green cornstalks and soybean vines put a wonderful mulch of the very best kind of fertilizer into the soil. This will emulsify the soil. If this soil has a clay subsoil, cultivate it at once with a disc harrow to pulversize it and keep it from getting hard on top.

Sow a winter crop to cover and protect the soil. The next spring plow the ground 6 or 7 inches deep, turning under your cover crop, then harrow thoroughly and plant your corn. Cultivate the corn shallow and when ready to lay by, plant soybeans again and harvest and plow the soil just the same as you did the year before, only plow it crossways from the way you plowed it the year before. This loosens up the soil so the roots can go down deep in fertile soil and the moisture can come up. I have raised a fine crop of corn in this way when it was a year of crop failure.

Plant alfalfa or any grain on this ground the following year, and you will see a real crop of grain. If the ground is worked this way for a few years it will make real virgin soil which will produce wonderful vegetables or any kind of fruit which will contain all the mineral and vitamin elements.

Those who have tractors can do this work easily with great satisfaction and big rewards. Everyone that has any land should work his vegetable garden this way; also the land on which he raises fruits. It pays big dividends to prepare ground in this fashion when you plan to plant an orchard or fruit of any kind. I have set out an orchard in this kind of soil and obtained growth in three years which would ordinarily have taken five or six years. This way of handling the soil holds the moisture and keeps the water from running off. There are many other ways to improve the soil.

If one does not have sufficient horsepower and machinery to cultivate the soil deep, he should get together with his neighbors and get the necessary power and machinery. Bring the deep soil up to the surface and thoroughly pulverize it, then the fine and tender roots will have a nice mellow bed in which to run in every direction and get their nourishment.

All the plants—wheat, corn, oats, flowers, fruit trees, in fact, all plants and trees—have many more roots if they have a nice finely pulverized bed of soil. This kind of soil will also produce a stronger plant which will yield better grains and fruits, very much more abundantly, and the planter will be more than doubly paid for all the work put in on the land.

(30)

It is of very great importance to have the soil worked deep enough so that the roots of all the plants, grains of all kinds, can go deep into the ground, not only to draw nourishment but moisture. It is wonderful for both wet and dry seasons. When it is wet, the water can go down into the soil, and when it is dry there is a deep mellow mulch of soil for the roots to penetrate deep enough to get the moisture from beneath. Therefore, when the soil is loose deep down, the moisture will come up, as it cannot do when the soil is hard and lumpy, nor will it dry out so quickly.

When the soil is loose and finely pulverized, the sun, oxygen, and other life-giving elements can penetrate deeply and give life and proper nourishment to the plants.

It is my desire to arouse the people to thoroughly cultivate their soil, plant at the right time, and thoroughly cultivate their crops. In so doing they will be well repaid for their labor.

Fruits grown in the shade and fruits raised on worn-out ground where commercial fertilizer has been used, have very little life-giving properties. Even wheat, many times, is raised year after year on the same ground without properly taking care of the soil. Now you can put all the sixteen minerals back into poor, depleted soil, by handling your soil right. Just as soon as your crop is harvested, plow the ground and sow it with soybeans, cowpeas, rye, or buckwheat. When the crop is full grown, drag it down, and plow it under, plowing deep. In the northern states it must be plowed under before it freezes. This will wonderfully help to make virgin soil. In the fall the ground should be plowed deep so as to expose it to the sun and air. Red clover which was formerly used so much for improving soil does not grow as well las it used to. But with soybeans the ground can be improved much more successfully and more rapidly than with other things.

It is very easy to raise hay in some of the Southern States where hay is scarce by sowing oats and cutting them just before they turn yellow when the oats are full grown and the straw is yet green. This hay, when cut, makes an excellent hay, which is real medicine for stock, and the grain splendid. I have kept work stock in good shape on this kind of hay.

In raising vegetables and garden truck, I have many times raised two and three crops on the same ground the same year. When one crop begins to get ripe you can work the ground between the rows, and plant your second crop so when you harvest the first crop, your second crop is well under way and so you can keep on raising two and three crops of some things.

It is well to have a good book on farming and gardening of which there are many on the market that are not expensive. There is a very excellent book called "Garden Guide," (the amateur gardener's handbook) by A. T. De LaMare, which can be obtained from A. T. De LaMare, Inc., 438 West 37th Street, New York, N.Y. This book is inexpensive, but is full of very valuable information written in simple plain language. Everyone who has a garden would do well to get one of these books. (I have not been paid for advertising this book.) Learn about the things that grow very quickly and which will produce a great amount of food in a short time on a small piece of land. In every state there is a government experiment station which has valuable bulletins on all kinds of farming subjects and many of them are free.

Farming and Gardening

Farming and gardening are intensely interesting when you learn to do them correctly. Many people might have an abundance of food now who have land, but do not make the right use of it. Here are some of my personal experiences:

To have early tomatoes in the extreme northern states where it is very cold and the season short, plant the tomatoes in February in a box in the house when you do not have a greenhouse or hotbed. Then transplant the plants two or three times before time to set them out in the field or garden. The transplanting makes them sturdy and produces large roots, so when they are set out they have lots of vitality and soon make a large plant which bears fruit much earlier. Later when it gets warm enough, plant the seeds right out in the garden or field, and do not transplant them at all. Plant a number of seeds in the same place, leaving the strongest plant and transplant the others.

For early lettuce: Sow in the fall early enough for it to make two or three leaves, then get some brush and throw over the bed. Put some straw or hay of some sort over this to shield it against the fierce winter. The brush and straw protects it against the snow, keeps it from packing solid and smothering the plants. In the spring after the hard frosts are over, remove the brush and straw.

For early onions: Plant in the fall. There are a number of varieties with which you can do this. The potato onion is an excellent variety for this. If you send to your seedhouse, they will send you directions for fall planting.

There are varieties of spinach which can be planted in the fall. Let the spinach grow three or four leaves the same as lettuce, before covering. This will give you spinach, onions, and other greens very early in the spring—much earlier than if you do all your planting in the spring after the ground gets warm enough. In the Southern States you can have greens the year around.

(33)

For early potatoes: Plant much earlier than they are usually planted. I have had potatoes frozen off three or four times, but they seem to grow right along. When they are small it does not hurt them to have the tops frozen off. Thus for early potatoes, I have had them three or four weeks sooner than if I had waited until potatoes are generally planted.

For early strawberries: Get early varieties and plant them on a southern slope or southeastern slope. Protect them with a little light straw; then when they start to bloom early the frost does not hurt them. When the danger of frost is over, rake the straw off, leaving some between the rows for mulching the strawberries. Plant the late varieties of strawberries on a northern or western slope. Cover them lightly with straw and leave on until quite late. This will produce a later crop. Then for a general crop, raise them wherever they grow best. Working it this way you will have berries for a much longer time. Get early, late, and ever-bearing varieties, thus you can have berries for a long season. I have kept a strawberry bed in good bearing condition for five or six years. After all the berries have been picked, harrow the ground with a fine toothed harrow, criss-crossing the patch as if you were going to harrow the plants out. This will take out the old plants, thus giving the new ones a better chance.

Keep planting various other garden truck at different times so as to have green shelled peas and beans nearly all summer long. You can plant green corn at different times and have roasting ears all summer. I planted some of the evergreen sweet corn so that it would produce roasting ears just before the frost. Then we would cut the corn, shock it up, and gather roasting ears out of the shocks for a long time after there had been many a hard frost. When you get father south where the winters are not so long and so severe, it is much easier. You can have an abundance of garden stuff all the year around as there are a number of greens and vegetables which will stand light frosts.

Everyone who has any ground at all should have a patch of ground cherries. They grow abundantly and make a very fine sauce.

In the fall when fruits and vegetables are cheap, can up a lot so you will have an abundance when you cannot go to the garden and get it. There are small canners and can sealers that can be used in homes where goods may be canned just as well as in the canning factories. Tin cans are very cheap, but it is really better to use glass jars as they can be used and re-used.

Many years ago I helped a man buy a canner. He had eighty acres of land with a heavy mortgage on it, which he paid off with the help of his canning outfit in just a few years. If you could listen to this man tell his experience with this canning outfit it would be extremely interesting. He said that one time he bought a large two-horse load of pumpkins for three dollars. He canned them and the proceeds from this one load of pumpkins was nearly thirty-five dollars. Aside from being very practical, it is a very interesting thing for the children. Give them a share in it and a part of the profits. Every farmer's child should have a garden space of his own, and the profits of that space should be his. When I was on the farm I had but very little to buy and always something to sell.

All farmers should produce an abundance of feed for their stock. I used to cut our grain as early as possible and do my best to get it threshed before it rained on the shocks in order to preserve the straw in the best possible condition. Grain also brings a better price when this is done, and the straw makes excellent feed, when it is well taken care of. Always save the cornstalks and do not let them weather out in the field. I always had plenty of feed for my stock which could not be readily turned into cash on the market. Thus my feed cost me very little.

We kept our stock in good healthy condition by cutting up red clover, pea hay, and well-preserved corn stocks, and feeding a little bran or shorts over it. They would eat this with great relish.

The farm is an intensely interesting place when you work it right. Children get interested in it if you give them some part, and let them have some of the proceeds. I was born and raised on a farm, as I have said before, and the farm has always been interesting to me. Many years afterwards I became interested in the manufacture of health foods. While I experimented extensively in raising food from the soil, I also experimented on a large scale in preparing food which could perfectly nourish the body. I have developed many nice foods and made palatable dishes which are really healthful, invigorating and life-sustaining. I have a regular experimenting outfit and am continually working to develop food to meet the needs of every disease of the young and old. Although I have worked at different things during my lifetime, no work is more interesting to me than work on the farm and in the garden—to take some barren land and make it fertile, straightening out and cleaning up the corners, planting seeds, cultivating and seeing the plants grow and develop, continually adding new and better varieties, trying to produce as early a crop as possible, and then have a continual supply all season long of fresh garden products, and growing new varieties of flowers and enjoy the old-fashioned varieties that we used to have when we were children. When we were youngsters, and later on young men and women in my parent's home, the farm was heaven on earth for us.

All the good things in the city do not equal the good things that my mother and my sisters would prepare. The pig panfuls of baked apples with fresh cream over them, and a good piece of old-fashioned coffee cake made from whole-wheat flour. Show me a dish in the city nowadays that beats that. And a dish of clabbered milk that comes out of the icebox on a hot day. Leave the cream on the milk, grate some genuine rye bread over the top of it, together with a little cinnamon and sugar, and then a soup spoon to eat it with. What have you that could beat that? So very delicious and palatable you could practically live and work on it. Those days we made it of cow's milk, but now we make it of soybean milk, which is far better. Also in those days we used cane sugar, but now we use malt sugar, which is infinitely better and like the juice in ripe fruits.

Then I often think about the wonderful dish of fruit soup which we relished so much, made of prunes, raisins, apricots, and various other fruits.

Another dish which we appreciated very much was new potatoes and peas. Mother would make some dumplings of whole wheat flour which we enjoyed better than any spaghetti that was on the market. Now we have soybean spaghetti which is still much better.

Then when I think of those wonderful pieces of baked squash, which we always enjoyed so much, made of those had squashes that we had to take an axe to split open, served with nice fresh butter, also parsnips, carrots, and vegetable oysters, cooked until nearly done and then put in the oven and baked with a little cream, my mouth waters.

When the strawberry season came on, those big dishes of dead-ripe strawberries fresh from the vines with a large piece of homemade coffee cake and some of that wonderful cream. Can you beat that in the city? The most of the strawberries sold in the city are picked too green and are almost worthless. They do not have that delicate flavor that they have when picked fresh and ripe from the vines. When fruit is picked fresh from the trees or vines, thoroughly ripened, it is without question an antidote for disease and premature death. Then when the cherries got ripe, oh! how we did enjoy climbing up in the trees and eating them.

We had three different varieties, red, white, and black ones. We liked the black ones best.

The we had an abundance of currants also; red, white, and black. When the raspberries got ripe, of which we had an abundance in the garden and also in the woods, we used to pick them by the water-buckets full and make juice of them. This is infinitely better than any soft drink that you buy in the cities, and does not contain any harmful ingredients as they do.

Both the red raspberry leaves and the juice is a wonderful medicine. It will break any kind of a fever. How we used to enjoy, when we were working out in the fields on a hot day, seeing Father or Mother coming with a big pitcher of raspberry juice, nice and cold. I do not believe there is anyone who goes to a counter for a soft drink that enjoys it like we enjoyed this. Sometimes they would come with a big pitcher of lemonade with fruit juice in it.

When we would pick the different berries, cherries, and currants my mother would allow us so much a quart, and then we would go down town on the Fouth of July and other special days, and mother would tell us how much she thought we should spend of the money we had. With most children nowadays, when they get hold of a little money, it burns in their pockets, and they are just seeking an opportunity to spend it for some knick-knack. Our great ambition was to try and see how big we could make our little pile so we could buy something worthwhile with it. I shall never forget when I was a little lad I had never had a jack-knife of my own, so I saved quite a little bit of money, and I wanted a jack-knife so much my mother told me I could buy one and told me just about how much she thought I should spend for it. I bought the knife, and my mother said she thought I did very well. Many times during the day I would put my hand in my pocket and take it out and look at it.

It was intensely interesting for us youngsters on the farm as the years rolled around. There was always something to look forward to. When the harvest was gathered, we always enjoyed the thrashing and harvesting, as the neighbors helped one another and we always had a great time during the harvest season—plenty of good things to eat and all kinds of sports. The children had many innocent sports on the farm. We saw the circus man keep three or more apples in the air at the same time and not let them fall to the ground, so, when we had spare time, we practiced it and got so we could keep four apples in the air without letting them fall to the ground. Both my younger brother and I were pretty good shots with the rifle. We would throw a bottle in the air, just as high as we could throw it, and when it began to come down we would shoot at it and break it in the air. Sometimes we would have other sports. We would run and jump, until we got so we could jump over a fence as high as our heads. Then we would jump off something quite high down on a straw pile and make two somersaults before we would strike the straw.

There were no automobiles in those days, but we had nice horses. My father would let us ride them sometimes.

We practiced until we could stand on them and gallop. There were so many interesting things that space will not permit me to mention them all, but suffice it to say that seed time was interesting—to watch the various things grow and have abundance of it on our own table. Harvest time was extremely interesting. Then we would get wood ready for the winter. Then there were times when there was not much to do and we would gather beechnuts, hazelnuts, and walnuts, then cranberries—and my sisters would make a fine cranberry jelly. We would make a barrel of sauerkraut and a barrel of string beans—these we sliced up and put up just about like sauerkraut. We made a big crock full of tomato jam. Now we make it without cane sugar.

In those days only seven to ten per cent of the people were in the cities, while now, there are some eighty per cent of the people in the cities, cooped up in tenements and apartments. The shows, movies and pleasures people have in the cities are not wholesome. They are physically and mentally destructive. The pleasures which we had on the farm were of a different nature and would make real men and women out of the people. They were elevating and inspiring, instead of degrading and debasing. The pleasures of the city do not make noble men and women, good fathers and mothers, good husbands and wives or good citizens. On the farm you do not have to be afraid to go out into the dark, nor do you have to be afraid you will not have something to eat. It is a very small matter to arrange to have something to eat, even if there should be a drought. It is a very easy matter to can up enough to have enough to eat for two or three years. Then if there is a crop failure you would not go hungry. You should also have enough wheat, rye, and barley to last two seasons should there be a crop failure.

Our place was often called "The Garden of Eden." Both my mother and father were lovers of flowers, and we had various trees and hedges, and plenty of fruit at all times. We children were always interested, as we had never learned to run the streets in the cities at night. We had our different little sports evenings, then we would go to bed. Mother and father always knew where we were at night. We never had that craving for money that young folks in the cities have, because they can never get enough to carry out all their plans and schemes which are so expensive nowadays.

Herbs

One of the most interesting things on the farm is herbs, both for food and as a medicine. When I was just a very small child, I used to gather red clover blossoms and our father would carry them in town to the post master who was afflicted with cancer. This was over sixty years ago, and I cannot remember the particulars, but I do know that my father took the red clover blossoms to him every year. The postmaster lived to be a very old man.

Then our groceryman had a daughter who was afflicted. What the trouble was I do not remember, but I very distinctly remember that we would gather the wintergreen, which grows very abundantly in that country, and my mother would take it to her. The outcome of that also I do not remember, as it was over a half a century ago.

I used to gather the mullein flowers and other herbs for an old doctor. We had what we called the draw-shave, a long narrow knife with two handles, one on each end. We used to shave off the rough bark from the white ash trees, slippery elm, birch, wild cherry, willows, pines, poplars, and a number of other trees, and then after we had the outer rough bark off, we would shave off the inner fresh bark which contained the medical properties, and dry them so as to have them ready for use. I do not know what people used them for then, but I know perfectly well what I am using them for now, because I have been using them

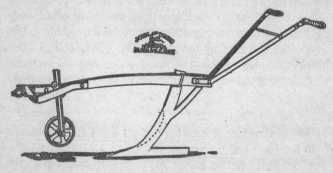

SUBSOIL PLOW

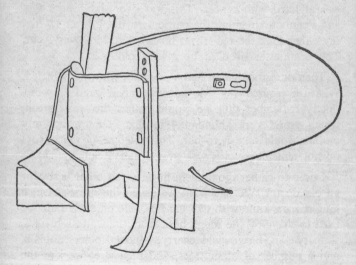

SUBSOIL ATTACHMENT

for many years and see wonderful results. I know from actual experience what they do for mankind.

Many of the things that occurred when I was a child are as vividly before my mind today as if it were only a short time ago.

Shown preceding is a regular sub-soil plow, that can be used on ground that has not been plowed to sub-soil 18 inches deep, or less. Follow with this sub-soiler and another team in the furrow that has been made by the regular turning plow, to stir the ground deeper. If you do not have two teams, unhitch from the turning plow, to the sub-soiler.

Next is an attachment that can be used on a regular turning plow. It can be set so that it digs the dirt 4 to 6 inches deeper than the turning plow goes. A heavy team is necessary to use the attachment with the turning plow; if your team is not heavy put on more horses. Or if you have a tractor, it will draw the regular turning plow with the sub-soiler without any difficulty, and even two plows could be used.

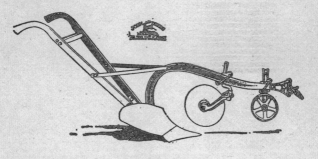

TURNING PLOW

This is a regular turning plow with a rolling, cutting coulter. If your plowing ground is covered with vines of any kind, or long hay or straw the plow cuts it in two, so that it will not drag in front of the plow.

The most effective way to work ground is to plow it 8 or 10 inches deep in the fall, and sub-soil it, then work it thoroughly with a disc harrow, and put a winter crop in, letting it grow until spring as much as it will, then plow it again crossways, turning under the winter crop, and sub-soil it crossways. The deep stirring of the ground in this way will give the moisture a chance to come up, and will also hold the moisture from rainfalls in the ground, and give the roots of your grains and corn a chance to go down deep.

People who have not already used this method will be surprised how it will increase the production of their grains or corn. I have raised a fine crop by this method when my neighbors had very little, or nothing. This is intensely interesting and profitable. Thoroughly pulverize your ground, because these fine roots cannot grow when there are hard clods of dirt, nor will they hold moisture.

CHAPTER III

HISTORY OF MEDICINE

Hippocrates, the "father of medical literature," as he was called, was, so far as we know, the first man who practiced medicine as an art; the following is a copy of the oath Hippocrates took.

"*I swear by Apollo the physician and Aescaulapius and health and all heal,* and all the gods and goddesses that, according to my ability and judgment, I will keep this oath.

"And this stipulation . . . To reckon him who taught me this art equally dear to me as my parents, to share my substance with him and relieve his necessities if required, to look upon his offspring on the same footing as my own brothers and teach them this art if they wish to learn it. *Without fee or stipulation.* Either by precept or lecture or any other mode of instruction, I will impart knowledge of the art to my sons and to those of teachers and disciples bound by a stipulation and oath according to the law of medicine, and to none others. I will follow the system of the regimen which, according to my ability and judgment, I consider *for the benefit of my patients* and abstain from whatever is deleterious and mischievous. *I will give no deadly medicine* to anyone if asked; nor suggest any such counsel and in the like manner I will not give a woman a pessary to produce abortion. *With purity and holiness I will pass my life and practice my art . . .* Into whatever houses I enter, I will go into them for the benefit of the sick and will abstain from any voluntary act of mischief and corruption. And further from the seduction of males or females, of freeman and slaves. Whatever in connection with my professional practice, or not in the connection with it, I see or hear in the life of men which ought not be spoken of abroad, *I will not divulge* as reckoning all such should be kept secret.

"While I continue to keep the *oath* inviolated may it be granted to me to enjoy life and the practice of the art, respected by all men in all times. But if I trespass and violate this *oath* may the reverse be my lot."

"HIPPOCRATES"

"Apollo, the Physician," was addressed as the "two-horn God," in Orphic hymns. There was only one original two-horned god, which was Nimrod, who founded the Chaldean monarchy. Nimrod was the original Appollo. Apollo "nimrod" was the mighty hunter who went before the Lord and was the husband of Semiramis. Aescaulapius, who was sworn by next was supposed to be the "father of medicine" at this time, and times past. Temples were dedicated to him in all the kingdoms of Greece and Rome. There were also temples erected to this same personage. The name is not in the Greek language, Egyptian, Assyrian, or Hebrew, but in the Chaldean language. There are three words which make up the word Aescaulapius, ASHE, SKUL, APHE. The words MAN, SKUL mean to instruct, APHE means snake. Aescaulapius means MAN-INSTRUCTING-SNAKE. In the Bible we are told that Satan was the only man instructing snake, the menace of all mankind. SATAN, Aescaulapius was never a man, but a creature that took it on itself to instruct the human race. Hippocrates was a man. It is proven that he lived upon the earth and died. Hippocrates is known as the "Father of medical literature." His treatises are filled with the practical knowledge of the difficulties of the human race and practical knowledge may be derived from studying his works at the present day. So far as history informs us, the first work of any importance referred to Hippocrates works. We find that he believed in the "effort of nature," and left many things to the "effort of nature." In his oath, he swore he would "give no deadly medicine" which means he would not give anything of a deadly nature. He was one of the "regular school," but he was a herbal practitioner. No minerals were used, unless salt was thought of by some physician. This same system was used up to the year 1500 A.D. No deadly medicines were given by respectable physicians. All through history we have evidence of what people did, but the evidence is there that no "regular" physicians were unwise enough to attempt any poisoning of the body.

Among others, and as prominent as anyone, was Scribonius Largus, who lived during the reign of Nero. He was a Roman. He wrote a book in which there was a formula made up of sixty-one ingredients, the principal one being the dried flesh of vipers. This formula was called *Therica* and was kept until about the eightheenth century. But the physicians who followed Hippocrates were satisfied not to give any deadly medicine. Those medicines were sought for by ignorant people who thought if medicine made the bowels active it was good and made them better, as people think of present-day cathartics. When doing this they defied the life force of the body.

In the year 1490 A.D., there was a physician in Germany, named William Bombast von Hohemhein. When his son was born he named him Theophratus von Hohemhein. The son was carefully taught in the same school as his father. He became dissatisfied with his father and teachers and went into the mines of Tyrol. There he saw minerals purified by the action of other minerals and he conceived the idea of purifying human bodies in the same manner. He began trying minerals on the bodies of his patients. We have no record of the result of his experiments, because there was none made. He called himself "Paracelsus," for what reason we do not know, unless to designate that he was above the Celsus who lived centuries before him. His ideas were those of a chemist about the human body. He salivated his patients when they had "actions of the bowels," and it seemed as though he knew what to do for them.

It is stated that he publicly burned the books of Galen and Hippocrates, and threw aside all their ideas and went in for chemically purifying the body by use of minerals. His own ideas were disastrous to him. He died in 1541, being only fifty of fifty-one years old. He did not live long, but he transformed the medical practice. After his death there were hundreds of people who took up his practice of giving minerals in place of herbs, roots, and barks.

As far as we can find in history, he was the first man who ever gave mercury, who made any profession of "medicine." He gave it in large and small doses. Up to the present day this form of giving minerals has increased until the majority of doctors in the civilized world use minerals to purify the body. The herbalists in Great Britain are called botanic practitioners. They are really successors of Galen and Hippocrates, and the regular doctors of today are successors of the descendants of Hohemhein of the fifteenth century.

From 460 B.C. to 1500 A.D., nineteen hundred years, we have no record of anyone giving minerals for the cure of diseases until Hohemhein had his mind turned into chemical channels by going into the mines at Tyrol, where he got the idea of purifying the body by the use of minerals. There was very little deviation from the beliefs and teachings of Hippocrates that in "nature there was strength" to cure disease.

In 1492, when Columbus discovered America, is seems that there is no doubt when he went back that either he or some of his men carried the germs of syphilis. There are people who have doubts that this disease originated here in America. The Italians called it a "French Disease," and the French people said it originated in Spain. Chancroids and gonorrhea were known from earlier times, and may have existed since the time of Egypt. I think it is safe to say that whether it originated in America, or wherever it originated, it was only a periodical increase in the violence of the disease. It was called the "new disease" in the early part of the fifteenth century. Hohemhein tried his mercurial compounds on his patients and in his works stated that it seemed to "drive out humor." That is the way that mercury came into general use in the treatment of syphilis.

It would not have hurt Freeman Bumstead's reputation as teacher if he had told the exact truth and given the facts as they were, that mercury was the invention of an ignorant mind, that human bodies are not subject to chemical laws, like minerals, and could be purified by another mineral, which invention led the world into the deception of dosing the body with a poison to combat another poison, but in reality substituted one poison for another in the body. Mercury takes away absolutely nothing, but places a far worse condition in the system than there was before. The giving of quicksilver (or Quack Salber) resulted in the calling of physicians who dosed with quicksilver "quacks."

In the early part of the eighteenth century, a German physician by the name of Hahneman, set forth the idea that it would be better to give smaller doses of medicines. He started giving medicines in powdered form, and in such small doses that it had little effect as a drug. He did not discard the old materia medica, but in addition to giving mercury, arsenic, and all other minerals, included some of the most filthy serums, unsanitary preparations from bees, bedbugs, snake poisons, etc. Anyone with intelligence, who would take a few minutes to think about the make-up of the human body, would realize that minerals and such unsanitary medicines could not prove a panacea for any of the ills of man that they seemed to think they would.

Hahneman was in the wrong when he ignored the fact that it is the strength of nature that restores the body, when he said "like cures like."

Herbs were the first medicine used by man. Allopaths are about five hundred years old.

In 1769, Samuel Thompson was born in Alstead, N. H. He was one of six children. He was often taken to the woods to help a botanic practitioner and a midwife by the name of Benton, to help gather herbs and plants. When Thompson was very young, he experimented with the herb Lobelia. He chewed it and swallowed the juice until he vomited, and called it the emetic herb. He went to school for one month when he was ten years old. When he became about twenty-four years old, he remebered the action of lobelia and started to make use of it. He had no education whatever, except his knowledge of herbs and roots, and their effect on sick people. When about nineteen years old he cut his leg and was laid up for some time, but, instead of cutting it off, he applied a poultice of Comfrey root, and saved his leg.

The saying, "History repeats itself," is certainly found to be true in the career of Samuel Thompson. He was an uneducated farmer, without medical training, knew nothing of Roman history, but he perfected the same treatment that was practiced by the Romans two thousand years before. Hippocrates also, who was the "father of medical literature," lived in poverty during his youth.

There is no doubt that Thompson proved the emetic qualities of the herb Lobelia, and his ideas were correct about the necessity of eliminating the waste materials from the body, to restore it to the natural condition of health. Thompson's idea was to cleanse the body. His idea of steaming the body is what the Russians have done from time immemorial. He steamed the body to get outward heat, and used herb stimulants to produce inward heat. And yet, in Gould's 1900 dictionary, he said that "sweating, lobelia, and capsicum were the principal agents relied upon in this school."

Many people followed the theories of Thompson after he died. His ideas of relaxation, stimulation, and use of astringents were taken up by many doctors because they were satisfied with the correctness of the results.

Dr. Curtis, of Cincinnati, Ohio, chartered one of the first of these colleges from legislature. W. H. Cook took charge of another, and when Dr. Curtis died, the institution was moved to Chicago under the name of College of Medicine and Surgery.

Before Thompson, the American Indians, as well as Indians of other countries, used all kinds of herbs, roots, and barks in the healing art, and are using them today. I have at times learned many valuable things from them. These Indians are using some of the same herbs for the same diseases as they did in Christ's time.

Many years ago Naturopath doctors were given permission to practice in England, and Herbal doctors are fast growing in popularity and favor with the people. English Royalty employs herbal doctors.

Along medical lines, England and many other countries are far ahead of the United States. In Germany, Frederick the Great established religious, political and medical freedom by this statement: that in his kingdom, "Everybody can go to heaven as he pleases."

CHAPTER IV

FRESH AIR AND EXERCISE

Through the lungs the system receives life-giving air. One may live for many days without solid food, and several days without even liquid food, but death comes in a few moments without air. The capacity for air can be greatly increased by proper exercising of the lungs, as has often been demonstrated in the treatment of consumption. Air is a simple mixture of numerous gases, but is chiefly composed of oxygen and nitrogen. Life is more dependent upon the regular and adequate supply of oxygen than any other element. The nitrogen of the air dilutes the oxygen, as in an atmosphere of pure oxygen we would live so fast as to be very short-lived. Experiments have shown that prolonged inhalation of air in which the proportion of oxygen is much greater than that in which it naturally occurs in the atmosphere, causes great disturbance of the system and finally death. Therefore, we know that the mixture called air is not an accidental compound, but one perfectly and admirably adapted to the needs of human beings as well as animals and plants.

The watery vapor in the air is necessary to enable the lungs to utilize the oxygen readily, as is shown by experiments that prove that dry oxygen is not as readily absorbed as that which contains the proper proportion of moisture. A great change occurs in the blood when it passes through the capillaries of the lungs. As the pulmonary artery brings the blood from the right heart to the lungs it is a dark purple color (its color is due to the carbonic acid or impurities which it contains), then when it leaves the lungs it is a bright red color having exchanged the poisons for oxygen. This oxygen is then absorbed by the red blood corpuscles and taken to every part of the system, and is assimilated in the capillaries of the tissues. The blood then gathers up carbonic acid and goes back to the lungs to be cleansed again. Other impurities are also given out in the lungs. The blood is slightly cooled and loses some of its water as it passes through the lungs. The amount of carbonic gas exhaled during digestion is greatly diminished by the use of stimulating foods, sugar, animal foods and more especially by wine, rum, beer, ale, cider, tea and coffee. Strenuous exercise increases the exhalation of carbonic gas to six times the ordinary amount.

The lungs can and should be greatly improved by systematic exercise. When the lungs are not well expanded habitually, they lose to a greater or less degree their elasticity. In many cases there is almost total loss of the power to really expand the chest, which is very necessary to perfect health development. When a person feels weary and exhausted from sedentary employment, the practice of deep breathing and prolonged respiration, with the spine erect and the chest well expanded, will prove very refreshing and will induce restful sound sleep. The great advantage of abundance of lung exercise is seen in the fact that professional singers suffer less from lung affections than others. The chest of professional singers is always better developed than in the majority of persons.

The detrimental effects of breathing impure air, especially in a room where there are several people, are headache, nervousness, dullness and aggravation of all diseases pertaining to lung affections. The headaches with which school children are afflicted are often caused by foul air. Consumption is most frequent in those whose habits, vocations, or occupations are sedentary, as they are usually kept in an atmosphere of foul air.

An old army surgeon who had charge of large hospitals during the war related a very interesting experience illustrating the importance of giving the sick, especially persons suffering with fever, an abundance of pure air. He said that in a large hospital he had at one time 320 cases of measles during the winter season. The hospital caught fire and burned to the ground, and the patients had to be placed in tents. All but one or two recovered. He said he had no doubt but that the number of deaths would have been thirty or forty at least, had the patients remained in the hospital.

Walking increases the inhalation of oxygen threefold. Regular exercise in the open air is one of the most important factors for preservation of health and prolongation of life. The degree of activity of life depends upon the amount of oxygen taken into our bodies. In cold weather we get a larger supply of oxygen than in the hot weather, and it makes us more active mentally and physically.Outdoor life in the cool fresh air of temperate zones gives a strong constitution and increases our resistance against disease.It is a well known fact that the inhabitants of temperate zones have more energy than those of the tropics. *A sound and vigorous body can only be produced by pure blood and healthy nerves.*

Oxygen, the elixir of life, is one of the best blood purifiers, and one of the most effective nerve tonics. It is simply provided by nature for all. Useful work in the open air will bring new strength and vitality, and give a happy and cheerful attitude of mind. If the poisonous waste matter which should be thrown off by exhalations from the lungs is retained, the blood becomes impure, and not only the lungs but the stomach, liver, and brain are affected. The digestion is retarded, the skin becomes sallow, the brain clouded and the thoughts confused, the heart depressed, and the whole system inactive and very susceptible to disease.

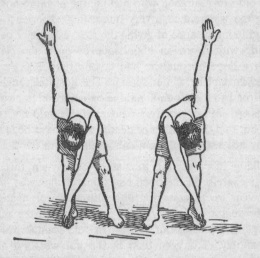

VALUABLE EXERCISE TO STRENGTHEN THE ENTIRE SYSTEM

Proper exercise in the open air and sunshine are among God's greatest gifts to man. It gives good form and strength to the physical organism, and all other habits being equal, is the surest safeguard against disease and premature death. It gives buoyancy, free from the extremes resulting from artificial life.

Every room and especially every sleeping room in the house should be well-ventilated throughout the year, both day and night. Have plenty of light and sunshine and air which is wisely mixed by our gracious God, in your houses to make you strong, healthy, and happy.

CHAPTER V

FASTING

There is much said throughout the entire Bible about fasting. We will consider some of its uses and benefits. God instituted fasting for both spiritual and physical blessings. The priests in Christ's day fasted twice a week. Throughout the history of the Bible the people fasted and prayed in order to gain victories. It has two purposes—the upbuilding of the body and the spiritual upbuilding of the soul. Christ fasted forty days to get the victory over appetite in man's behalf. On this point of appetite our first parents fell, and thousands have gone into an untimely grave because of indulgence of it.

I have made many experiments with fasting. I fasted for one day a number of times just to get victory over appetite and to gain spiritual strength, and have also fasted a number of times for three days. Once I fasted for twenty-one days, and worked from early until late and never rested during the day. Another time I fasted for twenty-three days, and worked every day. I could have fasted forty days, but was working too hard.

There are persons who advocate long fasts for health (and otherwise), but I warn everyone against long fasts, as they do not benefit physically, and are not a spiritual requirement. Short fasts for a day or two are very beneficial, both spiritually and physically, especially when plenty of water is taken in connection with deep breathing exercises. To abstain from rich food, and to eat but very little plain food, even for days and weeks, would be very beneficial.

This would give the system a chance to purify itself of poisonous substances.

At one time I with others was eating dinner at an outing and we noticed a man who was not eating. I went to him and asked, "Friend, have you anything to eat? We have plenty and some to spare." This man replied, "I am fasting. I do not care for anything to eat." I then asked him his reason for fasting. He said, "I used to have rheumatism so bad that I was unable to do anything. All the doctors and medicine didn't help me, and one day a man came to me and said if I would fast two days a week my rheumatism would leave me." I asked him who the man was who told him this. He replied that he did not know, that he had never seen the man before, and had never seen him since. He said, "I followed his instruction, and it was but a short time until my rheumatism was gone, and I have never had it since. This was a number of years ago."

I am thoroughly convinced that a great many people eat too much. Many eat food that does not give them proper nourishment. It is also true that many people are undernourished because they eat devitaminized food, improperly prepared, and improper mixtures of food which ferment and make poor blood of what they do eat. The weak, the lean, and undernourished must be very careful about fasting.

In Bible times when one fasted an entire day, it was counted that he had gained a victory. I know of different times when people fasted one day, and then in the evening after sundown they ate a lot of food. This would not be counted as fasting one day. Fasting means not to eat anything all day until the next day. A serious mistake is often made when too much food is taken after the fast, and much injury to the system is the result. A great deal of the effect of the fast is thus lost.

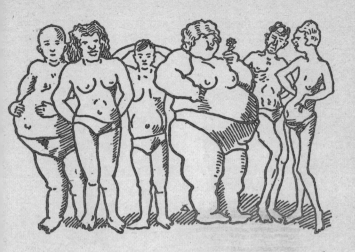

The above picture is a fair sample of the sights to be seen along beaches where thousands of people are bathing. When you eat the foods which are robbed of their lifegiving properties, you get into all kinds of shapes, as you see in the above picture.

But if we eat the food as God has made it with all the vitamins and mineral salts, as they are now called, we do not get nervous, irritable, unreasonable, and out of sorts. When the minerals and vitamins, which would keep the body symmetrical, are removed from the food, we grow all out of shape and proportion, and it makes us subject to all kinds of diseases, of which there are as many as there are different concoctions made for us to eat. When we feel so tired all the time, that which gives us pep and makes us courageous is not in the food.

I have seen many herds of horses, cattle, sheep and other animals, and they are all very much alike because they eat the food the way God has made it for them. Just stop and think! There is not anything in any of the meats which is not in the grains, hay and grass which the animals eat. Why eat it second-handed! Let's eat it in its pure original state, what do you say?

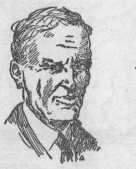 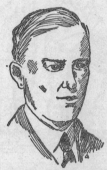

A diet of acid forming foods and combinations causes waste matter in the system, which in turn causes wrinkles and makes us old. I have seen just as radical a change in a person as you see in the picture above, a man with a skin wrinkled, yellow and old looking, after he was put on a right diet, and given sweet baths, and herbs to cleanse the blood stream and intestinal tract and colon. The change was so great that people who knew him said he looked twenty years younger. I have seen this done many times. I, today, am a living example of the above.

There is so much written about foods today that it becomes confusing. So much about calories, acid-forming foods, alkaline foods, etc., and one writer says this and one that, and I have heard people say many times they did not know what to eat any more. In the above picture we see a cow with a calf—this cow raised this calf in this pasture, was never out of the pasture, and had nothing to eat but the grass that grew in that pasture, and water to drink, and the calf had nothing but the milk she got from her mother, until she was large enough to eat the grass too. This calf was beautifully developed, had a well-proportioned body, nice hair, good solid bones, good sound teeth, good hoofs, and good eyes. Now there was not anything in the milk, which was not in the grass, and this milk produced this calf, that

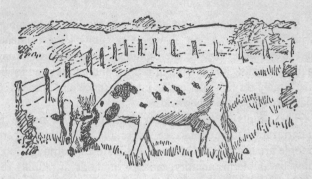

shows very plainly that all the vitamins were in the grass, and all the minerals, protein, and carbohydrates. Now it is just the same with all the food which God has given us, while it is true that different kinds of fruits, grains, and vegetables, have somewhat different properties, and I would not recommend that anyone should take any one particular food, and live on it to the exclusion of others. But if the natural life-giving properties which are in the foods as God made them, are not destroyed in their preparation, we wouldn't have to worry about calories, or alkaline and acid-forming foods. All natural foods have the right amount of alkalinity and acid in them, which the body requires to keep it in perfect health. I was born and raised on a farm in the northern part of Wisconsin, and we raised practically everything we ate, and we were a large family of children, and never sick, and we lived to be old people.

CHAPTER VI

EFFECTS OF DEVITAMINIZED, ADULTERATED FOODS ON THE BODY

Our health depends on how nearly we live in harmony with Nature's laws. An all-wise God put all the elements in the soil necessary for the buliding of our bodies. Wrong habits of eating and the use of refined and adulterated foods are largely responsible for the intemperance and crime, and sickness that curse this world.

The results of man's trying to improve on nature is deteriorating the human race, especially in America where people are accustomed to so-called luxuries. Although food may be ample in quantity, modern methods of refining remove the most important elements, and in many cases they are adulterated, and preservatives added to conceal their inferior quality.

Calories

Calories are not a sufficient foundation to determine the nutritive value of food. Foods which show a high caloric value, are often deficient in nutritive elements, and organic salts. In order to determine the true nutritive value of foods, it is important to study the composition of foods in regard to the amount of mineral elements they contain. *For perfect health we must have perfect digestion, assimilation, and elimination. The ignorance of the average person regarding the laws of his being is appalling.*

Adulteration of Foods

Many staple foods on the market are according to the present prevailing standards legitimate, and are widely advertised, but are most unhealthful and cannot be recommended from a health standpoint—foods such as, white flour, candies, white sugar, white rice, various canned and preserved foods, sulphured fruits, highly seasoned foods, etc. The majority of these foods are deficient in organic salts, and substances which are detrimental to health have been added to preserve or color them.

Deficiency Diseases

You cannot get mineral supply for your body from pills or bottles but out of natural foods the way nature prepares them.

God in his infinite wisdom neglected nothing, and if we would eat our food without trying to improve, change, and refine it, thereby destroying its life-giving elements, it would meet all requirements of the body.

Diseases Caused by a Deficiency of Minerals

Anemia	'Nerves'
Acid conditions	Neuralgia
(Auto-intoxication)	Neuritis
Appendicitis	Pellagra
Cancer	Paralysis
Colitis	Infantile paralysis
Constipation	Pleurisy
Convulsions	Pneumonia
Diabetes	Rheumatism
Dysentery	Rickets
Eczema	Sciatica
Heart Disease	Scurvy
Intestinal Diseases	Tetany
Malnutrition	Tuberculosis
Menstruation	Tumors
(disorders of)	Skin eruptions

Bread

When the miller removes the outer shell from the wheat and the germ from the center the necessary elements are taken away. White flour is mainly starch.

Nerves are nourished by the blood. The blood must be pure and contain all the elements necessary for nourishing the nerves, and every part of the body.

Health-Destroying Foods

Spices, mustard, pepper, vinegar, salt, condiments, salted meats, canned meats, salted fish, tobasco sauce, worchestershire sauce, gravies, fried or greasy foods, pastries, predigested foods, tobacco, very hot or ice cold foods, coca cola, all soft drinks, chewing gum, coffee, tea, cocoa, white flour and white flour products, can sugar and products. The organs that make our blood cannot convert spices, pickles, etc. into pure blood.

The Irish potato is a very valuable food, but not after it has been peeled, and boiled in a quantity of water, which is drained down the sink, leaving the potato lifeless, and minerally exhausted, and acid producing.

Food

The food question should be given its proper place in the medical world. We are made of what we eat, nothing else, and we should eat to increase strength and preserve health and life. All foods do not agree with everyone, but everyone should eat the natural foods that agree best with him. Disease and illness would be rare if every blood stream were pure, and the body was not full of waste matter and toxins. Poisonous waste matter in the system is the result of more food being taken than the body can assimilate or eliminate. Foods high in protein specifically cause this, such as, meats of all kinds, eggs, etc. You may eat anything for a while, but the results will inevitably follow. The use of starchy foods and tea contribute greatly to intestinal ills, constipation, leucorrhea, etc. Acid blood is one of the results of excess of sugar and starch. It is not always the amount of food taken that causes trouble, it may be wrong combinations, indigestible foods of all kinds, especially greasy and fried foods.

Overeating

Overeating or too frequent eating produces a feverish state in the system, and overtaxes the digestive organs, the blood becomes impure, and diseases of various kinds occur. It also produces excessive acid, and causes the gastric mucous membrane to become congested. Hyperacidity is a common result. An excessive intake of food is much more common than a deficiency. Over-fed people are much more likely to have cancer than under-fed. Cancer, Bright's disease, arteriosclerosis, high blood pressure, and apoplexy are some of the consequences of overeating.

It must always be remembered that what would be enough for a hard-working man would be a great excess for a man of sedentary habits of work.

The modern method of serving is very destructive. The bill of fare is arranged so that the most highly tempting dishes are presented last, such as pastries, ice cream, etc. This encourages excessive eating. After having eaten enough, this extra food is added which becomes a poison, and is a burden to the system.

When the bowels are full already, the second meal is compelled to lie in the stomach overtime and sour. Overeating makes the work of the stomach, liver, kidneys, and bowels harder. When this food putrifies, its poisons are absorbed back into the blood and consequently the whole system is poisoned.

Condiments

Condiments are simply added to make food taste better to a perverted appetite. The taste for condiments is a purely acquired one. Condiments of all kinds are repulsive to infants and everyone whose taste has not been perverted. They furnish no nutrition, and are very irritating to the delicate lining of the stomach and digestive organs. They favor a feverish condition in the system which is very injurious to health and cause dyspepsia and nervous irritability. Mustard and black pepper cause inflammation of the stomach and skin, habitual use produces intestinal catarrh and ruins the digestive juices. The idea that spices and similar substances aid digestion is erroneous. Condiments hinder rather than aid digestion. The oils found in condiments are all irritant, and when applied externally in a concentrated form will cause blistering, inflammation and irritation, and if the contact is prolonged will destroy the tissue. The effect upon the stomach is similar. When these poisons are absorbed into the blood they are brought into contact with every cell and fiber of the body. Often the delicate cells of the kidneys undergo a degenerative change from the use of condiments, their efficiency is impaired, and as a result we have Bright's disease and other disease.

Pickles

Pickles are indigestible, they resist the action of the gastric juice as would pebbles, and cause great irritation and chronic diseases. They are hardened by the action of the acetic acid, and sometimes the addition of alcohol. They arrest the action of the saliva and cause gastric catarrh. Acetic acid is an active poison. Stuffed olives, green olives, brandied fruits, etc., are in the same class. Salads in which vinegar is used is far from wholesome and must always be excluded from the sick or invalid diet, in all cases. Lemon should be substituted for vinegar in all cases. Lemon is an excellent tonic and cleanser for the system. "Germs of any kind cannot live in lemon juice."

Free fats undergo no change in the stomach. They stay in the stomach and prevent digestion until they enter the duodenum wheer the pancreatic juice and bile transform it so it can be absorbed by the system. Vegetable oils are also free fats and do not digest in the stomach. The growth-promoting vitamin which is sometimes associated with fat is bountifully found in greens.

Fats are easily digested in the form of nuts, ripe olives, and nut preparations. Nut butter is in every way superior to animal fat and butter, and contains no disease germs. DO NOT ROAST THE NUTS THAT NUT-BUTTER IS MADE FROM. Never roast nuts, as roasting ruins the oil contained in the nut. Vegetable oils, and such recipes as given in this book perfectly take the place of all animal fats and butter.

Fats produce a sense of satisfaction after eating, more than any other food, and therefore should be used sparingly. Fats are fuel foods and excess of fats encourages intestinal putrefaction, biliousness, obesity, congests the liver, etc.

Chapter VII

FRUIT DIET

All fruits contain acids which are necessary for the proper elimination of various toxins, poisonous acids, and other impurities

Natural acids are highly alkaline.

The value of a fruit diet cannot be over-estimated, especially in sickness, ill health, or whenever the body is filled with poisons. Germs cannot grow and live in fruit juices. Typhoid fever and cholera germs cannot resist the action of fruit juices such as lemon, orange, pineapple, strawberry, apple, and grapefruit. A fruit diet will disinfect the stomach and alimentary canal. Fresh fruits are more effective for this purpose than stewed fruits.

Citric, malic, tartaric acids are powerful germicides found in fruits.

Malic Acid is found in pineapples, apples, quinces, pears, apricots, plums, peaches, cherries, currants, gooseberries, strawberries, raspberries, blackberries, elderberries, grapes, and tomatoes.

Citric acid is found in strawberries, red raspberries, cherries, red currants, cranberries, lemons, limes, grapefruit, and oranges.

Tartaric Acid is obtained from grapes and pineapples. Tartaric acid is important in treating all diseases of hyperacidity, such as lung diseases, sore throat, indigestion, etc.

Oxalic Acid is found in plum,s tomatoes, rhubarb, sorrel, yellow dock, spinach, and is especially good for constipation and an inactive liver.

Lactic acid is found in buttermilk and clabber milk, also soybean buttermilk. It is good in treatment of termentation, and putrefaction and in treating hardening of the arteries it is especially good.

It is better to use fruits uncooked. Never sweeten them with cane sugar.

A fruit diet is an excellent cure for chronic constipation, also for reducing. Fruit gives the body strength and energy. Fruits are solvents, and should always be abundantly used in an eliminating diet.

Fruit is an ideal food. It develops more slowly than other products, therefore, for a longer time receives the beneficial effects of the sunlight, and air.

Dates, raisins, and figs and many other dried fruits have become staple foods in civilized countries. Dates and raisins are high in natural sugar which is very easily assimilated. Figs both fresh and dried, especially Black Mission Figs, are rich in bone-building elements.

Chapter VIII

MEAT-EATING

Meats of all kinds are unnatural foods. Flesh, fish, fowl, and sea foods are very likely to contain numbers of germs. Meat contains bacteria. This bacteria infects the intestines causing colitis, and many other diseases. They always cause putrefaction.

Research has shown beyond all doubt that a meat diet produces cancer in some cases. Excessive uric acid is caused by meat-eating. Excessive uric acid causes rheumatism, Bright's disease, kidney stones, gout, gallstones. I have treated cases of severe headaches with which the patients had suffered for many years and every remedy had been tried without relief, but when meat was excluded from the diet, they obtained most gratifying results.

Uric acid excreted from the urine comes from two sources: (1) Uric acid taken into the body in meat, meat extracts, tea, coffee, etc. (2) Uric acid formed in the body out of nitrogenous foods. A diet of potatoes is excellent to rid the system of exccessive uric acid.

It is an established fact that meat protein causes putrefaction twice as quickly as vegetable protein. There is no ingredient in meat which cannot be procured in better quality in products of the vegetable kingdom. Meat is an expensive second-hand food material and will not make healthy, pure blood, or form good tissues.

The argument that flesh must be eaten in order to supply the body sufficient protein is unreasonable; it is found in abundance in beans, peas, lentils, and all kinds of nuts.

The nutritive value of meat broths is practically nothing. They always contain uric acid and other poisons.

Nuts perfectly take the place of meat. With the exception of the peanut, and chestnut, the average nutritive value of nuts is about two-hundred calories per ounce. This is double the value of an equal quantity of sugar or starch.

Almonds: One-fifth of the weight of the almond consists of protein, and it is of the very finest quality. The almond affords a most delicious oil, which is highly digestible. Almond butter can be made into a delicious milk or cream, which, with the addition of a little sweetening, resembles cow's milk in appearance and nutritive properties.

Hickory Nut: A pound of hickory nut meats is equal in nutritive value to more than four pounds of average meat. Two-thirds of the weight of the hickory nut is easily digested oil.

Pecan: The pecan is a valuable nut, high in nutrition.

Walnut: A pound of walnuts contains almost fifty per cent more protein than the same quantity of beef. The English walnut differs slightly from the black walnut, in that it contains more fat and less protein.

Butternut: The butternut also contains more fat than the black walnut, but has the same amount of protein. The butternut contains about three per cent carbohydrates, therefore, is very valuable for persons suffering from diabetes.

Peanut: When thoroughly dried the peanut contains fifty per cent more protein than the best beefsteak. Further, half its weight is an excellent oil. Emphasis must be placed on the fact that the salted, roasted peanuts, as found on the market, are over-roasted, and indigestible. Unroasted peanut butter is easily digested and highly nutritious. The protein of the peanut is equal to the protein of milk and eggs as a tissue-building element. A very fine milk can be made from unroasted peanut butter. Peanuts are also used extensively in malted nuts, and vegetable meats.

Cocoanut: A most excellent substitute for butter can be prepared as follows: Cut the meat of the nut in strips, grate it or grind through a meat grinder. Soak in several times as much water as you have cocoanut, using warm water, let set for two or three hours. A rich cream will rise to the top. Skim off and work into a butter with an ordinary butter ladle.

It is better to eat nuts in an emulsified form such as nut butters. When eaten otherwise, they must be thoroughly masticated, so that no little hard pieces will enter the stomach.

Small particles of such concentrated foods cannot be acted upon by the digestive juices, and often pass undigested into the alimentary canal.

Nut butters prepared without roasting are superior in nutritive and hygienic value to the best cuts of meats and to dairy butter and cheese.

The protein of nuts is of greater value for the renewal of the body cells than the protein derived from the muscular tissues of a dead animal with all its waste poisons.

Composition of Edible Portion of Nuts.

	Protein	Fats	Carbo-hydrates	Ash
Almonds	21.0	54.9	17.3	2.0
Beechnuts	21.9	57.4	13.2	3.5
Brazil Nuts	17.0	66.8	7.0	3.9
Butternuts	27.9	61.2	3.4	3.0
Chestnuts, Dried	10.7	7.0	74.2	2.2
Chestnuts, Fresh	6.2	5.4	42.1	1.3
Cocoanuts	5.7	50.6	27.9	1.7
Cocoanuts, Shredded	6.3	57.3	31.6	1.3
Filberts	15.6	65.3	13.0	2.4

Composition of Edible Portion of Nuts.

	Protein	Fats	Carbo-hydrates	Ash
Hickory Nuts	15.4	67.4	11.4	2.1
Peanuts, Raw	25.8	38.6	24.4	2.0
Pecan Nuts	11.0	71.2	13.3	1.5
Pistachios Kernels	22.6	54.5	15.6	3.1
Black Walnuts	27.6	56.3	11.7	1.9
English Walnuts	16.7	64.4	14.8	1.3

The pecan, filbert, English walnut, almond, hickory, chestnut are abundant in growth-promoting vitamins.

The nut should not be used as a dainty; it should be a staple article of diet. The popular idea that nuts are hard to digest has no foundation. The habit of eating nuts at the end of a meal, when in all probability more food of a highly nutritious nature has been eaten than is necessary, is very injurious. It is an equally injurious habit to eat nuts between meals. Improper mastication is a common cause of indigestion from the use of nuts.

Peanuts should be heated slightly to remove the skin. Other nuts may be blanched and crushed without roasting. Over-roasting makes the nut very difficult to digest.

Nuts should be eaten as a part of every heavy meal, and made a substantial part of the bill of fare. As their merits are appreciated they will be used in this way.

Nuts contain more iron than any other food stuff; they also contain a high content of lime.

Chapter IX

FOODS

Baking Powder: Baking powder contains two chemicals: bicarbonate of soda; and tartaric acid. These two chemicals do not neutralize each other in any way so as to destroy or render them harmless, and there is left in the bread a substance identical with Rochelle Salts sold at the drugstore. For an illustration: Two teaspoonfuls of baking powder used to a quart of flour leaves in the bread 165 grains of Rochelle Salts, that is, 45 grains more than contained in Seidlitz powder. This has no nutritive value, but retards digestion, and gives the eliminative organs extra work to throw off the poison.

In 1908 there was a great stir made about the poisonous effects of baking powder. A direct appeal was made to President Theodore Roosevelt, and he appointed a committee to investigate the physiological effects of baking powders.

After this investigation, Bulletin No. 103 was issued by the Agricultural Department, which contained the final determination concerning baking powders by this committee. "In short, the board concludes that alum baking powders are no more harmful than any other baking powders, but that it is wise to be moderate in the use of foods that are leavened with baking powder." There is nothing in that statement which proves that baking powders are harmless; it simply says that one baking powder is no more harmful than another, but the physiological action of baking powders was of such nature "that it is wise to be moderate in the use of foods that are leavened with baking powder."

Our present phosphate beds are exhausted, but phosphate is still needed for the making of pancake flour and manufacture of baking powders. Aluminum compounds are used extensively with phosphates in the manufacture of fully one-half of all the baking powders manufactured in the United States. In the Manual of the Parke-Davis Company, one of the largest pharmaceutical houses in America, they state concerning aluminum: "Powerful astringent, (causes animal tissue to contract) rarely used internally, except in Painter's colic." Most baking powders on the market now are real poisons. They eat the lining of the stomach, or damage it until congestion and inflammation follow. Soda decreases the pancreatic juices, which are used to digest protein, fats and carbohydrates.

More than one hundred million pounds of baking powders are used in the United States every year, and less than one million pounds can be said to be free from DANGEROUS POISONS.

Cow's Milk: Cow's milk is not suited for human consumption. Half the invalids in the world suffer from dyspepsia, and milk should not be taken. Milk causes constipation, biliousness, coated tongue, headache, and these are the symptoms of intestinal auto-intoxication. Soybean milk, and nut milks are excellent substitutes, and have practically the same analysis, and the danger of disease is removed.

Common Salt: Salt should be used very sparingly. It contains chloride of sodium, which is an inorganic mineral and cannot be used by any cell structure of the body. It irritates the stomach and blood stream, is indigestible, and hinders the digestion of other foods. It is one of the causes of rheumatism, dizziness, cancer, scurvy, by putting harmful minerals into the system.

Sodium salts are plentifully found in fruits and vegetables, such as tomatoes, asparagus, celery, spinach, kale, radishes, turnips, carrots, lettuce, strawberries, and many others.

When salt is omitted, a person soon enjoys the flavor of the food more, as the main taste of people who use any quantity of salt is a salty one. Without salt more food flavors may be enjoyed. Salt must not be used in dropsy, hyperacidity, Bright's disease, gastric ulcer, obesity, and epilepsy.

The true science of eating and feeding should be thoroughly understood by all—what elements the system requires in order to build and repair, how best to supply them, and how to prepare them in the most appetizing manner and without destroying their life-giving properties.

The human body is a finely constructed machine, and transforms energy from the food supplied. As the automobile burns gasoline, the human body burns food. Every machine known is constantly wearing, and requires renewal of parts; just so, the body must have proper food to build new tissues and to repair worn out ones.

COMPOSITION OF THE BODY: Over 60 per cent water, also contains many mineral elements in different amounts.

Carbohydrates: Supply energy.

Cellulose: Is the framework of fruits and vegetables and supplies bulk, which aids in normal intestinal peristalsis, and stimulates the bowels.

Fats: Supply energy in a very concentrated form, and are also fuel foods.

Mineral Matter: Supplies building materials, and helps regulate the body processes. Mineral salts are necessary for blood making and tissue building.

Proteins: Supply energy, oxygen, hydrogen, nitrogen, sulphur, phosphorus and a little iron.

Water: Supplies building material, and regulates the body's processes. Makes up the principal part of all the body fluids and secretions, and helps make it possible for the body to regulate its own temperature.

Vitamins: Found in raw and fresh vegetables, fruits, and grains next to the outer coverings of grains, and the peelings of fruits and vegetables, also in the heart of grains and fruits.

Foods Rich in Protein: Peas, beans, lentils, nuts, milk, eggs, cereals, cow peas, soybeans, peanuts, nut preparations, wheat. These build tissue.

Foods Rich in Fat: Butter, cream, egg yolks, butternuts, ripe olives, vegetables, oils, pecans, English walnuts, olive oil, pine nuts, and all nuts. These furnish fuel.

Foods Rich in Carbohydrates: Malt sugar, malt, honey, ripe fruits, starchy vegetables, such as potatoes and cereals. These furnish energy and fuel.

Foods Rich in Protein and Carbohydrate: Peas, beans, lentils, peanuts, milk, oatmeal, wheat, furnish fuel and tissue-building material.

Starchless Vegetables: Carrots, young beets, celery, cucumbers, tomatoes, soybeans, buttermilk, squash, turnips, rutabagas, onions, okra, Brussels sprouts, artichokes, furnish bulk.

Starchless and Sugarless Vegetables: Lettuce, spinach, and all greens, tomatoes, celery, radishes, beans (string), cabbage, cauliflower, eggplant, endive, asparagus furnish bulk.

Foods Which Supply Minerals

Iron: Spinach, egg yolks, dried peas, dried beans, whole wheat, prunes, watercress, celery, milk, cabbage, oats, lettuce, raisins, apples, English walnuts, lentils, and all greens.

Phosphorus: Legumes, egg yolks, milk, prunes, baked

potatoes, nuts, whole cereals, cottage cheese, especially soybean cottage cheese.

Calcium: Milk, whole cereals, eggs, cabbage, parsnips, citrus fruits, nuts, legumes, and soybean milk.

Magnesium: Cherries, apples, nuts, figs, raisins, turnips, prunes, milk, legumes, spinach, whole cereals, soybeans, natural brown rice.

Potassium: Cherries, potatoes, parsnips, turnips, apples, plums, red cabbage, eggplant, cucumbers, soybeans.

Sodium: Strawberries, apples, asparagus, cauliflower, spinach.

Chlorine: Spinach, cabbage, turnips, cauliflower.

Sulphur: Spinach, cabbage, cauliflower, onions, egg yolks.

Lime: Cottage cheese, egg yolk, milk, greens of all kinds, legumes, soybeans.

Fluorine: Cauliflower, cabbage, asparagus, potatoes, spinach.

Silica: Barley, oats, cabbage, onions, and oatmeal.

Iodine: Agar-agar, all garden vegetables, beans, peas, fish.

Use of Mineral Salts

Calcium: Builds bones and teeth. Whole cereals and fruits, especially citrus fruits, provide this.

FLOURINE AND SILICA ARE ALSO NEEDED FOR TEETH AND BONE.

Phosphorus: Builds bones, brain, and nerves.

Potassium: Necessary in the construction of cells in the body. Potatoes, also cherries, contain a large amount.

Sodium: Necessary for the proper constituency of the fluids of the body.

Sulphur: Necessary to the structure of the living tissues of the body.

Diet, for health, is of much more value than medicine.

There is today a greater menace to civilization than that of war. The name of this menace is Malnutrition.

We eat too much, and most of what we eat is poison to our system. "Half of what we eat keeps us alive, the other half keeps the physicians alive."

As well as eating too much, we do not masticate our food thoroughly. As most of our diseases can be traced to improper food, the medicine for all ailments is a correct, well-balanced diet.

Refined White Sugar. Sugar drains out all the mineral salts of the blood, bones, and tissues.

The fundamental principle of true healing consists of a return to the natural habits of living.

A fresh fruit diet is of greatest importance.

All citrus fruits are more or less laxative.

List of Laxative Foods

Prunes	Raisins	Turnips
Dates	Bran	Squash
Figs	Bran Muffins	Parsnips
Oranges	Bran Bread	Carrots
Apples	Whole Wheat Bread	Olives
Bananas	Spinach	Olive Oil
Pears	Celery	Walnuts
Peaches	Lettuce	Butternuts
Grapes	Okra	Cauliflower
Grapefruit	Onions	Pumpkin
Watermelon	Buttermilk	Blueberries
Lemons	Agar-agar	Cherries

Constipating Foods

White Bread	Blackberries
White Rice	Boiled Milk
Barley	Hard Boiled Eggs
Browned Flour Gruel	Meat
Browned Flour Gravy	Cheese

Chapter X

DIET

A true diet is not based on calories but on the organic elements that sustain and give life. Our most common and serious diseases are caused by wrong eating and drinking. This has been proven by numerous scientific experiments in recent years. Food is a substance which when absorbed by the blood stream will nourish, repair, and furnish life force and heat to the body, but if in its preparation and refining, the life-giving elements are taken away, it cannot furnish life force, but it will clog the funcitional activity of the body and will result in many disorders.

Many diseases are nature's effort to free our system from poisons and congestions resulting from wrong eating and drinking. But always when we assist nature to expel impurities and re-establish right conditions in the system, we can overcome diseases.

The whole nation needs more vitamins, better cooks, more care exercised in the preparation of our food, and less spacious hospitals.

Since Eve first surrendered to appetite, man has been growing more and more self-indulgent, until health is being sacrificed on the altar of appetite. God gave our first parents the food he designed the human race to eat. Only after he had destroyed the world by flood did he give permission to eat of flesh foods as all vegetation was dead, but then only of clean animals as given in the Bible, Lev. 11; but animal foods are not the most healthful for man; recent scientific research and experiments have proven this beyond doubt. The diet given in the beginning did not include flesh meats.

LEARN HOW TO AVOID AND OVERCOME SICKNESS BY CORRECT EATING AND LIVING.

Oatmeal

The common oatmeal, which we can get in every grocery in the land, is a most wonderful food, but is not properly prepared by many and terribly abused by the majority of people. It is one of the finest foods for growing children that we have, but the way the oats are eaten many times spoils the real quality of the oats. When milk and sugar are put on the oats, it causes it to ferment in the stomach and thus you lose the benefit of the oats. There is a great misunderstanding with many of the people about the steel-cut oats and the finely flaked oats. There is not a hair's breadth difference in the steel-cut oats and the finely flaked oats as far as food value is concerned or the life-giving properties.

"The chemical analysis of rolled oats and steel-cut oats is identically the same, because quick-cooking rolled oats is nothing more than steel-cut oats run through heavy rolls revolving at a great rate of speed. We guarantee a minimum of 15 per cent protein, and a minimum of 7.5 per cent fat, a maximum of 1.9 per cent fiber, 66 per cent nitrogen free extract, and 77 per cent carbohydrate.

"Rolled oats is one of the few—if not the only one—cereal food that carries the germ of the grain, and that is important."

The above is quoted from a letter from G. M. Hidding, General Manager of the Purity Oats Co., of Keokuk, Iowa, May 27, 1936.

This is the analysis of the finely flaked oats: Water 7.8; Protein 16.1; Fat 7.3; Carbohydrates 68; Potassium 13.1;

Sodium 3; Calcium 2.8; Magnesium 5.2; Iron .3; Phosphorus 18.2; Sulphur .3; Silicon 24; Chlorine 7; Fluorine; Iodine .01; Ash 2. The flake oats is so much easier handled by the most of the people because it digests much quicker, and it takes much less time to cook. The steel-cut oats ought to cook at least four hours in a double boiler, while the finely flaked oats takes only three minutes—a great saving in fuel, and further a great saving to our old weak stomachs. Many stomachs cannot handle the steel-cut oats very well because it is too coarsely granulated, and takes so much longer to digest and often will sour in the stomach before it is digested. A fine way to prepare oats is just the way it is given on the package. I myself eat it just that way with some zwieback and some nice soybean butter on the zwieback. I enjoy it very much, more so than many years ago when I used milk and suger on it. Something dry should be eaten with it so you get plenty of saliva mixed with it, like zwieback or some whole wheat crackers.

An excellent way in which to use steel-cut oats is the following: Combine equal parts of steel-cut oats and sterilized bran. Cook six to ten minutes, then set aside five minutes before serving. A considerable part of this will be imperfectly cooked; therefore it is not readily acted upon by the saliva and intestinal juices, but passes on into the colon, where it will aid in the destroying of putrefactive poisons caused from the decomposition of proteins and other poisons.

Oatmeal can be used in many ways. When oatmeal is not spoiled in the preparation or used in wrong combinations, it is one of the finest foods we have to prevent disease. I read in a daily paper many years ago that the Great Northern Railroad had a very urgent piece of road to make. They hired a big crew of men and worked them fourteen hours a day. Instead of giving them ordinary water to drink, they gave them oatmeal water to drink, and the paper stated that not one man was laid off on account of sickness, and it stated that never before has there been such a wonderful experience in the history of railroads. I could tell some wonderful experiences along that line, but space will not permit. Oatmeal water should be more frequently used than it is. It is a very good medicine for the sick. Take the finely flaked oats and put two heaping tablespoonfuls to a quart of water. You can make it stronger or weaker to suit your taste. Let it simmer for half an hour and then beat it up with a spoon or egg beater, and strain it through a fine sieve. This makes an excellent drink for anybody and especially the sick. If desired, you can add just a pinch of salt and a little soybean milk. Another recipe for making oatmeal water is: Take a heaping tablespoonful of oatmeal to a quart of water and let it simmer for two or two and a half hours in a tightly covered pan, and then strain it. This makes a very refreshing, cooling drink when it is cooled off in the ice-box.

I quote the following from *Diet a Key to Health,* by R. Swineburne Clymer, M.D., "Oats, steel-cut or Scotch. Silicon 24.0; Phosporus 18.2; Potassium 13.6, Magnesium 5.2. One of the richest silicon carries known and if properly combined with fruit or vegetable eliminants, is the ideal basic food for children during the winter months to prevent infection from all zymotic diseases."

It is not too much to say that oatmeal, if combined with other foods so as to prevent congestions and the formations of toxins and acids due to the acid reaction, would do more to prevent contagious diseases than all the serums thus far invented or that ever will be. Oatmeal is neither artificial nor a substitute. It is a natural agent for the supply of those elements which by their antiseptic properties make contagious infections impossible.

Besides this antiseptic quality, oats are rich in the phosphorus required by the child for the formation of brain and nerve and elements required by the mind in study.

Wherever a large amount of silicon is required, prescribe oatmeal, or, if this is not practical, due to digestive disturbances, then the extract, "Avena Sativa."

The following are extracts from a letter dated April 21, 1936, which I received from F. L. Gunderson, Biochemist, Nutrition Laboratory of the Quaker Oats Co., Chicago, Illinois:

"We are very glad to inclose a description of the manufacturing process for both standard and quick type of rolled oat flakes. Many people have the erroneous idea that the hulls of the oat grain are comparable to the bran of wheat. That is not correct. The hulls (or flowering glumes), of the wheat grain envelope the whole kernel rather loosely and consequently go into the straw stack at threshing time. In contrast, the glumes of the oat grain are wrapped a bit more securely around the kernel, and remain on the oat kernel as an individual wrapped until they are removed in the rolled oats mill. After removing the hull from the oats, the kernel from which rolled oats are made possesses all of the bran, middlings, endosperm, and germ portion natural to the grain. Whole oat kernels (oat groats), steel-cut oats, large or "standard" type rolled oat flakes, and small or "quick" type rolled oat flakes are all *whole grain* products. In the sense that refined is sometimes used as an antonym for whole-grain, there are no refined oat foods. The very botanical and physical structure of the oat grain, together with the universal oat milling processes are such that all oat foods are whole-grain products. The composition of steel-cut oats, large flaked oats, and small flaked rolled oats is identical if made from the same type of grain."

"With regard to the vitamins of oats, our own tests, as well as those of other well known research people, indicate that there is no destruction in the manufacturing process."

Quaker Oats, Mother's Oats, Quick Quaker Oats or Quick Mother's Oats

Description: Flaked oats made from the best quality of large oats with the hulls removed.

Method of Manufacture: The oats go through an extensive cleaning process in which corn, wheat, barley chaff, and weed seeds are removed. The oats are then carefully sized to uniform diameter by grading in special machines, the light oats, double oats, and pin oats being removed to feed. The oats are again graded to uniform length, about five grades being obtained. Only the plump sound oats of good size go into either of these four products. The clean graded oats are roasted and partially dried, after which they are cooled and passed to a large burr stone where the *Hulls are torn from the GROATS.* The oats mixture is next bolted to remove any flour, and the hulls are then removed in special air separators. Any unhulled oats are removed in cell machines and the cleaning process is continued until the groats are free of hulls and unhulled oats. For production of the two brands of "Quick" rolled oats the groats are at this stage steel cut. The clean groats pass to the steaming chamber where they are partially cooked with live steam and from which they pass to the rolls where the groats are formed into flakes. The rolled oats flakes are cooled in a current of air to about 110 degrees F., following which the product is immediately weighed and packed by automatic mechanical equipment.

Foods, Devitalized Cause Disease

Many people suffer almost continually from hidden ailments, the cause of which they are unable to determine.

They know they feel very miserable, and are subject to frequent headaches, indigestion, poor appetite, and many other troubles.

There is a cause for all such disturbances. Deficiency of necessary elements in the body is usually the cause of many such troubles. The human body is composed of sixteen or more elements, and a shortage of any one or more of these elements impairs the functioning of the entire system. There is no real definite organic breakdown in such cases generally, but the body is not functioning properly. An insufficient supply of any of these important elements is the major cause of a great many ailments. These minerals are supplied from properly prepared foods, but the American diet is very deficient in many of these important elements.

The refined, degerminated, demineralized, and devitalized foods are a curse to humanity. The miller in making white flour takes out the vital portion, or the part that makes a new plant—the wheat germ, and also the bran, or part that contains the minerals and vitamins which supply our bodies with blood-making material. Many other of the daily foods upon which we live from youth up, likewise have been treated in the same manner.

Foods that are improperly prepared lose much of their food value. It is very essential that foods be eaten in the natural state as much as possible. Too much cooking injures foods. There are certain food elements that are destroyed by even a small amount of heat, and for that reason such foods as can be eaten raw should be served often. Green leafy vegetables, such as cabbage, spinach, romaine, dandelion, carrots, lettuce, endive, celery, and many others contain those substances that the human body must have to function properly. A lack of such elements in the daily food is a species of starvation and will end disastrously.

Such vegetables as carrots, tender beets, parsnips, cucumbers, potatoes, young turnips and others like them should not be peeled. A stiff brush, or wire doughnut, is excellent to clean such vegetables so they need not be peeled. The highest mineral content of such foods lies just under the skins; therefore, this is lost if they are peeled.

Neither should any of the water from vegetables be thrown away. It contains valuable mineral salts and should be used. In cooking leafy vegetables, just enough water should be added to keep them from burning, and they should not be cooked longer than is absolutely necessary. Spinach or beet tops should never be cooked over eight or ten minutes. If beets are cooked with tops, it takes much longer to cook the beets than the tops, so the beets should be diced fine and put only enough water to keep them from burning. Use the stems, but cut them in quarter-inch lengths and add to the beets after they are about half done (about thirty minutes). Cut the leaves fine, and when the beets are about done, add the leaves, for it takes only a few minutes (about ten) to cook them. The salt should be added after the stems have come to a boil, and a little of Kloss Soybean Butter diluted with water to the consistency of cream should be added just as the fire is cut out, or it can be added when they are served. It takes about forty-five minutes to cook beets in this manner.

Never put soda in your vegetables to tender them. Neither should it be used in cooking dried peas, beans, corn, etc., even if it does shorten the length of time to cook them. The common use of soda biscuits and corn bread made with baking powder and soda is largely the cause of pellagra and other deficiency diseases, *because it destroys much of the vitamin content of foods.* Disease cannot get a foothold when the body is in the best condition.

The following is a list of the devitaminized foods, quoted from a bulletin put out by the Department of Agriculture, and which was reprinted from Cereal Chemistry, Vol. XII, No. 5, September 1935, compiled by Dr. J. A. LeClerc, Senior Chemist, and his associates. The consumption of devitaminized foods is astounding, and everyone should avoid the use of these commonplace, devitaminized foods:

FOOD	Yearly Consumption In U.S. (1931) Million Pounds	Per Capita Consumption 1931 Pounds
Refined sugar	12,017,000,000	98.5
Corn starch	158,000,000	1.3
Polished rice	719,000,000	5.9
White flour	20,825,000,000	170.7
Corn syrup	707,000,000	5.7
Corn sugar	780,000,000	6.4
Candy	1,439,000,000	11.8
Hominy and grits	341,000,000	2.8
Rye flour	292,000,000	2.4
Corn meal	2,598,000,000	21.3
Corn breakfast food	378,000,000	3.1
Macaroni and water noodles	451,000,000	3.7
Corn and cottonseed oil	1,403,000,000	11.5
Poultry	2,940,000,000	24.1
Beef, veal	6,893,000,000	56.5
Mutton and lamb	866,000,000	7.1
Lard and lard substitutes	2,720,000,000	22.3

Chapter XI

ALUMINUM UTENSILS

Aluminum poisoning is so prevalent that I feel it is a part of my duty to give my experience and warn people against the use of aluminum.

Some years ago we bought a nice supply of aluminum cooking utensils. Among them was a teakettle which was constantly standing on the stove with some water in it. I would drink two or three cups of this water every morning and then some more about an hour before dinner. I developed terrible bowel trouble. I tried all kinds of remedies, which generally effected a cure, but herbs or anything else did no lasting good. I tried to find the cause but it seemed that everything failed. The doctors made all kinds of explanations of my condition, but they were all far from the cause.

The condition grew worse and worse until I said to my wife: "Unless something helps me, I will surely die." One day I described my condition to a person who told me that the description was similar to the distress aluminum poison would cause. I immediately began to search into the aluminum proposition. I got different books treating on aluminum poisoning and went to Washington to search for what the Government had on the subject in the Food Department and found in those books experiments that different doctors had made on animals. I also learned that they held post mortems on those who had died from supposed aluminum poisoning. They found that the organs, like the liver, spleen, and kidneys, contained aluminum. They found that everyone who had any practical experience in it condemned aluminum as cooking utensils. In the Jefferson College at Philadelphia many experiments have been made on aluminum, the findings of which are available in the Food Department at Washington.

I have boiled water in aluminum kettles, and then some in granite ware. I poured some from each kettle into two different glasses. The particles of aluminum could easily be seen in the water boiled in the aluminum kettle. Many others have made the same experiment.

Everyone who knows anything about aluminum knows that aluminum is poison. It gives off very easily when food is cooked in it. I have seen heavy aluminum dishes which were all pitted on the bottom. Of course, this aluminum had all gone into the food which was cooked in these utensils.

One could write at length on this subject, but I have asked Doctor Chas. T. Betts, of Toledo, who has had long practical experience with aluminum, to write his experience, and this article is quoted as follows:

ALUMINUM COOKING UTENSILS
By Dr. Chas. T. Betts,
320 Superior Street
Toledo, Ohio

"Before I became ill, the question of poisoning by aluminum compounds never interested me. We had a splendid assortment in our home of aluminum cooking utensils in which we took great pride in thinking them the finest available. It was not long, however, after we began using them that my health was reduced to such a serious condition from some kind of poisoning that a journey was made to Colorado, seeking air, water, sunshine, or what not, in the hope that life might be prolonged.

"My first attention to the possibility of aluminum being poisonous or probably not fit for cooking purposes came when it was noted that the water from the soda spring at Manitou was effervescent when in contact with an aluminum cup which I used for drinking purposes, and that the same water had no such chemical action in a glass container.

"The above observation brought recollections regarding the activity of aluminum, or what is better known as the chemical action of the metal upon foods which had been prepared in our home. I remembered that peeled potatoes if allowed to stand in an aluminum dish overnight would become yellow and when cooked would look somewhat shriveled and have dark streaks through the inner part.

"The cranberries when cooked in an aluminum dish turned to a darkened color, with quite a few of the berries turning black.

"Bread or pie dough when mixed on a sheet of aluminum acquires a grayish color. The pot becomes darkened when cabbage is boiled in it. Tomatoes, apple sauce, rhubarb, cherries, grapes, etc., will clean an aluminum dish beautifully within five minutes, or as soon as they are brought to a boil.

"Ordinarily, well water boiled two hours will look rather milky and cause a dark coating over the inside of the aluminum dish.

"Another observation of particular note was that a butterscotch pie filling, boiled a few minutes in an aluminum dish, turned from a rich brown to a dark green color and that a mayonnaise dressing would turn from a light yellow to a brown color.

"Lemonade made in one of these dishes has a very bad taste if allowed to remain standing in the metal for any length of time.

"Coffee remaining in an aluminum coffee pot has a puckery or metallic taste.

"When you drive your car with an aluminum throttle, your fingers or gloves will become blackened by the metal rubbing off.

"Hydrogen gas is formed by boiling well water, or when heat is in contact with an aluminum dish. This can be noted on cold aluminum by the bubbles all around the sides of a pail. They form as far down as the bottom of the receptacle. If the batter of an angel food cake is stirred in an aluminum dish a few minutes, the finished product will have dark streaks through it. Whites of eggs will turn green if stirred ten minutes in an aluminum pan.

"A few other experiments brought to the writer's attention more vividly the possibility of being poisoned by these utensils. It was found that ordinary foods other than protein (beans, etc.), will not adhere to the metal. Cake, pancakes, and waffles do not stick to aluminum, and the use of butter or oil is not needed. (Alum baking powder sprinkled upon an iron utensil will prevent sticking of the dough.)

"Tarnished silverware can be made bright and shiny within a few minutes by putting the ware in an aluminum dish. Partly fill with water, add a little bicarbonate of soda, and bring to a boil. It will be found that all bubbles on wild beer will instantly disappear when the beverage is placed in an aluminum dish.

"When water is boiled in an aluminum dish for one-half hour and placed in a glass, a light, feathery substance can be seen with the naked eye, and precipitation takes place in the bottom of the glass after cooling. An interesting experiment can be noted by cleaning an aluminum dish with lye or bichloride of mercury. After this is done, a fine dust will cover the inside of the utensil within a few minutes.

Aluminum chloride is produced when salted bacon is fried in an aluminum spider after the grease has congealed. Vegetables cooked until dry will be covered with a white dust.

"It was further noted that it is impossible to make hard soap in an aluminum dish. Persons become sick after they eat sea foods which have been cooked in such ware with milk. The same effect was noted after eating custard which had been allowed to stand in an aluminum dish for some hours before serving. The most frequent cases of group poisoning came from serving salted fricassee of chicken, pork, or veal, which had been cooked and allowed to remain standing in the aluminum vessel for twelve hours.

"Recipes are given in various papers apparently by aluminum organizations advising the public how to clean the utensil that has acquired a dark coating. The following is one that was found in the *Toledo Blade,* Toledo, Ohio:

"Lightning Workers"

" 'Cook your rhubarb or fresh tomatoes in a discolored aluminum pan. They will accomplish more in five minutes than you could do by scrubbing for an hour.'

"It was discovered that agents were selling 'Lightning Silverware Cleaners.' Investigation proved that the lightning workers were nothing more or less than a small piece of aluminum which was to be inserted in boiling water together with the silver, with a little soda added. This does the trick beautifully.

"Many persons throughout the land noted the effects of food upon aluminum and of aluminum upon food. These observations were made in various localities, so that a discussion of national prominence arose regarding the possibility of such culinary ware being unfit to use for cooking purposes.

"Many believe the metal which dissolves from aluminum dishes is either filth or dirt. The metal is not a food substance, and it cannot become a constituent part of the human body. It is evident that it contaminates food with poisonous effects. That food values are damaged or destroyed is noted by the best available scientists in America; that the color of cooked foods shows adverse chemical changes when cooked and stored in aluminum; that various chemical poisons are formed according to the kinds of foods cooked when their salts become mixed with the metal or when seasoning agents are employed like salt, cooking soda, etc. It was observed that a poisonous gas 'hydrogen' is formed by them which permeates the room in which they are used.

"The above observation caused the writer to investigate what is in the record at Washington upon the subject, particularly the physiological effects to the human when the drug is ingested called 'alum' (aluminum) which is the generic term applied to all of these poisons resulting from mixing the acid metal aluminum in the hydroxide from which the salts of foods cooked therein or when the metal is in combination with the body digestive juices.

"The Government made a thorough investigation upon this particular point from 1925 to 1930. The Federal Trade Commission, Docket 540, took more than four thousand pages of closely typewritten testimony from 158 witnesses in a period of five years, after which an official report was made by Edward M. Averill. Many of the witnesses were professors, deans, biologists, and toxocologists from many colleges, some of which are the highest schools of learning in America.

"The following is the language used in part by Averill as his findings:

" 'The evidence in this record does not prove that they are harmless.'

" 'The evidence in this record does prove that there are substantial grounds upon which to predicate an honest opinion that they are harmful.' "

"We have evidence of a real nature, understandable by anyone, as a further proof that the aluminum, which dissolves from the utensils, has evil effects upon the body when consumed with foods. Our American people are banqueters. They love picnics and have extensive church gatherings at which they come to enjoy food, to worship or have a good time. Often these are turned into places of grief, anxiety, and death. The following is a report of an extensive group poisoning at one of these church dinners held at Punxsutawney, Pennsylvania, reported in the *Sun-Telegraph*, Pittsburgh, Pennsylvania:

"200 Church Diners Poisoned"

" 'Punxsutawney, Pa., Dec. 3—Two hundred people who attended a chicken supper at the First Baptist Church today are recovering from ptomaine poisoning. A dozen or more are seriously ill, but so far there have been no deaths.

" 'Women of the church prepared the supper at their homes and served it in the church auditorium, and every person who partook of the supper became ill.

"Physicians stated that the entire supply of gravy had been poisoned as the result of one of the women leaving the gravy in an aluminum container too long before taking it to the church. All the gravy was collected into one container to heat, and in that way the entire supply was contaminated."

"The question is often asked, 'Will aluminum cooking utensils cause gas in the stomach?' It was found that some American manufacturers of baking powder use a total of many thousand tons of aluminum annually, mixed with an alkaline substance—soda. This combination does make gas. If aluminum will make gas in a dish on the table, as when baking powders are used, aluminum from cooking utensils will certainly make gas in the stomach or bowels when it comes in contact with the same kind of chemicals—the alkaline juices of the body.

"The writer regained his health, sufficiently within eight weeks after he stopped eating the poison from his aluminum cooking utensils, to resume practice, and has enjoyed good health for many years since. All that is asked of the sick is that they do not use aluminum utensils or alum baking powders for a period of eight weeks and note results. If no improvement is observed, they can be used as before. This would surely not be a hardship on anyone seeking health."

CHAPTER XII

COOKING UNDER STEAM PRESSURE

We hear much about steam pressure cooking. Some condemn it, and some recommend it. I will give some of my practical experiences, proving, I believe, its value. I have had much experience with steam cooking for many years, and have the honor of securing the first patent on a home steam pressure cooker ever granted in the United States. This cooker is now used over practically the entire civilized world.

Some time ago I read a long argument against steam pressure cooking. The doctor who made this argument is well known in the United States, and I therefore, shall not mention his name. His experiment proves that he is not a competent judge of steam pressure cooking. He spoke of having cooked wheat, corn, oats, barley, rye, buckwheat, and sunflower seed two hours under thirty pounds of steam pressure. These cooked grains were fed to such animals as rats, guinea pigs, etc. These small animals became sick and paralyzed in a few weeks. From these facts the doctor concluded that steam pressure cooking is detrimental to food.

I have operated canning factories large and small, and have visited many other large canning factories; but have never yet heard of anyone cooking food under thirty pounds of steam pressure for two hours, nor for one hour under any such pressure. People used to cook navy beans and corn under ten to fifteen pounds of pressure for one hour. Most all steam pressure cooking is done at about five pounds steam pressure, which is ideal. In California a law was passed not long ago forbidding that certain foods be cooked under any more than five pounds steam pressure.

There is no kind of cooking, either in a kettle or in the bake oven, that preserves the life-giving properties better than closing the foods up tight in a steam pressure cooker and cooking until thoroughly done. I have had the privilege at different times of feeding groups of people where everything was cooked under steam pressure. We use the steam pressure cooker in our home with most gratifying results.

Potatoes are very delicious cooked in this way. Medium sized potatoes will cook in twenty minutes in a steam pressure cooker under five pounds pressure. When you take them out they are dry and mealy, and have an excellent flavor, if the potatoes had a good flavor to start with.

Spinach is wonderful cooked under steam pressure. It retains all of its life-giving qualities, when cooked under a low pressure, say five pounds, for ten minutes, depending somewhat on the condition of the spinach. A canning recipe book comes with every steam pressure cooker, giving all the details on how to cook each food, and how to handle the steam pressure cooker.

The following table shows the comparative amount of heat developed to each pound of pressure on the pressure cooker:

Steam Pressure Lbs. per square inch as shown on steam gauge.	Degrees of Heat Fahrenheit (Boiling Point of water is 212° F.)
1	216
2	219
3	222
4	225
5	227
6	230
7	233

Steam Pressure Lbs. per square inch as shown on steam gauge.	Degrees of Heat Fahrenheit (Boiling Point of water is 212° F.)
8	235
9	237
10	240
11	242
12	244
13	246
14	248
15	250

The steam pressure cooker is one of the finest cooking utensils that has ever been invented. You can cook everything without putting water on it. You can put several different dishes in the cooker and cook them all at the same time. The food will retain its natural flavor. Another advantage is that breakfast food or any other food can be cooked in a steam pressure cooker without having to stir it, and it does not have to be watched as it will never burn.

There is no way to cook foods that preserves the life-giving properties of vitamins and flavor more perfectly than under steam pressure. At the same time it is a great fuel saver. After the food starts to cook, it requires only a little fire to keep up the temperature. It also requires less attention than any other way of cooking, because food will not stick to the kettle, or burn. After you have set the pressure where you want it, you can go away and leave it to cook as long as necessary.

Chapter XIII

DISEASE OF ANIMALS

Meat eating is becoming more and more dangerous on account of the steady increase in disease among animals. Some time ago I had a nice flock of registered Jerseys, and one morning we noticed in the paper that in the adjoining county there were thousands of heads of cattle which they were obliged to kill on account of disease, so I decided to sell my drove of stock and keep three of the best milk cows. About six or eight months later, one morning a neighbor said to me, "Did you hear that Anderson had sixteen cows die yesterday and could not do anything for them?" So I decided to sell two of my three cows and just keep "old Lizzie," which was a registered Jersey. Her milk tested six and a half per cent butter fat. She never had anything but the very best of feed and the very best of care possible. A few weeks later she became sick and refused all food. I told my wife not to use the milk for a day or two, hoping there would be a change for the better, but there was none. Old Lizzie walked as if she was afraid to step on her feet and made queer movements with her lower jaw, and all at once she fell over and was dead. We decided then that we would never use any more milk.

Some time after this we noticed in the paper that there were four or five states in which the chickens as well as the cows were so diseased that for a long time they were not permitted to ship any eggs or butter or livestock. While we had not eaten any milk for a long time prior to this, we stopped using milk, meat, or eggs, and have not used them since. We found an abundance of good things which take the place of these. A few years prior to this I was up in the northern states near the clear water lakes, and found millions of fish dead on the water. On being examined they were found to have a live worm along the spine which killed them. Not long ago while in San Diego, California, I was told by reliable persons that not far from San Diego the dead fish were so thick on the water that the steamers had a hard time to run through them.

For many years I have spent much money and time to produce articles of food which most perfectly take the place of meat, milk, eggs, and butter. These articles taste very palatable, are easily digested, furnish perfect nourishment, and are very inexpensive, costing only a fraction of the amount paid for animal products. You will find all of them given in this book.

Chapter XIV

HISTORY OF WATER CURE

Water has been used from time immemorial for remedial purposes. It is not a modern discovery. The books of the oldest medical authors make numerous references to the use of the bath in combatting disease, and to its good effect. The learned Greek, Hippocrates, who lived about five hundred years before Christ, was the first man who wrote much on the healing of disease with water. He is referred to as the "father of medical literature." He used water extensively, both internally and externally, in combatting disease.

At a very early period the Egyptians practiced bathing considerably, as you will find in sacred history. If Pharoah's daughter had not gone down to the river to bathe, Moses would never have been found in the rushes. Ancient Egyptians' pictures, found in the tombs, showed people preparing for a bath. Bathing held a prominent place in the law that was prepared by Moses under divine instruction for the government of the Hebrew nation. The relation of the bath in the treatment of leprosy would naturally lead us to believe that it was used for curative effects. And it would be impossible to believe that an agent held in such high regard as a preventive of disease, should not be esteemed as a useful remedy.

The ancient Persians and Greeks erected stately and magnificent public buildings devoted to bathing. Darius the Persian's baths are spoken of as being especially remarkable. The Romans surpassed all other nations in the costliness and magnificence of their bathing facilities. Some of their greatest works of architecture were their public baths. The baths were supplied with every convenience for increasing the use and luxury of bathing. Kings and emperors struggled for superiority in perfecting and enlarging those sanitary institutions. Some of them were large enough for twenty thousand bathers to enjoy simultaneously. At one time the number of public baths in Rome reached the mark of nearly one thousand. Even Nero, who was a public disgrace, did at least one good act when he erected a beautiful public bath.

Two noted Latin physicians, Celus and Galen, praised and glorified the bath as being invaluable—that was almost two thousand years ago. Galen said that exercise and friction must be used with the bath to have a perfect cure. If only the regular physicians of a century ago had followed the practice of Galen as described in his works, what a lot of suffering would have been saved. Doctors would have refreshed and revived their patients who were fever-stricken, with God-given water, instead of giving drugs, quinine, etc., and letting them be consumed by the fevers that parched their lips, disorganized their blood, and many times ended their sufferings with their lives. The Emperor Augustus was cured by water remedies of a disease which had thwarted all other remedies.

The Arabians have always been looked upon as a wandering horde of wild men, but about one thousand years ago they had physicians among them that were some of the most learned men of that age. They were very sensible and enthusiastic about the efficiency of the bath. Rhazes, one of the most prominent of them, described a method that would scarcely be outdone by the present-day water treatment. The baths were used in pestilences.

In Constantinople the Turkish baths were used extensively in the 15th century.

In the year 1600 public vapor baths were numerous in Paris. They were connected with the barber shops, as are many in this country at the present time. Dr. Bell, of Paris, stated that in connection with the city hospitals nearly 130,-000 baths were given in one single year to outside patients. Undoubtedly, those in the hospitals were steamed and bathed as well. What a marked contrast with the present day hospitals in this country where the use of water is most sadly neglected. Such neglect is inexcusable.

The Germans in olden times were very fond of bathing, according to the records of history. During the Middle Ages, when they had the leprosy plague, it was a religious duty to bathe because of the national faith in bathing. History tells us that Charlemagne held court in a huge warm bath.

From the very earliest part of the 18th century water was used. Floyer published a history of bathing where remarkable cures were made by means of bathing, and he recommended them for numerous diseases. A Mr. Hancock, who was a minister, published in 1723 a book called *Common Water the Best Cure for Fevers*. Another book, published by someone else, was called *Curiosities of Common Water* and was published in 1723, in which it was said to be an "excellent remedy which will perform cures with very little trouble, and without charge," "may be truly styled a universal remedy." The French and German writers were also advocating the use of water as a remedy at this same time.

In 1840 to 1850 Victor Priesnitz, of Germany, led in the use of water as a curative. He met with considerable opposition from the doctors, when he took some of their patients and cured them after they had given them up. He had an accident in which three of his ribs were broken, and he treated himself with applications of cold water with success, and then tried it on others in a similar manner. His success encouraged him, and although he was an ignorant peasant, he learned various means to apply water to the body to suit different diseases. His success increased and in a few years he was famous world-wide. He succeeded in restoring hundreds of people to health who had been pronounced incurable. His friends claimed he was a great discoverer, but he really discovered nothing that had not been known for at least a century, if not thousands of years before. But he was an ignorant peasant, as before stated, and had no anatomical knowledge, which caused him to fall into many errors, as some cases related. Water is one of the most powerful and yet simple remedies which can be applied by an intelligent mother, who knows the effect of hot and cold, which we will deal with a little later.

The water cure spread to America about 1850 and until about 1854 prospered greatly, but the doctors would not stand for this, as they did not want the people to get hold of any remedy which was practical and non-expensive, that could be used in any home. About 1870 they had successfully prevented the water-cure practitioners from practicing in New York by a medical law. New York City was headquarters, and as soon as it was stopped there, its use was abandoned nearly everywhere for a while.

North American Indians use baths for many diseases. They have original ways of giving both water and vapor bath, the vapor bathing being the most commonly used, followed by plunging into a stream.

The native Mexicans use a hot-air bath. They confine themselves in a brick house, heated by a furnace on the outside. They seem to have implicit confidence in the efficiency of the bath to destroy disease, always using it when ill, with success.

Dr. Benedict Lust published *Sebastian Kneipp Water and Herb Cure*. Sebastian Kneipp cured the Archduke Joseph, of Austria, of Bright's disease in 1892.

Sebastian Kneipp, who was a Catholic priest, of Bohemia, Europe, gained a high reputation because of his success with the water cure, and he also had his patients return in so far as was possible to nature. He used the herbal remedies. His success was great, because he used natural remedies.

If you cleanse and nourish the body properly, and leave nature to itself, it will renovate and heal the body.

Of late years people have come to believe that there are remarkable virtues in certain spring waters. The claims that these waters are possessed of a wonderful healing virtue is not true. The healing virtue is in the moist heat that is gotten from it. The whole thing in a nutshell is that the use of water, combined with abundance of fresh air, sunshine, exercise, rest, recreation, and pleasant surroundings, effects a cure.

Unfortunately, in the early days the reputation of water as a remedy was injured because people, such as Priesnitz, used it to extremes, did not understand the body, or the uses of hot and cold water, and the useful and powerful reaction that can be brought about when it is properly used in this way. People were led to believe that it was a cure-all, and that cold water was the only remedy no matter what the condition or disease. In all cases rest, pure air, nourishing and simple food, sunlight, and exercise are of equal importance. Water is not a specific, but is one of the most valuable of many excellent remedies. This is true not only of water, but of other natural remedies. There may be a specific remedy for a specific disease, but not one, and one alone for all diseases. Several remedial agents must be combined, to suit the conditions, and not one used to the exclusion of all others. But as will be shown later, water is an important agency in the treatment of every disease, correctly applied, with other remedies.

Chapter XV

WATER

Water is one of the most abundantly supplied elements of nature for remedial uses. The blood and brain of the human body are composed of about four-fifths water. The fluid secretions and excretions are more than nine-tenths their weight in water.

The chemical composition of water is represented by the chemical formula, H_2O, which means that it is composed of two gases, hydrogen and oxygen, proportionately, two volumes of the former and one of the latter. Both are odorless, colorless, tasteless, and transparent. Oxygen is the greater supporter of combustion in life. Hydrogen is one of the lightest gases known.

Use of water.—Water exists in the form of ice when below 32 degrees F. When at 212 degrees F. or above, it is changed into vapor. Between 32 degrees F. and 212 degrees F. it is a liquid. Water possesses the greatest amount of heat required to elevate temperature to a given number of degrees, of any substance. Water also absorbs more heat by elevation than any other substance. When passing from the ice to the liquid state, it absorbs a great amount of heat from the objects it comes in contact with without any elevation of temperature. Water conducts heat much more readily than air, and communicates its heat to bodies with which it comes in contact, but it also abstracts heat when at a lower temperature.

Rain water.—Rain water comes the nearest to being pure water of any attainable. But it is unwholesome because it gathers many impurities as it falls. Filtered rain water and distilled water are the purest forms.

Hard water.—When water is hard, it will not produce a lather with soap. The hardness is due to salts of lime, gypsum, and chalk, and others, which makes it unfit for use externally, and especially internally.

Mineral water.—These waters contain solutions of salts of magnesia, iron and others, as well as iodine, arsenic, and sulphur, which give them a medicinal taste and they have been much used for cures of chronic ailments. These waters are absolutely unfit for drinking or cooking purposes. They contain no particular value for cleansing. One would naturally know that water which is unfit to cleanse the outside of the body, could not be of much benefit as an internal application.

With the exception of pure air, there is no other element of nature that is as important in sustaining life as pure water, or has as important a relation to the human system. A person can live longer on water alone than if deprived of it. A large proportion of our food, in variance to the type, contains from fifteen to ninety per cent water.

Water undergoes no change in the body, but is absolutely essential to the performance of the vital functions, as it enables various organs to perform their work so that life is maintained. The circulatory system is one that is especially dependent upon water. Water is the solvent which floats the blood corpuscles, nutritive, and waste elements which the blood is carrying. By the aid of water, nutritions enter the blood and are conveyed to fibers of the intricate human mechanism, where repair and growth are needed.

There is no other element which is so adapted for this exact purpose as water. It circulates through the most delicate capillaries, without friction, and even passes through membranes into parts that are not accessible by openings.

Water is continually passing away from the body from some organ of elimination, either skin, kidneys, or lungs. If the kidneys become obstructed, we all know there is serious trouble. The dry air entering the lungs all the time absorbs moisture from the pulmonary membranes. Therefore it is necessary to supply the body with plenty of pure water at all times. The average person eliminates about five pints of water in twenty-four hours, and an equal new supply must be made in order to preserve the fluidity of the blood. People whose work is of laborious nature which necessitates profuse perspiration naturally require more water than others.

It will also be noticed that the diet has a great deal to do with the amount of water demanded by nature. People who eat largely of animal products, and use salt, pepper, spices and condiments, require considerably more water to dissolve and cleanse the system of these unhealthful things. People who use mostly fruit, vegetables, grains and avoid the use of stimulating foods and drinks, require less water, as a great many vegetables and fruits are composed of more than half water.

Water is the only substance which really quenches thirst. Other beverages quench thirst in proportion to the amount of water they contain, and are unwholesome to the extent of the injurious elements that are added.

The skin performs several important duties for the body, the most important being excretion. That fact would be easily demonstrated if a coat of paint or varnish were applied all over the body, for a person would die almost as quickly as if a dose of poison had been given. The millions of little sweat glands are actively and constantly engaged in separating from the blood impurities which if retained would cause disease and death.

The skin also is an organ of respiration. It absorbs oxygen, and exhales poisonous gases, although most of this work is done by the lungs. In some lower animals, all work of respiration is done by the skin. The skin not only absorbs oxygen but absorbs liquids to a great extent. If a person stays in a warm bath for some time the weight of the body may be considerably increased. Seamen, when deprived of fresh water, wet their clothing with the sea water and the skin absorbs the water part.

The skin helps greatly in the regulation of temperature. It is non-conducting and dense, which prevents to a considerable degree the escape of necessary body heat. When the body becomes over-heated from strenuous vital activities, fever, or external heat, the skin relieves the tissues by favoring escape of heat. This is exactly what happens in fever, when you give plenty of water, and bathe the outside of the skin, excite perspiration, etc. The moisture evaporates through the perspiratory glands out upon the surface. It is a powerful, cooling process.

The skin may also be called the organ of touch. It is the most extensive sensibility organ of the body, and is very closely connected with all the great nerve centers. That is why water treatments are so efficient and have such a good effect in nervous diseases.

Every opening of the body to the surface is in line with mucous membrane. Mucous membrane lines the air passages and lungs, also the urinal and genital organs, and the whole alimentary canal. The mucous membrane resembles the skin in structure, as it is made up of several layers like the skin. It also secretes and excretes. It excretes foul material (as the exudation in diphtheria) and secretes useful substances when in fluid state.

The importance of the skin as an eliminative organ is evident by the offensive odor of perspiration, which has the distinct odor of tobacco, if the person uses it in any form. This also proves that the skin not only eliminates, but eliminates poisons from the body as well. Every movement we make destroys a portion of the living tissues. When they are dead, they are poisonous and must be removed. Some of the poisons in the system are very deadly, such as poisons from the urine, bile ducts, gall bladder, etc. They must be eliminated quickly, and here the marvelous use of water is again exhibited. Pure water dissolves these poisons whenever it comes in contact with them and is brought by the current of circulation to the proper organs—liver, skin, kidneys, and lungs—and the poisons are expelled.

The skin has millions of pores from which flow constantly a stream of poisons from the disintegration of the body. As we perspire these poisons are left on the skin. As time passes, more and more are left there. If the skin is normally active, it would take three or four days for these poisons to form a layer, which could be compared to a thin coating of varnish. Unless the person bathes properly and often, they would continue to accumulate and increase until it would undergo a process of decomposition.

We all know that a person who does not bathe often has a very unpleasant and unpardonable odor about them, but this offense is not equal to the evil done to oneself. This accumulation obstructs the work of the millions of little pores, and some of the poisons are reabsorbed, thus poisoning the system. Frequent cleansing with water will keep the skin wholly free from poisons. It is easily understood why so many people have torpid skins, because it is not uncommon to find people who have never taken a real, general bath in their lives, and the most of them do not practice it enough. A cleansing bath every day is best, but at least three times a week. You wash your face and hands every day. Why not the entire body? A cleansing bath three times a week will keep the skin supple and clean. The bath should be as indispensable to a woman as the mirror. Many very refined and fastidious people who spend many hours in dressing, etc., and women in using creams, lotions, and make-up to beautify the portions of the skin exposed to view would be quite shocked to learn the true condition of the unwashed skin. We do not say that this is true of every one, but it is true of a great many.

Inactivity of the skin is one of the main causes of all skin disease, coupled with an aggravated condition caused by wrong dietetic habits. The relation between the skin and kidneys is very close, and inactivity of the skin is very often caused by kidney disorders, nervous disorders, rheumatism, gout, and dyspepsia. It is a common cause of lung affection.

The value of water as a preventive of disease was recognized by ancient peoples, and baths were used to a far greater extent than in modern times. Moses, who was the great Hebrew lawgiver, commanded his people to be scrupulously clean, and made bathing a part of their religious duties. His example was followed by Mohammed, who required his people to bathe before each of the five daily prayers. "Cleanliness is next to godliness."

The Greeks regarded the bath as a very essential means of securing physical health. Daily baths were practiced by them, from the youngest to the oldest. The Romans made a luxury of the bath.

The most renowned physicians from Hippocrates down to Galen, Selus, Boerhaave, and also others such as Sebastian Knieppe, Melville C. Keith, and many more agree that bathing is an invaluable means of preserving health. Nevertheless, as people have become more enlightened and more civilized, bathing has been more and more disregarded.

During the dark ages in Europe, the bath was unknown, to which fact Michelet, a noteworthy historian, tells us that, in his opinion, accounted for the terrible plagues and pestilences of that period.

They felt the need of something and started using poisonous drugs. Bathing is a natural instinct, and all nature shows the importance of baths. Rain is the natural shower bath. The influence of it is shown in the fresher, brighter and more erect appearance of all living plants. Birds and animals do not neglect their morning baths. If man's instinct were not perverted by the habits of civilization, he would value the bath highly and bathe freely as do the more humble creatures whose instincts are still true to nature.

Man's intelligence has made it possible for him to become grossly perverted in almost everything—food, appetite, bathing, etc. Man does not go astray from nature because he lacks intelligence or instinct, but because he wishes to gratify his own desires.

Many are afraid to use one of God's greatest blessings —pure water—because they have never experienced its beneficial effect.

CHAPTER XVI

WATER — EFFECTS AND TREATMENT

Water benefits the system in three distinct ways. When taken into the stomach and intestinal canal, it is received into the blood and increases its volume. Then fullness of the circulatory vessels is increased (They are never expanded to their fullest extent.), allowing room for a change in the volume of their contents. Blood is more fluid, and the circulation is quickened by its dilution.

Excepting air, water is the most transient of any element taken into the body. It is eliminated four way, namely: lungs, skin, kidneys, intestines. By its dissolving action, the poisons that are separate from the tissues are dissolved. Then the volume of the blood is increased, more water comes in contact with the waste matter in every part, therefore, undesirable waste is removed, as is proven by the increased urinary secretions, and increased activity of the skin (perspiration).

Free water drinking increases the elimination of the mucous membrane of the intestinal tract, which is an important organ of secretion. The result of the increased action is that it renders the contents of the intestines more fiuid, thus helping the universal trouble—constipation. It also removes from the blood its foulest materials, rendering the blood cleaner for the building up of tissues, and in this way aids both waste and repair.

The use of water aids all vital processes by increasing change of tissues. It is a false idea that bathing renders a person more susceptible to colds. Colds are caused by disturbance of circulation. Frequent bathing makes the skin active, thereby increasing the circulation. A person who takes a daily cold morning bath has an almost perfect immunity from cold, and is not nearly so susceptible to changes in temperature. Colds contracted after bathing are the result of neglect of precaution.

Disease does not exist without some disturbance to the circulation. In health, each part of the body receives its due share of blood. Therefore, in any disease one of the first things to do is to balance the circulation. Applications of cold water contract the minute blood vessels, and thus the amount of blood is lessened. Or the same may sometimes be accomplished by applying hot water to some other part of the body, so that the surplus will be drawn there, and thus relieve the suffering organ.

Hot applications must be applied to the part where there is not enough blood, while at the same time you can apply cold applications to some other part to send more blood to the other part. Very often the two can be combined thus advantageously, because one part of the body cannot contain too much blood without some other part being deprived of its due proportion. So that while a cold application is required at one part, a hot is required at another.

Regulation of bodily temperature is closely associated with circulation, and the two are controlled by the same remedies given in the same way. A part which contains too much blood usually causes a high degree of temperature, or other extremely unpleasant symptoms. A cold application will relieve both. (See Treatment of Fevers.)

When you wish to reduce the temperature of any or all parts, the water must not be extremely cold, as the reaction will bring more blood to that part. Use warm or tepid water, just a few degrees below body temperature. This can be continued in any instance for some time without injury, or until the body is reduced to normal temperature. Many times one or more organs become torpid or inactive—the skin and liver in particular. When the blood vessels become inactive, congestion results. Alternate hot and cold applications, continued for thirty minutes or more, will relieve congestion more quickly than any other remedy. Fomentations given as hot as can be borne, with cold sponging, and drying between each fomentation, is the best method.

All pain is caused by disturbance to the circulation, because the overfilled vessels put pressure upon the nerves. Relief will be obtained from hot applications, as they relax the tissues, and the nerve fibers will be relieved of pressure, and the circulation will then be increased so as to relieve the congestion.

A large majority of diseases are caused because of obstruction in the various organs. Usually the obstruction is the accumulation of natural waste matter of the tissues, or the taking of foreign materials, such as one absorbs in hard water, and indigestible food. The warm bath removes external obstructions, and water used internally will remove internal obstructions because it is the best solvent that we have. Obstructions in the stomach are easily removed by emetics. (See Emetics.) Obstructions in the bowels should be removed by enemas. (See Enemas.)

In fevers, cholera, etc., the blood is usually abnormally thick, which causes difficult circulation, and the tissues do not obtain nourishment. There is positively nothing but water that can remedy this condition. If water will not stay on the stomach, the skin will absorb a great deal by lying in a tub of water the proper temperature—depending on the difficulty. Hot and cold fomentations applied to the abdomen will often relieve headache. They seem to affect the whole system. Fomentations applied to the abdomen and spine will relieve general nervousness, and numerous other ailments. Ice applied to the spine is an excellent remedy in cholera and several other nervous diseases. A full, warm bath may be given with equal success.

Water is one of the most powerful means of affecting the human system in either health or disease.

Effects of cold water.—Cold baths, or applications given below a temperature of 85° F., cause instant contraction of the small arteries, because of its influence on the sympathetic nervous system. If cold applications are continued, the part will become bloodless. Moderately cool or cold applications, continued for some time, will more or less permanently lessen the supply of blood, until the part becomes thoroughly warmed again. A very brief cold application will cause only momentary contraction, which is followed by relaxation; then there will be an increased supply of blood to the part. The effect of cold application, prolonged or short, is exactly the opposite. When cold is first applied, there is a slight increase in the rate of pulsation, but this soon subsides, and there is a marked decrease. It is better to make the application warmer at first and then decrease the temperature gradually so that there will not be a shock, or chilly feeling, and the same results will be obtained. This applies especially to nervous persons, as the sudden application of cold is always a shock. When you reduce the temperature of the body, the action of the heart is also proportionately reduced. A great many times the real temperature is reduced, but the skin glows, and feels warmer. The only accurate way to determine temperature is by thermometer.

Effects of hot water.—Hot baths, or applications, should be given above a temperature of 98° F. A short local application causes increased circulation. As with cold water, the effects differ according to the length of the application. A full hot bath causes increased pulsation. A bath given from 106° to 108° F., will increase the pulse from normal to between 100 and 120 beats in a short time. A bath several degrees hotter, up to 112° F., will increase the pulse more than 150 beats a minute. When giving an extremely hot bath, always keep cold to the head, and every fifteen or twenty minutes sponge the entire body with cool water. This will avert faintness. Extremely hot baths are seldom required. It is better to have a temperature, as a rule, around 102° F.

There are very few agents which will so rapidly and powerfully excite and stimulate as the hot bath. The undesirable results of hot baths are because of irrational or incautious use. But these same results are proof of its power.

Effects of Warm Water.—A warm bath is between 85° and 92° F. A warm bath never exceeds the temperature of the body. Warm baths decrease the temperature, pulse, and respiration, as do cold baths, but differ otherwise, as there is no shock in a temperate bath.

Therefore it is not followed by any reaction.

Warm baths greatly increase the action of the skin, viz., perspiration, absorption. When a warm bath is continued for two or three hours, the weight will be increased as the skin absorbs a great deal of water. The general effects of a warm bath are mild and soothing, doubtless because of close approximation to the body temperature. It supplies favorable conditions for the performance of natural and usual functions.

Therefore, we see that when water is applied at a proper temperature, it is the most natural and powerful means of depressing or increasing the vital activities of the body.

Water applications are wholly of a sympathetic character, and all parts of the body are closely connected together by the sympathetic nerves. The skin and the mucous membrane are closely connected as has been shown.

There are many ways of administering water of all temperatures, each producing some modifications or general effect of a given temperature.

Amount of Water Needed Daily

The average person does not drink enough pure water. At least six glasses must be taken daily. More is better, depending upon the kind of food eaten. Cool water is good, but ice water should not be taken. Babies and delicate patients should be given water as carefully as food.

When one drinks an abundance of pure, fresh water the blood and tissues are bathed and purified, thereby being cleansed of all poisons and waste matter. Water is also an essential constituent of the tissue cells and all body fluids, such as digestive juices, etc.

Water dissolves nutritive material in the course of digestion, so that it can be absorbed into the blood, which carries it to various parts of the body to repair and remove waste.

Water keeps all mucous membranes of the body soft and prevents friction of their surface.

Water aids in regulating body temperature, and body processes.

Make a special effort to have pure water; soft water is preferable.

Chapter XVII

WATER — ITS EFFECT IN SICKNESS

There are very few agents that possess as many remedial properties as water. Anyone treating the sick should try to accomplish the greatest amount of good with the least expense to the vitality.

Sedative.—Sedative drugs diminish the action of the heart. They affect all the nerve centers controlling the heart, and their action is very often uncertain. Water is very much more efficient, and its use is never followed by hurtful after effects.

There is not one drug that will decrease the temperature of the body as quickly and efficiently as water. The pulse can be reduced from forty to twenty beats in a few minutes by the use of a cool or cold bath. To decrease heat, apply below 98° F.

Anodyne.—Anodyne will lessen the nervous sensibilities, thereby relieving pain. Hot water fomentations applied will always give relief, and have often been used when drugs failed. A warm bath will invariably soothe and rest an extremely nervous person and produce restful sleep.

Antispasmodic.—Water is unrivaled as a remedy in hysterical convulsions, infantile convulsions, puerperal convulsions, and cramps.

Astringent.—The use of cold water in arresting hemorrhages is well known by all physicians.

Laxative.—The use of water in many ways is most effectual in correcting constipation, but never causes violent or unpleasant symptoms that attend and succeed the use of purgatives.

Eliminative.—Water is a perfect eliminator. Dissolves all poisonous waste materials and foreign elements in the blood, thereby aiding their elimination.

Diaphoretic.—It produces profuse perspiration.

Alterative.—For many years mercury has been considered the most noteworthy alterative of the materia medica. However, it must yield its place to water, as the only thing it ever does is destroy the elements of the blood, but water not only destroys the waste elements, but increases the circulation and construction.

Tonic.—Water used properly will increase the circulation, and the temperature very quickly and powerfully. The tonic effect of a cool bath is well appreciated by everyone.

Stimulant.—Hot baths are the most efficient stimulants. They will stimulate the circulation so as to increase pulse from 70 to 150 in fifteen minutes.

Derivative.—One of water's most important properties is its powerful cleansing effect. No application can equal water in efficiency and certainty of action. Water will work wonders. Its use has been terribly neglected to the great detriment of the human race. Its merits have been well demonstrated and generally acknowledged for years.

Here is one of my favorite personal water treatments which I enjoy myself very much. It is douche spray. I have the operator stand maybe ten or fifteen feet distant if we have the room and have the stream of water come with a force strong enough so it will just hurt slightly. To begin with I have the water a little warmer than the temperature of the body or as warm as I can comfortably stand it and have him start on the back of my head and go up and down my spine clear down to my feet. Then I keep turning and he sprays well on the side of my neck and face clear around,

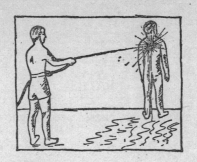

up and down, and so I keep turning around and around and have him spray right in my face. Then I turn my head down so it will hit on the top of the head and all over the head and keep turning until I am well warmed up. Then I turn around and have him turn the water a little cooler than the body temperature and start on the back of the head again and go up and down the spine clear to the feet and keep turning myself so he strikes every part of the body. I hold the feet up so it strikes the bottom of the feet and keep turning until it gets around the entire body. We keep this up for ten or fifteen mintues, striking every part of the body from the top of the head to the bottom of the feet. I enjoy this treatment very much.

Chapter XVIII

BATHS

Baths are divided into classes, according to the temperature, as follows:

1. Very cold .... 32° to 55° F.
2. Cold .... 55° to 65° F.
3. Cool .... 65° to 80° F.
4. Tepid .... 80° to 92° F.
5. Warm .... 92° to 98° F.
6. Hot .... 98° to 104° F.
7. Very Hot .... 104° F.,and above

Rules for Bathing

1. Never take a full bath within two hours after meals. Local applications of water may be made in a shorter time, such as foot baths, fomentations, compresses, and even sitz-baths.

2. Always use the thermometer when possible in preparing baths for the sick. The method used to test water for babies by placing the elbow in the water will sometimes help when a thermometer is not available.

3. Temperature of the room should be between 70° and 85° F. Patients or invalids require it warmer. There should always be good ventilation, but no drafts.

4. Do not use either extremely hot or cold baths for very old, feeble, or extremely nervous patients.

Although it is permissible when just warm enough to start perspiration, never take a cold bath when extremely fatigued or exhausted. It is better to start with tepid and increase to the cold water.

5. Never allow more than three or four days, at the most, to elapse without a warm cleansing bath. A cold morning bath is an excellent means of stimulating the whole nervous system as well as preserving bodily cleanliness.

6. Bath attendants should carefully avoid giving shocks to nervous people, or those affected with heart disease, or apoplexy.

7. The best time for hydrotherapy treatments is about three hours after breakfast.

8. Cold baths should not be taken during menstruations. A warm sponge-bath is best.

9. Always use the purest and softest water obtainable.

10. Baths should always be given of an agreeable temperature to sick persons, unless giving some particular treatment for effects.

11. When symptoms of faintness appear, apply cold to the head and face, give drink of cold water, or lower the temperature of the bath by adding cool water.

12. As a precaution against taking cold, always decrease the temperature of the bath before finishing if the person is not strong enough for a shower or cool sponge bath.

13. Cold baths should always be brief, unless given for a specific purpose to a portion of the body.

14. It is extremely important that the patient should be carefully dried. Never leave a patient chilly. Rub him until warm.

15. It is well to have patients exercise a little before and after bathing.

16. Rest after bathing will add to its beneficial results. It is best to lie down and keep covered.

Baths are one of the most powerful means of affecting the human system in either health or disease. Weak patients should have sponge baths, or if necessary, sponge baths in bed. If susceptible to chilliness, sponge one portion at a time, dry, cover, etc.

Turkish Baths

Turkish baths are given to produce profuse perspiration. Plenty of water should be taken before, during and after the bath to make up for that which is lost by perspiration. The chief agent is hot air. The temperature varies from 105° to 140° F. There are usually unpleasant sensations, but as soon as the patient begins to perspire, these disappear.

After the patient has perspired thoroughly, he is taken to a room of about 90° to 100° F., where the attendant thoroughly rubs and manipulates the body to remove all the dead skin, after which the whole body is thoroughly lathered and rubbed, either with the hand or a brush. A shower is given, and then the patient is immersed in a tub of cool water. The spray is all that is necessary, however. The patient is then dried, wrapped in a sheet (a blanket sometimes being necessary), and lies down in a room where the temperature is 70° or 80° F.

Besides being powerful to produce perspiration, the Turkish bath wonderfully stimulates elimination. It is a king of remedies in acute or chronic rheumatism, jaundice, malaria, syphilitic diseases, obesity, dropsy, rheumatic gout, skin diseases, eczema, and hydrophobia. It will break up fevers, typhoid, etc.

The Roman bath is quite similar to the Turkish, with the exception that after the patient has been dried, he is thoroughly rubbed with some sweet oil. This is excellent for persons who are very susceptible to colds.

How to Give a Turkish Bath Without a Cabinet.—Use a common No. 3 washtub. Tilt with a two-by-four or block of wood. Fill with hot water; also fill a large pan for feet. Place blanket on edge of tub, place patient in tub with his back on the blanket, and feet in pan of hot water. Cover well with a sheet, which should be tight around the neck. Take water out and add hot water until the patient perspires profusely, giving him plenty of water to drink. This is preferable to a pack if the patient can be moved.

Electric Light Bath.—This bath is simply artificial sunlight. The advantage is that the patient is not subjected to a hot atmosphere, yet it produces profuse perspiration. It is a fine tonic, and is good for use where it is desired to increase the activity of the skin, which it penetrates.

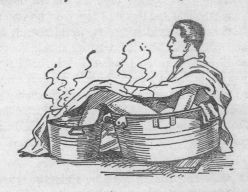

SITZ BATH

Sitz Bath.—The sitz, or hip-bath, is one of the most useful. A common tub may be used, placing under one edge something that will elevate it three or four inches. A regular tub made for this purpose has the back raised higher than the front to support the back, the sides slanting down to support the arms. The water should cover the abdomen. The temperature should be suited to the condition of the patient.

The hips and abdomen should be rubbed well by the attendant. The patient must be covered with a sheet or blanket during the bath, and several blankets must be used if sweating is desired. Begin the bath at a temperature of 90° to 95° F. The sitz-bath is useful in men's diseases, piles, genital and urinary diseases and disorders, constipation, dysentery, diarrhea, congestion in the abdominal or pelvic regions. It is absolutely indispensable in uterine and many diseases peculiar to women. It is very valuable and effective in nervous affections and in diseases which involve the brain, such as cerebral congestion.

Foot Bath.—The vessel used should be sufficiently large to have the feet and legs well covered with water to the knees. The hot and cold is a very useful remedy in chilblains and cold feet. The temperature should range from 100° to 120° F. The cold water should be 50° F., or less. Keep the feet and legs in the cold water for not more than two minutes. By alternating, this will produce a powerful reaction. The feet should always be rubbed while in the bath. The foot bath is most useful in neuralgia, headache, toothache, catarrh, colds, cold feet, congestion of the abdomen and pelvic organs.

Leg Bath.—This can be done by sitting in a bath tub. It is useful for chronic ulcers of the leg, swollen knees and ankles, varicose veins, and will also relieve headache and palpitation of the heart.

Tub Baths for Cleanliness.—Full tub baths are the most beneficial baths that can be taken, and are also very pleasant. The full bath should be taken at least two or three times a week, thoroughly scrubbing the entire body using a good soap, Ivory being one of the best. This will open the pores and make the skin glands active; then poisons can be eliminated from the system. When this kind of bath is

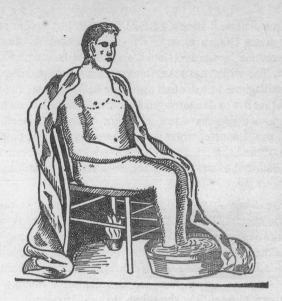

VAPOR BATH

given in diseases, if the patient is rubbed thoroughly while in the water, good results will be obtained.

A hot, full bath is a specific aid against colds, if taken as soon as they are contracted, making sure that the person does not become exposed or chilled afterwards. For rheumatism, neuralgia, gout, colic, sciatica, gall-stones, etc., the bath must be taken very hot, so that the person perspires. Do not make the water hot to start with, but keep increasing the heat. For comfort and good results, when the person becomes too warm, have him stand up and shower off with cool water, or rub body with towel that has been dipped into cool water. If the person has heart trouble keep icebag over the heart. Keeping cold compress on the head or around the neck will do much to avoid faintness.

In sickness, it is best to take the bath just before retiring. Baths have a tonic effect. The temperature must be determined by the individual, and should be suited to the case. The writer has taken many cases where persons had been diagnosed by doctors as having heart trouble, and was told that it was dangerous to give them a hot bath, and has given such persons warm tub baths freely with beneficial results. Of course, when there is heart trouble, or palpitation of the heart, great care much be taken when beginning the bath not to have it too hot, or leave the patient in the tub too long.

Eye Bath.—Applications of water and other solutions to the eye may be applied in many different ways. A brief application can be conveniently applied by placing the solution in the cup of the hand, holding over the eye and blinking, thus bringing the eye directly in contact with the solution. Small glass cups are also made for holding the solution. The solution should be changed frequently.

In giving applications of anything to the eyes it is essential first to know what the difficulty is, what caused it, and then apply the best thing to remove the cause.

When membrane which lines the eye lid and covers the eye ball becomes inflamed, or there is inflammation of the external structures, cold or cool applications are required. Inflammation of the cornea, or the pigmented membrane behind the cornea, perforated by the pupil, requires hot applications. Compresses made of two or three thicknesses of linen should be used, and changed every five minutes. Cool applications are excellent made in this way. Fomentations are the best method of applying heat. They should be as hot as can be borne. If they give relief, continue for a half hour or more. In case it increases the pain, stop immediately.

Alternate hot and cold applications will give relief in most cases. Leave the hot application on the longer, applying the cool for only a few minutes.

An eye bath of pure cold and hot water is infinitely superior to the patent eye washes on the market.

Daily eye baths of tepid water will benefit those who must use their eyes a great deal in working, or who read a great deal. Many people ruin their eyes from neglecting to give them proper care and rest. An excellent eye wash is made by steeping one teaspoonful of golden seal, two heaping teaspoonfuls boracic acid powder, and a half teaspoonful of myrrh in a pint of boiling water.

Ear Bath.—Applications are made to the ears by use of fomentations, compresses, douches, sprays, or poultices Fomentation and compresses are useful in inflammatin of the structures of the ear, and abcesses, and will restore the hearing in many cases.

Syringing of the ear should not be practiced, as it often results in irreparable injury.

The douche is a valuable means of removing foreign susbtances and insects. Warm douches are good to remove hardened ear-wax, and thus restore the hearing. When taking the douche, lean the head over a basin, so that the water can freely run in and out of the ear.

Nose Bath.—Close the mouth when drawing any liquid substance into the nose, or when injecting it by means of a fountain syringe. Always apply gently, violent applications often causing great pain and irritation. Never give injections with a piston syringe, as this often forces the susbtance into the Eustachian canal, and produces deafness. As a rule, the temperature of nose baths should be tepid or warm.

Salt Glows.—Wet two pounds of common coarse salt with water. Have the patient stand ankle deep in warm water. The body should be wet. Begin with the arm, applying the wet salt. Have the hands on each side of the arm, and rub vigorously with to-and-fro movements until the skin is aglow. Rub the whole body in a like manner. The salt glow is a vigorous circulatory stimulant.

Chapter XIX

COMPRESSES AND FOMENTATIONS

Compresses.—A compress is composed of several folds of cloth. When a cool compress is desired, wet the compress in the exact temperature desired, and place upon the part, wringing just so that it will not drip, and change every five minutes. A cold compress is prepared by placing crushed ice between the folds, and is very good. This, of course, does not need to be renewed so frequently.

In applying compresses to delicate parts, great care should be taken not to injure the part, a very thin compress being much better in such cases.

In applying warm compresses, cover the hot compress with a dry cloth, flannel being preferred.

The effects of a compress are very similar to those of a poultice.

The wet girdle, leg pack, wet sheet pack, chest pack and wrapper, and half pack are simply large compresses.

Fomentations.—Fomentations are local applications of hot and cold given alternately to relieve pain, to increase the circulation, etc.

To Make a Fomentation.—Take one half of a single bed cotton blanket and fold twelve inches wide. Take one-half a single bed woolen blanket. Have a large pan, the size of a dish pan, or bucket of boiling water. Dip the cotton blanket in it up to three or four inches of the ends, and keep the water boiling. Wring the folded blanket out of the water, have the flannel blanket spread out on a table, and lay the steaming cotton blanket on it, folding twice on

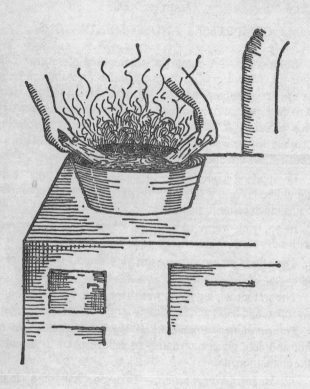

(1) Heating the Compress

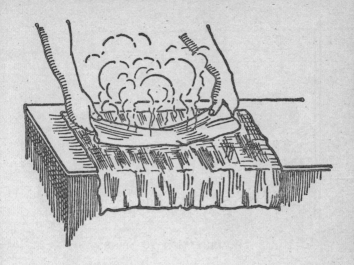

(2) WRAPPING THE COMPRESS

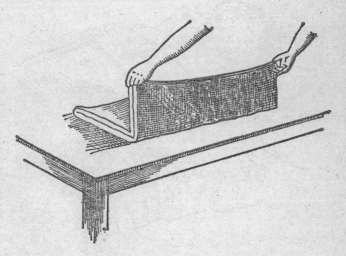

(3) FOLDING THE FOMENTATION

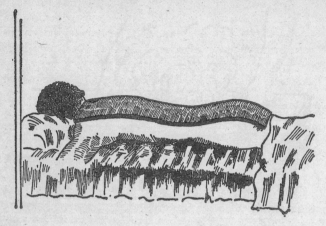

FOMENTATION TO SPINE

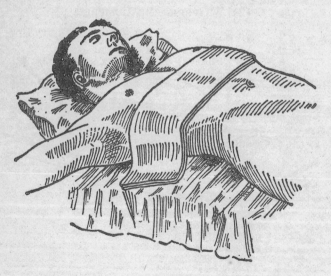

FOMENTATION TO STOMACH, LIVER, AND SPLEEN

one side, and once on the other. Apply to the patient as hot as can possibly be borne, running the hand under the fomentation on the skin as often as necessary. When you have run the hand under a couple of times, lift the fomentation, then quickly and vigorously run in a towel dipped out of cold water. Leave the fomentation on until it is comfortable, then sponge with the cool towel, and apply another. It is good to sponge with the cold towel several times during a fomentation.

Three fomentations are usually applied, one following the other. Keep the patient covered between fomentations, or it is better to have two sets of fomentation cloths, and have another ready to apply immediately upon removing one. Patients are usually better able to stand more heat upon the second application. Dipping the hand in cold water will enable the attendant to wring the fomentation much hotter than he would otherwise be able to do.

Fomentations may be applied for a period of from fifteen minutes to one hour, according to the case.

Fomentations should be employed in acute inflammations, local pains and congestion, neuralgia, toothache, and pleurisy.

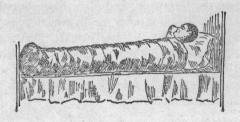

BLANKET PACK

How to Give a Blanket Pack. Have two double blankets, part wool, one single blanket, part wool if possible. Then have a large boiler or kettle of BOILING water, and a small basin of very cold or ice water is preferable, to be used in making compresses for the patient's head.

Give a hot foot bath while the blanket pack is being prepared. If the patient is able to sit up, have him sit by the bed to give the foot bath, if not, have the patient lie on one side of the bed with his feet in hot water. It is well to give a hot herb tea at this time to aid in producing perspiration, such as, yarrow, boneset, sage or catnip.

Place one double blanket on the bed, this one to be wrapped over the wet pack, then take the other double blanket and fold the two longer edges over until they almost meet in the center, then fold one side over the other. This will form a long strip the full length of the blanket. Put the folded blanket in the boiling water. (Do this carefully, so as not to disturb the folds.) leaving about ten inches of each end of the blanket out of the water, so that two persons can take hold and twist the blanket in opposite directions until all the water possible is wrung out. The blanket must become thoroughly saturated with the boiling water. After the blanket has been wrung out (wring as dry as possible), place it on the bed, open, and place the patient in it as quickly as possible, as it cools rapidly when opened. Wrap the patient first in the hot wet blanket, then the single blanket, and then the dry double blanket. Be sure the feet are well wrapped, and the dry blanket securely wrapped over the wet one. Wrap the blanket so that the arms are next to the blanket and not the body.

Chapter XX

MASSAGE

Massage is a systematic rubbing and manipulation of the body. Massage prevents stiffness, promotes circulation, and brings health and tone. By massage the muscles are exercised as fully as possible without exhaustion, and the blood is propelled to greater activity.

Massage is one of the most valuable of remedial measures. When used in combination with water, it accomplishes amazing results. It assists in building of the blood and rebuilding of the tissues in general.

Common sense and consideration for the condition of the patient must be used. For those who are weak or delicate, massage should be light until muscles become accustomed to the treatment, then more pressure and force may be used.

Give massage after hot bath or fomentations. Lubricate the skin with olive oil or cocoa fat. Always stroke toward the heart. When possible have a high table, so that the attendant does not have to stoop. The patient should lie flat on the back with all muscles relaxed. The patient must draw up his knees to relax the abdomen when it is being massaged. After massaging the arms, stomach, and legs, the patient should lie face downward for the back treatment.

When desired, one may start by giving the scalp a brisk rub with the fingertips. Massage the face with a rotary motion, beginning with the chin and working upward to the ears.

Arms.—Commence at the finger tip and stroke upward to the shoulder. Start with the finger tips and rub each finger joint separately with a circular movement. Grasp the arm with the two hands and manipulate, the thumbs away from each other, as if dividing the muscles from the bone. Do this the whole length of the arm. Next, wring or twist the muscles in the same way that one would wring a wet cloth. This drives the blood from the muscles and stimulates the nerve centers. Next, knead the muscles by placing one hand on the under side and one on top, grasping firmly, and using the balls of the thumbs to roll the muscles with a slow rotary motion from left to right. Now start again at the finger tips, and commence a series of squeezes, working on each muscle with a firm quick grasp. This tends to accelerate the flow of the blood to the heart. Pound with the sides of the open hand, fingers extended. Now whip the arms with the finger tips, using a light short stroke. This is done by shaking the hands from the wrists.

Chest.—Lay the hands flat. Give rotary motion from left to right. Grasp the flesh near the short ribs, working the muscles upward by a rolling motion.

Abdomen.—Draw the knees up to relax the muscles. Place hand flat on the bowels near hips, using wrist force. Roll the hands firmly, but gently, toward the tips of the fingers, using a rotary motion from left to right. Great benefit may be derived from massage in cases of torpid liver, constipation, etc.

Legs.—Treat in the same manner as the arms, using extra force on the deeper muscles. The deep muscles will stand thumping, hacking, and slapping that arms cannot.

Back.—Commence with the back of the head and neck. Massage the base of the brain and down the spinal column very thoroughly. The main movements employed are stroking, pounding, kneading, and percussion.

In giving the massage, there should be a free action from the wrist, the tips of the fingers and balls of the thumbs being used most, except in the pounding and slapping. The movements should always be firm. A half-way-given massage is worse than none at all.

Movement of Swedish Massage

Arms.—Lubricate from wrist to shoulder.

Friction from hand to shoulder.

Fulling from shoulder to hand once.

Spiral friction from hand to shoulder, twice to each side of the arm, beginning on the inside of the arm.

Knead from hand to elbow three times, friction. Repeat.

Rotary kneading to elbow.

Rolling, down three times, alternating with upward friction.

Friction from hand to shoulder.

Percussion from shoulder to hand.

Hacking, spatting, down and up each side, once.

Joint movements—bend and then pull the arm, then move around in a circle.

Vibration and stroking.

Chest.—Lubricate.

Friction.

Fulling down one side and up the other.

Friction.

Beginning on neck, palm kneading, twice.

Friction.

Percussion, tapping, hacking, spattting.

Stroking.

Abdomen.—Lubricate.

Deep breathing.

Reflex stroking.

Deep vibration.

Side and circular shaking.

Percussion, tapping, hacking, spatting, clapping on colon.

Knead colon twice.

Friction.

Fulling up and down each side, and up and down the rectal muscles.

Rotary kneading twice to each side, alternating with friction.

Stroking.

Leg.—Lubricate.

Friction up.

Fulling down.

Spiral friction up, twice to each side of the leg, beginning inside.

Circular friction up.

Rotary kneading to foot, leg and knee, three times, alternating with friction, repeat.

Back.—Lubricate.

Friction.

Fulling down one side and up the other.

Friction.

Knead spine with thumb.

Give rotary kneading to both sides twice, alternating with friction.

Heavy friction down spine, twice.

Circular heavy kneading down each side of spine, twice.

Knead shoulders with palm. Knead down each side of spine with palm.

Grasp the muscles up and down the spine.

Heavy wringing up, down, and crosswise.

Percussion, hacking, spatting, clapping.

Stroke entire back. Finish with at least ten light friction strokes to back.

Special Abdomen Massage for Constipation.—Lubricate. Have patient breathe deeply. Reflex stroking, deep vibration, circular shaking, percussion to colon, tapping, hacking, spatting, clapping. Heavy friction four times, fist kneading to colon four times, knead colon with heel of hand and fingers, friction, mass kneading, rolling, fulling, friction, rotary kneading as in general massage, percussion to lumbar spine.

Fulling.—Place hands on both sides of the arm, rolling backward and forward, up and down the arm.

Stocking.—Lay hands flat on the part of the body being massaged. Move hands slowly downward. Stroking is a sedative when gently applied to the spine. Stroking the abdomen increases the activity of the bowels and should always follow the course of the colon. Place the hands low down on the right side, and down opposite the point of starting. One or both hands may be used.

Clapping.—Clapping and percussion are practically the same thing. Clap the surface with the palms of the hands.

Chopping.—This is similar to clapping, except that the sides of the hands are used. The blow should be quick, using little force. Strike the surface with the edge of the finger, keeping them apart, so that they clap together with each stroke. Strike alternately with each hand.

Chapter XXI

HIGH ENEMAS

There are several different kinds of enemas, such as ordinary enemas taken to relieve the rectum and lower colon; astringent enemas, taken in diarrhea, dysentery, etc.; and nourishing enemas, given in wasting diseases, unconsciousness and other conditions where it becomes necessary to administer food by rectum. But high enemas as recommended in this book, are taken to thoroughly cleanse the entire length of the colon. All you need to take a high enema that thoroughly cleanses the colon, is a four-quart enema can with an ordinary rectal tip.

It is best to take it lying down. Lie on the floor, or in the bath tub. Use four quarts of water, or herb teas. It is not usually possible for a person to take the entire four quarts at one time, at first. When beginning, take a small amount of water, expel, then take more, and so on until you have used the entire four quarts, retaining as much each time as is possible. As soon as the colon is clean, you will be able to retain the full four quarts. You must try again and again until this is possible. When taking the high enema, assume different positions, also roll from side to side, so that the water is allowed to pass in, as sometimes there is a kink in the colon, and many times just a change in position allows a great deal more water to flow in.

There are some cases where there has been a diseased condition of the colon for some time, or some other difficulties which might make it impossible to ever retain this amount of water. In those cases, take as much as possible.

CHAPTER XXII

NURSING

Characteristic of a True Nurse

1. Faithful, intelligent and efficient care of the sick is often responsible in a large measure for recovery.

2. Consideration and kindness characterizes a nurse. Irritability, thoughtlessness, and inconsiderate acts are inexcusible. Nurses must be kind in thought, word and deed.

3. Cheerfulness—a bright and sunny disposition brings life, hope and cheer into the sick room. The sick room is not a place for a gloomy, morbid nurse.

4. Unselfishness—untiring devotion to the interests of the patient are required of a nurse. She should be willing to sacrifice herself in behalf of her patient, not regarding personal comfort and convenience.

5. Anyone who is upset by trivial circumstances or who is excitable in trying times should not be a nurse. Good judgment and calmness will tend to inspire confidence in her intelligence.

6. A nurse must always be patient. People who are ordinarily thoughtful and considerate frequently are unreasonable in the extreme when sick, and demand attenion, often unnecessarily. A nurse should always be firm to secure compliance with her instructions.

7. A nurse should be able to divert the patient's mind from undesirable and depressing thoughts, without making it apparent. She should be discreet and impersonal in her con-

versations. Reading to the patient is excellent and should be done whenever permissible. Avoid exciting, tiresome, and any objectionable topic, either in reading or in conversation. Regulate the matter of visitors without giving offense. Good sound common sense is needed at all times.

8. A nurse should observe the changes in the condition of the patient. She must observe anything that is giving discomfort to the patient and change it if possible as many times the patient will not say anything for fear of annoying the nurse too often.

9. Physical soundness is most essential in a nurse—good hearing, good vision, and a good sense of smell.

10. A nurse should wear noiseless shoes. Uniforms should not be so stiff as to make a rustling noise with every movement.

11. The nurse should speak distinctly and softly, never in loud tones, but whispering is very objectionable, and is always annoying to the patient. The patient's questions should be answered discreetly, never in a manner that could convey the impression that there was something to be concealed that he desires to know.

12. A nurse's hands should always be warm, clean, and the nails well trimmed. Gentleness and firmness should characterize the touch.

13. General neatness of personal appearance should be strictly regarded.

14. All tasks should be accomplished quietly without confusion and noise. This does not mean to move around on tiptoe, which would invariably be annoying to the patient.

Don'ts

Never sit and tap with the foot or fingers.

Prepare quietly for bed or the night after the patient is ready for sleep.

Try to time the giving of food, treatment, drinks, etc., so as not to disturb the patient when settled for a nap.

Do not continually ask patients how they feel and whether they would like something done for them.

Do not let direct rays of light shine in the patient's eyes.

Avoid unnecessary noise with dishes and papers.

Do not hurry them with meals, but encourage them to masticate thoroughly.

Avoid jarring the bed.

When sitting in a rocking chair, do not rock incessantly. It would be very annoying to the patient.

How to Keep a Chart

At given times during the day the temperature should be taken, usually morning and evening. Use a self-registering thermometer, thoroughly disinfected each time it is used, and see that the mercury is below 96 degrees. If it is not, shake it down, being careful not to hit the thermometer against anything. When taking the temperature the thermometer is usually held in the mouth beneath the tongue for three minutes with lip tightly closed; or under the armpit five minutes. If taken under the armpit, the arm should be held close to the body to prevent the air from striking the thermometer. When taken by mouth a cold drink should not be given for at least 20 minutes before taking.

Care must be used when taking children's temperature that they do not bite the thermometer. With children it is usually better to take temperature by the rectum. Temperature is normally 98½ degrees, although higher in the early evening. Fever rarely rises above 105° F., and then the patient is in a perilous condition. In some diseases the temperature may rise above 107° and recovery still take place as in inflammatory rheumatism, hysteria, etc., while in others such as inflammation of the bowels, above 105° F. would indicate great danger.

The Pulse.—The pulse is usually felt at the wrist, over the radial artery, and coincides with the beating of the heart. When it cannot be continued distinctly at the wrist, place the hand over the heart. The average pulse rate in adults is about 72 beats a minute, and in children from 72 to 120. Pulse is usually faster in sickness, though sometimes slower. At times it may reach 140, then something must be done at once to lower it. (See Fevers in the Table of Contents.) The character of the pulse is as important as its frequency, which varies considerably. At times it will be weak, irregular, rapid, slow, or intermittent.

Respiration.—Normally the respiration is one-fourth the number of pulse beats. It is important to observe not only its frequency but whether it is noisy, irregular, painful, difficult, or abnormal in any way.

Coughs.—When a cough is present, it should be noticed at what times it is worse, how frequent, duration, and the character. When there is expectoration, the color, whether profuse or scanty, frothy, bloody, thick, etc., should be noticed.

Discharges.—Note bowel discharges of patient and report the size, frequency, color, consistency, and general odor, the color, quantity, and odor of the urine, the nature of sediments, the frequency, etc. In saving a specimen for examination, save the first specimen in the morning. In case of retention in the bladder by which the bladder will become distended and the urine dribble away, a catheter must be used.

Miscellaneous Symptoms.—The way a patient speaks, whether nervous, restless, rational, irritable, the strength of the voice, the hours of sleep, the locations and character of pain or pains, and whether diminished or aggravated by pressure, whether constant or intermittent, stationary or movable. The condition of the tongue, whether clean, furred, coated, etc.; the eye, whether there is swelling of the lids, undue sensitiveness to light, alteration in size of the pupils, color, etc.; the skin, as to warmth of body, color, moisture and general appearance; the expression, whether pinched, anxious, wan, peaceful or otherwise; the general attitude and demeanor of patient—all this information should be charted. Record charts can be obtained at most drug-stores.

GENERAL CARE OF PATIENTS

How to Make a Bed

The mattress should be firm and the sheets large enough to permit them to be well tucked under its edges so they will stay smooth. It is usually desirable to protect the bed by rubber sheeting placed under the lower sheet.

Place a sheet folded lengthwise across the bed over the lower sheet in the middle of the bed. This is called a draw sheet. Tuck the ends well under the mattress on each side. To change the lower sheet loosen sheet at both ends and sides. Have patient roll to one side of bed, if possible. Fold soiled sheet up to patient, follow up by the clean sheet folded and the outside edge firmly tucked under side and ends of mattress. The patient can roll back to the other side of the bed on the clean sheet. Then remove the soiled sheet and tuck the clean one in on the other side and ends of the mattress. The draw sheet can be placed at the same time the clean sheet is placed.

Change the upper sheet by folding crosswise. Tuck the clean sheet in at the foot of the bed and draw into position, the soiled sheet then being drawn to the foot and removed. Strict attention should be paid to having the under sheet perfectly smooth, not only for the patient's comfort, but to prevent bed sores. See that there are never any crumbs in the bed.

Changing Clothing

In changing a patient's clothes, remove the sleeves first. Lay the clean garment face down on the patient, with the top toward his feet. The sleeves are then put on, and as his head is slightly raised the soiled garment can be slipped over the head and the clean one put on at the same time. If the patient is at home and cannot be raised at all the garment must be cut down the back. Then as one sleeve is taken off the clean one replaces it, and the garment can be gradually tucked under the shoulders and body, and the other sleeve changed. Since some patients are very susceptible to changes in temperature as garments are being changed, it is necessary to have a light wrap at hand to throw around the patient's shoulders.

Bathing

Only a small portion of the body should be bathed at a time, and should be thoroughly dried. Use a good soap.

Temperature and Ventilation

The temperature of the room should be kept at about 70° F. In some diseases it may be necessary to keep the temperature higher, and in others lower. The air should always be moist. If there is a hot air furnace or stove, keep a dish of water on the radiator or stove. If the nurse sleeps in the room with the patient, it should be large and well ventilated.

Disinfection

Lysol or any good disinfectant may be used. The aid of a disinfectant helps materially in keeping the air pure.

It should be diluted in water and kept in vessels for receiving discharges.

Disinfection of Clothing

In infectious diseases, all washable clothing, sheets, etc., should be boiled in a covered boiler for a least one-half hour. They should be placed in disinfectant solution immediately upon removal. Handkerchiefs should not be used. Pieces of soft cloth, disposable tissues or paper handkerchiefs should be used and burned.

All sweepings from the room should be burned.

Eating utensils must be boiled, using a good strong laundry soap.

General Instructions

1. When choice is possible, a bright, sunny, airy room is best in which to nurse the sick—if possible, a room remote from the rest of the house so that noise will not annoy the patient.

2. The room must be kept clean and neat. The sweeping should be done with a dampened broom or dust mop. Dust with a damp cloth to avoid raising dust.

3. In serious illnesses keep the paitent as quiet as possible. It is better to keep from them unpleasant happenings in the household.

4. Prepare and serve food daintily. Feed patient slowly. Give liquids by using a glass drinking tube or drinking straws.

5. Visitors' calls should be brief and not be permitted to weary the patient. It is better to have one caller at a time than to have two present at once.

6. Never jar the bed by knocking against it.

7. When fanning is desired, it should be gentle.

8. The nurse should never dress or undress in the same room with the patient.

9. A nurse should have an opportunity to spend an hour daily in the fresh air and sunshine, and should not for any length of time be on both day and night duty.

10. In fevers, give water freely, a sip every few minutes, but not too much at one time.

11. For nausea sips of very hot water or small pieces of chipped ice swallowed whole sometimes give relief.

12. Prepare for a seriously injured patient by having a warm bed with plenty of hot water bottles. In case of a severe shock, keep the head low, stimulate freely, and rub the extremities briskly.

13. In cases of fainting, keep the head low, loosen the clothing about the neck and waist, give plenty of fresh air, bathe the face with cold water, and let the person inhale smelling salts or ammonia cautiously.

14. Heart failure must be treated as a shock. Give small doses of red pepper. Either peppermint, scullcap, or lily of the valley tea is very good. Take as much as needed. A cold towel rub, given by bathing one part of the body at a time and drying thoroughly, is excellent.

15. Soak sprains immediately in very hot water. This will relieve to a great extent the pain and swelling; then apply Liniment (See Table of Contents.) freely.

16. Bleeding from the nose which cannot be checked by pressure on back of neck and cold water, may often be stopped by syringing the nostrils with cold salt water. (See herbs for hemorrhages.) Raise the arms above the head. Apply cold water to nape of neck and end of nose.

17. Extra covering should always be available during the early morning hours when a patient's vitality is lowest.

18. Bedpans should be warmed before using. Place folded towel on pan under patient.

How to Give an Enema in Bed

The bed should be well protected by rubber sheeting. Expel all air from the enema tube by letting some water run through before inserting. The enema tip should be well lubricated with soap, vaseline, or oil. Have patient lie on back, knees flexed. Insert the tip and let the water run slowly. When there is pain, shut off water and let patient roll from one side to the other, and resume after a few moments' rest. Four quarts can be injected if care is used, and can be retained from ten to fifteen minutes. After withdrawing the tip, fold a towel and press tightly over the anus for a few minutes to aid in its retention. (Look in Table of Contents for Enemas.)

Vaginal Douches

Place patient on the back, hips well elevated. In cases of congestion it is best to use one gallon of water as hot as possible. (Look in Table of Contents for Herbal Douches.)

Chapter XXIII

FRUITS

God planned in the beginning that fruit should form a large part of our diet, and if we would practice that now, it would mean very much to our health. While it is true that fruit, like other things, has deteriorated very much since creation, yet if we would take care of it and eat it in a proper way, it would prove an untold blessing today.

In the beginning man was told to dress the trees. This was for a wise purpose. Every tree should be pruned and dressed so that the sun will shine on the fruit at least part of the day, if not all day. If there are too many limbs and leaves, and the fruit grows altogether in the shade, it has much less food value, flavor, and life-giving properties. The seed of fruit and vegetables grown in the shade for two or three years will not germinate. It has to a great extent lost its quality and life-giving properties. Therefore all fruit trees should be pruned so that sun and air have free access. Another thing that should be remembered is that fruit before it is ripe is in the starchy state; in this condition it has but little food value, and is hard to digest. But as fruit ripens, it turns into grape sugar, especially when ripened in the air and sun, and requires practically no digestion. Fruit which is grown in the shade or is picked before it is ripe is better cooked than raw. A great deal of the fruit that is shipped is picked before it is ripe. While it does ripen to some extent after it is picked, it is never the same as it is when ripened on the tree.

If fruit is picked before it is full grown, it is practically worthless as far as real food value is concerned, excepting, perhaps, the banana, which is a very peculiar fruit. It can be picked green and will continue to ripen and develop its sugar. It should never be eaten until every particle of green disappears, and the outer skin begins to turn brown, and the pulp has become mellow. Most bananas are eaten altogether too green, and while still in the starchy state. When the banana is fully ripe, it develops twenty-five per cent of grape sugar, which requires very little or no digestion. Any infant or invalid can eat them when mashed up.

Some time ago the writer was in a fruit store looking for a bunch of bananas that suited him. The storekeeper said: "I like bananas, but I cannot eat them." He said: "Yesterday about eleven o'clock I got very hungry and ate two bananas, and they made me so sick that I had to go to bed." The writer asked him to point out what kind he ate. He had eaten bananas that were in the starchy state, and had probably not masticated them properly. Without proper mastication, bananas will form gases and putrefy and cause trouble. Let me emphasize again, *never* eat a banana until it is thoroughly ripe.

In buying prunes, buy a large size, for the large prunes have practically no larger pit than the small ones. The smaller the prunes, the less meat you have, and the more pits. A large prune when soaked overnight in cold water can be eaten without any cooking, and is very delicious. You can do the same thing with figs, apricots, or peaches when you get a good grade. When you do cook them, a very little cooking is all that is needed. Remember that the fruit before it is ripe is in the starchy state and requires cooking and digestion, and after it is thoroughly ripened it requires no cooking and little digestion. The juice is ready for assimilation.

Unripe grains are the opposite of unripe fruits. The grain before ripe is in the milky state, or grape sugar state and could be digested without any cooking. That is the way the grain was eaten in the beginning, and no doubt that is the way the disciples and Jesus ate it. But when it ripens, it turns into starch. We have no fluid to digest raw starch properly, and therefore grains should be thoroughly cooked.

"All the elements of nutrition are contained in the fruits, vegetables and grains." *R. & H.* 1883, No. 19.

However, the juice of oranges, grapes, pineapples, and grapefruit may be taken when pure with no sugar added. These juices can with good results be taken as a drink between meals to quench the thirst.

There are several reasons why we should not drink with the meals and eat so much soft food. First, we hear so much about alkaline foods and that they are all right to be eaten, but an indisputable fact is that the saliva is highly alkaline and much more so than any of these alkaline foods. And the fact is if we eat our food dry, getting it thoroughly saturated with saliva, it alkalinizes the system more than all the alkaline foods combined that we know. And second, when the food reaches the stomach there comes the digestive juice known as the gastric juice. In order for the gastric juice to properly do its work it needs the saliva and then as the food leaves the stomach there comes the pancreatic juice and the bile. They cannot do their proper work without the saliva and the gastric juice. If many of these little points were observed, you would see a marvelous improvement in your health. And then another point is: When you take so much fluid with your meals and also the soft foods, it dilutes these various digestive fluids so they are too weak and have not the proper power to digest the food as God had planned they should. There is perfect law and order in our system, and when we violate these, we have to suffer the consequences.

Many years ago when we made tests on these things, we found that half a good-sized lemon would destroy typhoid germs in a glass of water and the healthy gastric juice in the stomach is four times as strong as the lemon juice. Here is where the Scripture is fulfilled that when we eat or drink any deadly thing, it shall not hurt us. I would not advise anyone to take carbolic acid, or any of these concentrated poisons and think that is what the Scripture tries to convey—that these digestive fluids would counteract them, but this nevertheless is true that if you see to it that your blood stream is pure and you eat the foods that make your digestive fluids pure or normal, then your system will be able to resist typhoid, diphtheria, smallpox, tuberculosis, and the deadly fever germs. And then God has provided still further preventive, non-poisonous remedies, like the gentian root, the calumus root, the valerian root, and the black currant juice and leaves, and many others. These are God's harmless preventives, and anyone can take them in abundance. God never intended that man should take any poisons which are Satan's production. God cannot hear our prayers in recovery of the sick when we use Satan's poisonous remedies, which always do the system harm for God's remedies never leave a harmful effect on the system. Nature is God's physician for suffering humanity, healing without money and without price. There is no law against one's being his own doctor, which would prevent one's going into a garden and eating the right fruit and then plucking some of the leaves, and making a tea of them and drinking it.

Do not fail to read the wonderful medical properties of the various trees in this book. These are life-long experiences by seeing the wonderful results day by day of what these things really produce. When only a youngster, I used to gather the leaves and bark for my mother and father, and for some of the herb doctors.

CHAPTER XXIV

THE ELIMINATING DIET

All the good food that may be eaten cannot do the body any good until you have eliminated and cleansed the body of excess acids and mucus. The intestines retain these poisons and they are one of the main causes of disease and old age. By the eating of an abundance of alkaline or base forming foods, one can rid themselves of these poisons and acids. The eliminate these unnatural, unhealthful conditions, and make it possible for the food eaten to be assimilated and absorbed by the system, the body must be flushed and cleansed. The eating of these foods will bring about a natural rejuvenation, by constantly supplying the blood stream with the natural elements of which they are originally composed, as found in natural foods, eaten raw or cooked so as not to destroy their minerals or life-giving properties. You will be feeding the entire body, not stimulating it. Lev. 17:11, "The LIFE is in the blood," and in the same chapter, fourteenth verse, "For the life of all flesh is in the blood." Health and happiness depend upon the blood stream containing all the sixteen elements; when one is missing, disease results in some form. To make the blood stream pure and health producing, eat food in its natural state as far as possible, drink freely of pure water, bathe frequently, exercise in pure air and sunshine and use non-poisonous herbs that were given for the "service of man." Ps. 104:14.

In most of the civilized world we are able to do this almost any time of year, as we have the citrus fruits the year around, and also fresh vegetables.

(159)

We repair our homes, buy new parts and have our automobiles repaired, and give other machinery that we may be using constant repair. Just so, we must repair our bodies by supplying them with natural elements and minerals to build and repair parts that are constantly being worn out.

The blood stream which circulates through every cell in the body, if pure and alkaline, will dissolve and carry away all poisons. No disease can exist in a pure blood stream.

How Long Should One Stay on an Elimination Diet?

This depends entirely upon the individual. If you have been sick, or eating unnatural foods for years, or almost a life-time, you will have to eliminate many times, that is, eliminate a week, or longer if you are stout or overweight, and then eliminate again. One pound a day may be lost by faithfully eating just the eliminating foods, and this that is lost is mostly waste and poisons. Very little that the body really needs or that produces health will be lost, as these foods supply all the elements and minerals needed to build the body. Also if one has taken patent medicines, drugs, serums, etc., it will take longer to eliminate these poisons from the system. When all pains and discomfort in the body are gone, the poisons will have been eliminated; until they are, you will have to eliminate again. Everyone could safely eliminate seven days in every month. Very little healthy tissues will be lost. The most that is lost is unhealthy tissues and waste, and the sooner you rid your body of these, the better for your health.

Do not use when taking the eliminative diet the following: Milk, cane sugar, gravies, butter, free fat of any kind, macaroni, spaghetti, tapioca, corn starch, meat, tea, coffee, chocolate, ice cream, pastries of any kind, cane sugar products, white flour products, all kinds of liquor and tobacco.

Use all kinds of fruits liberally.

If fruits do not seem to agree with you, take one-fourth teaspoonful of golden seal in one-half glass water, twenty minutes before you eat.

Chapter XXV

MINERALS FOUND IN THE BODY

The following is a list of the elements found in the normal body: Hydrogen, phosphorus, chlorine, calcium, oxygen, carbon, magnesium, sodium, nitrogen, flourine, potassium, silicon, iron, iodine, manganese.

All these elements are bountifully supplied in natural foods, if not destroyed in their preparation. All life is furnished from within and must be replenished by living organic minerals in foods. Inorganic chemicals obtained from the drugstore are dead, and while they may stimulate for a time, they can give neither life nor health.

Natural chemicals especially are needed for the purifying cleansing process.

Water.—Lemons, fresh pineapple, limes, peaches, grapefruit, oranges, tomatoes, and all juicy fruits.

Postassium.—Poor circulation and constipation denote a lack of potassium. Potassium foods should always be used in abundance in female troubles. All leafy vegetables, watercress, parsley, swiss chard, tomatoes, mustard greens, beet tops, spinach, endive, dill, dandelions, watermelon.

Sodium.—Sodium is very solvent. Abundance should be eaten in cases of rheumatism, hardening of the arteries, kidney stones, gall stones, stiff points, acidosis, and diabetes. Spinach, okra, cucumbers, carrots, celery, beet roots, apples, huckleberries, gooseberries, strawberries.

Iron.—Organic iron is very important; it removes waste products, and assists greatly in cleaning the blood stream.

Inorganic iron should never be taken as it is an irritant to the kidneys. Red and white cabbage, spinach, beets, lettuce, raw carrots, cherries, currants, blackberries, strawberries, loganberries, onions.

Sulphur.—Sulphur is especially needed in eliminating blood diseases, skin diseases, eruptions, pimples, etc., also rheumatism. Foods containing sulphur aid in reducing. Cabbage, asparagus, Brussels sprouts, raw celery, cauliflower, onions, radishes.

Sulphur foods stimulate the liver, and poromte the flow of bile.

Chlorine.—Chlorine is a great destroyer of poisons. In pyorrhea, Bright's disease, and gangrene there is always insufficient chlorine. Chlorine foods also greatly assist in keeping the intestines clean.

Raw white cabbage, spinach, radishes, fresh asparagus, parsnips, unpeeled cucumbers, raw carrots, watercress, spinach, lettuce, onions, raw or cooked plain, turnips.

Magnesium.—Magnesium is nature's laxative. Foods containing magnesium are especially beneficial to persons suffering from auto-intoxication and constipation, also stiff joints and cracking joints. Apples, potatoes, barley, string beans, blackberries, blueberries, cabbage, celery, Chinese cabbage, cocoanuts, dandelion greens, oatmeal, oranges, plums, prunes, radishes, rice (natural brown or wild), and watercress are rich in magnesium.

Manganese.—A strong purifier and effective neutralizer of body acids. Peppermint leaves, endive, dandelion greens, parsley, senna leaves, watercress, mustard greens, etc.

Oxygen.—Oxygen is a dissolver, and is found everywhere in the air, fruits, and vegetables. Everyone needs more oxygen. When the blood passes through the lungs, it is purified by oxygen. Abundance of oxygen assists elimination greatly. So, above all things, breathe deeply. Use grape juice, orange juice, grapefruit juice, sweet apple juice liberally. Oxygen hastens elimination and burns up poisons.

All the above elements when taken in abundance will cleanse the blood stream. Therefore, the greater the quantity taken of these foods the sooner the body will be cleansed. Drink water copiously between meals, eat at least two grapefruit a day, six oranges, and three lemons. Eat a large raw vegetable salad each day. Have one meal of cooked vegetables per day, cooked properly. Do not use cane sugar with your fruits or lemonade, as it destroys the good benefit of the fruit. Do not mix the fruit juices.

Fresh pineapple, ripe peaches, cherries, plums, pears, apples, ripe strawberries, blueberries, rapsberries, are excellent, but all fruits must be ripe before being picked, else they have not the eliminating qualities.

The eliminative diet is not a fast. It is a feeding process. It feeds the body through the blood with the necessary life-giving minerals that everybody needs. The eating of fresh fruits and vegetables in quantities prevents the shrinking of the stomach and intestines, and also prevents lines and wrinkles in the face and body.

Best Vegetables.—Spinach, celery, carrots, parsley, tomatoes, asparagus, mild green onions, red or green cabbage (best raw), lettuce, cucumbers, radishes, okra, eggplant, etc. (See Potassium Broth in Table of Contents.)

Persons wishing to eliminate that have ulcerated stomach and cannot take fruits should drink two quarts a day of this broth. This is also excellent for invalids.

It is highly necessary that the bowels move freely. If they do not completely evacuate at least two or three times a day you are constipated. It is wise to cleanse them once or twice a week with an herb enema.

We have five organs of elimination—skin, lungs, bowels, kidneys and liver.

The bowels will be greatly improved by these foods and the help of non-poisonous herbs.

The lungs eliminate poisons freely when we practice deep breathing and exercise.

The skin cannot eliminate poisons when it is dry and inactive. There are millions of pores that breath and eliminate poisons; therefore a daily bath should be taken by everyone, and during the eliminating, it is excellent to take an Epsom salts bath every other day. Use three pounds of Epsom salts to a tub full of water. Drink plenty of water or broth while in the tub. Massage the body while in the tub. Salt glows are also highly beneficial. Rub the body thoroughly all over with half common salt and half Epsom; this increases the activity of the skin and the circulation. Finish with a cool shower or sponge off, rubbing vigorously with Turkish towel.

Take moderate exercise in the open air.

Eat nothing but fruits and vegetables. Strictly eliminate bread, oils of any kind, butter, white sugar, canned fruits, potatoes, cakes, eggs, or any food that is not mentioned in the eliminating diet.

Many people do not understand why they cannot have other good, wholesome natural foods. This is because they would upset the reaction of these cleansing foods. Do not taken any starchy foods, sugars, proteins, as these things congest and clog the system.

When the cells of the body are clean, they function normally and harmoniously; therefore the whole body is rejuvenated and the vitality restored.

Cook all vegetables with as little water as possible, using only salt for seasoning.

Before beginning to eliminate, cleanse the system with herb laxative. This will rid the body of much waste matter and mucus, and prevent such a great stirring up.

Immediately after taking the elimination diet eat sparingly of easily digested foods, such as baked potatoes, green lima beans, tender peas, corn, tomatoes, carrots, etc.

Chapter XXVI

HERBS

The great remedial properties of herbs and juices of fruits and vegetables have been recognized and appreciated since time immemorial. Only since Theophratus Van Hohemhein started using chemicals have people been looking for medicines chemically and artificially prepared. People have been diverted from the true healing remedies by superfluous advertising, and false science has succeeded, as chemical poisons are quick-acting, and people have been deceived for a time. But in this day, and for some time previous, people seeing the effects of drugs, etc., and the evil after effects, are looking for something better.

"When the Saxon invaders entered Great Britain they took with them much knowledge concerning herbal healing. It is well known that they made frequent use of the dandelion, comfrey, nettle, burdock, and other common wayside herbs in treating the sick. The Saxons girls were taken into the fields by their parents and taught names and healing virtues of the plants, and so a knowledge was planted that grew until it became customary to have an 'herb garden' in England. What a blessing it would be to the homes of this land if our children were taught the value of raspberry leaves, thyme, sage, peppermint, yarrow, and dozens of other wayside herbs. More than half the sickness and deaths in early life would be unknown, and chronic sufferers would be a curiosity. Only those who know the value of herbal remedies can appreciate the wonderful effects of a knowledge of the herbs we tread underfoot daily would produce.

"With all our boasted knowledge, we have to admit that the North American Indian, the Indians of other countries and the natives of other countries, in their native state, unskilled in letters, without any knowledge of anatomy, physiology, or chemistry, prevent and cure with simple herbs many diseases which baffle the best efforts of the medical schools."

Herbal healing was the first system of healing that the world knew. My parents, originally from Germany, brought with them much knowledge of these simple herbs, as told elsewhere in this book. I gathered many of them when a small child, and was taught their use.

WHY USE HERBS? They are Nature's remedies, and have been put here by an all-wise Creator. There is an herb for every disease that a human body can be afflicted with. The use of herbs is the oldest medical science. Herbs were mentioned in the Bible from the beginning of creation. Much has been written about herbs all down through history, to the present day.

The Bible on Herbs

The first thing Moses taught the Israelites was to clean their premises, wash their clothes and their bodies, and to leave all the harmful articles and the lustful diet of flesh which they were eating in Egypt. He taught them to live on simple, nourishing food, and use herbs for their medicine. He taught them that the grass was caused to grow for the cattle, and herbs for the service of man.—Psalms 104:14.

The Prophet Ezekiel said that the fruit of the tree was for man's meat, and the leaves for man's medicine.—Ezekiel 47:12.

The Great Apostle Paul said that if you are weak, eat herbs.—Romans 14:2. Further he said: "If any man defile the temple of God, him shall God destroy."—1 Corinthians 3:17.

Daniel said he would not defile himself with the portion of the king's meat, nor with the wine.—Daniel 1:8.

The wisest man that ever lived said: "Better is a dinner of herbs where love is, than a stalled ox and hatred therewith."—Proverbs 15:17.

Samuel, one of God's foremost prophets, when he was training young men for the ministry or the priesthood, taught them the use of herbs.

When God had created this world and made a beautiful garden, He put the tree of life in it, the leaves of which were for the healing of the nations. The Lord told them to eat freely of this tree, because that tree was especially designed to keep them well. This trees corresponds with the tree of life that is found in the Paradise of God, of which the redeemed are going to eat freely. When man was driven from the Garden of Eden and had no more access to the tree of life, God added herbs to man's diet and God expects that we shall partake of them to keep us from getting sick. They are one of God's remedial agencies for afflicted humanity and his plan was that everyone should raise herbs in his garden and gather those that grow wild everywhere and use them, when needed.

This is what my parents did and many others. We never were sick, and we never had a doctor. If we would only come back to God's original design for the human family, sickness would be rare instead of common.

"Thorns also and thistles shall it bring forth to thee; and thou shalt eat the herb of the field." Gen. 3:18.

"And Ahab spake unto Naboth, saying, Give me thy vineyard that I may have it for a garden of herbs, because it is near unto my house." I Kings 21:2.

"They were as the grass of the field, and as the green herb." 2 Kings 19:26.

"For they shall be cut down like the grass, and wither as the green herb." Psalms 37:2.

"How long shall the land mourn, and the herbs of every field wither?" Jer. 12:4.

"For the land, whither thou goest in to possess it, is not as the land of Egypt, from whence ye came out, where thou sowedst thy seed, and wateredst it with thy foot, as a garden of herbs." Deut. 11:10.

"And God said, Behold, I have given you every herb bearing seed, which is upon the face of all the earth, and every tree, in the which is the fruit of a tree yielding seed; to you it shall be for meat." Gen. 1:29.

"And one went out into the field to gather herbs, and found a wild vine, and gathered thereof wild gourds his lap full, and came and shred them into the pot of pottage: for they knew them not." 2 Kings 4:39. This Scripture teaches everyone that is using herbs that they should learn to know the herbs growing around them, so they will not gather the poisonous instead of the non-poisonous herbs.

CHAPTER XXVII

MEDICAL TREES

When I study the herbs, flowers, roots, barks, and the leaves of the trees, and see the wonderful medical properties they contain, the marvelous benefits that are derived from their use, I feel that the word "wonderful" is inadequate to express the real truth. The phrase, "the mighty miracle working power of God" is none too strong. If you had seen the things that have actually been done by the use of these herbs in connection with hygienic measures, you would not think for one moment that these statements are overdrawn. As I go out into the woods and see the lofty trees, I feel like taking off my hat in reverence to God for the wonderful medical properties in these various trees for the healing of man as well as for their use for building houses in which to live, furnishing fuel with which to cook our food, and heat to keep us warm.

OAK

The inner bark of the lofty oak has wonderful healing properties, as do the leaves, and acorn cups. A tea of the bark, and the powder of the cups are excellent for bleeding at the mouth, spitting of blood, and to stay vomiting, or other fluxes, in both man and woman. The powder of the acorn made into a tea resists the poison of venomous creatures. A tea made from the acorns and bark resists the force of poisonous medicines, and will also check the involuntary passing of the natural seed. It is also excellent for ulcerated bladder and bloody urine. The distilled water of the buds, before they become leaves, can be used either outwardly or inwardly for inflammations, burning fevers, and infections. The water of the leaves is especially excellent for whites. It is also very useful in the following diseases: Leucorrhea, womb troubles, piles, troubles in the rectum, hemorrhages, varicose veins, to normalize the kidneys, liver, and spleen, goiter, hardened neck, tumors, and swellings. DOSE: 1 ounce of the bark steeped in a pint of water. Use one teaspoonful three or four times a day for dysentery or diarrhea. Inject for leucorrhea. Use also as a gargle for sore throat and catarrh. Use the powdered bark on ulcers. It is astringent and antiseptic. Good in enemas for colon trouble, in gonorrhea, gleet, and leucorrhea. Also good for stomach troubles and goiter.

PINE

In the stately pine I see wonderful properties which are useful for *bronchial* and *catarrhal troubles, rheumatism,* kidney troubles, coughs, throat troubles, influenza, tonsillitis and croup.

POPLAR

In looking at the tall poplar tree, I see wonderful properties in the bud, bark, and leaves. They are useful in the following diseases: *Rheumatism, chronic diarrhea, cholera infantum, intermittent fever, jaundice, liver, kidney troubles, hay fever, diabetes, influenza, neuralgia, la grippe,* and used externally for *cancers, bad ulcers, gangrenous wounds, eczema* and *sciatica.*

CEDAR

In the beautiful cedar there are splendid medical properties for *coughs, fevers, pulmonary catarrh, rheumatism,* and *scurvy.*

The leaves and twigs, when boiled in white vaseline or cocoa fat, make an excellent salve.

BALM OF GILEAD

The beautiful balm of Gilead, which we admire so much for its wonderful fragrance, has excellent properties in the bark and leaves for cough, colds, lung troubles, kidney, and urinary troubles. When the buds are boiled in olive oil, cocoa fat, or some other good oil, they make an excellent salve. The buds and the bark are also excellent for scurvy as a stimulating tonic and to increase the flow of urine. The bud is especially good for the healing or soothing of inflamed parts, the healing of fresh cuts or wounds, and as a gargle for sore throat. The buds are very valuable for coughs and colds. When I was a child, we gathered the buds before the leaves burst out, and made a tea of them which could be used to gargle for various throat troubles. To add an equal part of any one of the following herbs will add to its efficiency: chickweed, coltsfoot, horehound, hyssop, liquorice, lobelia, ragwort, anise, or red sage.

BALSAM

The balsam evergreen tree, which we used for Christmas trees, which raises big blisters on the outside of the bark, is filled with very wonderful medicine, called balsam fir. The twigs and the bark have these wonderful medical properties that are good for rheumatism, kidney trouble, gleet, inflammation of the bladder, and urinary compliants.

HEMLOCK

The hemlock is the common tree which is used to tan shoe leather. When I was a child, I used to gather little hemlock twigs for my father for various purposes. They are used for kidney and bladder troubles, will increase the flow of urine, are successful in the treatment of leucorrhea and prolapsus of the uterus, to use internally as a douche. For diarrhea it can be used as an enema. It is very good to bathe sores and ulcers on the outside of the body. The powder can also be put in shoes when the feet are tender and have a bad odor. It is good to use as a gargle and mouth wash as it is a powerful astringent and disinfectant.

EUCALYPTUS

The wonderful eucalyptus tree, from which eucalyptus oil is made, has a wide range of uses. The leaves and bark are very useful in fevers, and acute and chronic bronchitis in its various forms, *asthma,* and similar ailments.

MANOGLIA

The magnolia tree, which is so much admired for its beautiful and fragrant flowers, has wonderful medical properties which are little known to man. The bark is very effective for many ailments. In the first place, it will do the work of quinine, proving more effective than quinine, and leaves no evil effects behind it. Quinine leaves evil effects whenever taken. The medical properties of magnolia will cure the tobacco habit, when taken with other hygienic measures. (Look in Table of Contents for Tobacco Habit.) It is good for fever, dyspepsia, dysentery and erysipelas.

BEECH

Another valuable tree is the beech, which is admired as a shade tree, and for its wonderful nuts. Its leaves and bark contain wonderful medical properties for stomach troubles, ulcers, liver, kidneys, bladder, diabetes, to produce appetite, and is an excellent tonic.

The leaves are soothing to the nerves and stomach and are astringent. Very useful in swellings and soothing to sores and wounds for both man and beast. It is cooling and healing. Make a tea by taking a heaping teaspoonful to the cup of boiling water and let steep one-half hour. Bathe sores of all kinds freely and often. It is antiseptic and will make old sores clean and heal them if bathed often. Take three or four cups a day; one, one hour before each meal and one upon retiring. It is a fine remedy for diabetes.

BIRCH

The bark and little twigs of the birch tree have a splendid flavor similar to that of the wintergreen. We used to gather it and use it with wintergreen and spikenard in making a health drink. It has wonderful medical properties for bowel troubles, rheumatism, gout, for purifying the blood, and to expel worms. It is splendid for boils and sores taken internally and applied externally.

SLIPPERY ELM

We all admire the wonderful slippery elm tree. In my childhood we used to go out with a large knife called a drawshave, and shave off the outer rough bark and then cut off the inner bark in big strips, and carry it home for medical use. It contains various properties which are entirely harmless, and of which even small infants can partake to prevent suffering. Slippery elm is excellent for bowel and bladder troubles, lung troubles, diarrhea, stomach and kidney troubles, boils and inflammations, ulcerated stomach, and bronchitis. It should be in every home, and will save those who use it from much suffering and many doctor's bills. (Look in Table of Contents for Slippery Elm.)

LINDEN OR BASSWOOD

The linden or basswood, is an old-fashioned, well-known household remedy. The inner bark, leaves, and flowers are used. It is useful for colds as the tea taken hot promotes perspiration and is excellent to cleanse the system of slime and mucus, especially to cleanse the kidneys, bladder, and stomach. It is also excellent for female compliants, for poultices on boils, and other painful swellings. It is valuable for coughs, for use as a gargle, for hoarseness, sore throat, epilepsy, and headaches.

CHESTNUT

The inner bark and leaves of the chestnut tree are used for their medical properties, and the nuts are used for food. They are low in protein, high in carbohydrates and starch, and contain mineral matter such as phosphate of potash, magnesia, and some sodium and iron.

BUTTERNUT

The bark, leaves, and root of the butternut tree are used for medicine. It is a tonic and a splendid laxative, soothing to the system, and will expel worms from the intestines. It is an excellent remedy to take for chronic constipation, is a splendid liver remedy, and is good for fevers of all kinds, colds, and la grippe. The nuts are splendid for food and are high in fat and mineral matter.

IRON WOOD OR LEVER WOOD

The iron wood tree, also called lever wood, has a number of splendid medical properties. Use the inner bark and the inner red wood of the tree. In order to use the bark or inner red wood, you would have to shave it, or cut it up into small chips, and boil them for fifteen or twenty minutes. A good time to gather the bark is in the latter part of the summer. It is a good tonic and a splendid blood purifier, is very beneficial to the stomach, and for use in dyspepsia, neuralgia, fever, ague, scrofula, and as a nerve tonic.

PEACH

We go to the orchard and find the peach tree with its delicious fruit for food, and leaves that are a most healing and specific remedy for jaundice, dyspepsia, fever, stomach troubles, worms, and are useful to stop vomiting or morning sickness in pregnancy, and as a laxative. Gather plenty of peach leaves and always keep them on hand.

APPLE

The apple tree, with its delicious fruit, also has valuable medical properties. The bark is most useful for gravel in the bladder, as a tonic, and for bilious and intermittent fever. It is an old-fashioned home remedy. The apple tree itself has medical properties, being rich in potassium, sodium, magnesium, and iron salts, which contribute to the building of blood and bone. It is rightly called the King of Fruits. Those who have too much acid should select sweet apples, which have little acid, and those who have not acid enough can eat sour apples. Old people and very small babies can eat a mellow apple if it is scraped, and do well on it. Apples are very high in food value and life-giving properties. They should not be eaten between meals, but one can make an entire meal of them. If you have good teeth, eat the peeling, core, and seeds and chew them thoroughly. Apple is especially good for diabetes and is also excellent for the liver and kidneys as well as being beneficial in hyperacidity. An exclusive apple diet for a while would prove of great benefit to the system. If anyone would drink a glass of good apple juice an hour before each meal, it would prove of great benefit, but it must be made from good, sound apples. The ordinary apple cider is not fit to be used.

CHERRY

In the orchard we also find the cherry tree. Not only does it furnish us one of the most delicious fruits, but it has splendid medical properties. The cherry contains malic acid, and is high in life-giving properties. The bark is one of our most wonderful remedies to loosen phlegm in the throat and chest for tuberculosis, coughs, bronchitis, heart troubles, stomach trouble, dyspepsia, fever, and high blood pressure. It is also a most wonderful voice conditioner for singers and speakers, clearing out the throat and chest and toning them up; it makes you feel that you want to sing. Some of this cherry bark ought to be in every home. There are a number of species of the cherry tree all having very much the same medical properties.

HICKORY

The hickory tree is a well-known tree, noted for its strength, and toughness of its wood, used for making axe handles and wheels of vehicles of various kinds and many other things where a strong wood is needed.

The inner bark and leaves have medical properties; they are laxative, and useful in purifying the system, also good for washing ulcers, and sores, for diarrhea, and kindred troubles. Very useful in colitis. Take a heaping tablesspoonful to a quart of boiling water, let simmer fifteen minutes, strain off, and use as an enema.

To take internally, use one teaspoonful of the granulated bark or leaves to one cup of boiling water, let simmer thirty minutes, strain off, and drink from one to three cups a day.

TAMARACK

The tamarack tree is a tall, slender tree. There is a gummy substance which runs out of the bark which I used as a child to chew as gum. It has a very good flavor, better than other gums on the market. Of course I do not recommend chewing gum as it is injurious to the system. The inner bark made into a tea is good for bleeding of any kind, for the spitting of blood from the lungs or throat, and for bleeding hemorrhoids. Is good for lessening too profuse menstruation. A good medicine for liver troubles, jaundice, and the spleen, also the colic. Is very effective for poisonous insect bites. Good for the spleen when enlarged and hardened, for pains in the ear, and inflammation of the eyes. Bathe the eyes with the tea, using an eye cup or medicine dropper and drop some of the lukewarm tea in the ear, will relieve earache. Is an excellent wash for gangrene or old running ulcers and will help overcome the itch and kill nits and lice. A tea made from the ashes is very healing to burns and scalds. A splendid medicine for a person subject to melancholy and jaundice. If there is constipation, add a little buckthorn bark and calamus root, making a tea of same, use the inner bark. Of the granulated bark or leaves take one heaping teaspoon to the cup and take one-half cup four or five times a day, more or less as needed. If buckthorn bark and calamus root are used, take a teaspoon of each, and mix with the teaspoon of tamarack. Use a heaping teaspoon of this mixture to the cup of boiling water, steep thirty minutes, and take as much as needed.

ALDER

Of the alder tree, both the leaves and bark are used. Use the leaves when you can get them. Very useful for swellings of all kinds. When you can get the green leaves, crush them and lay them on painful swellings. Will relieve the pain and take down the swelling. Make a poultice, crush the leaves. The green leaves, or dry leaves made into poultice will allay the inflammation in a swollen and painful breast. Take a heaping tablespoonful to a pint of boiling water. Let steep half an hour. If used for poultice, take just water enough so the leaves are moist. The fresh leaves are excellent for burning and aching feet, when laid in the shoes under the bare feet. Also good to bathe the whole feet in strong tea.

CINNAMON

The cinnamon tree is a wonderful tree. The cinnamon contains many wonderful properties, besides its beautiful flavor. It is stimulating, and prevents gas and sour stomach. It warms up the stomach. It expels the gas from the stomach and bowels and is somewhat laxative. It is somewhat astringent and therefore is good in diarrhea and stomach complaint and will relieve the pain of griping. We sometimes put it with other herbs to prevent griping and give them better flavor.

Dose.—Take a rounding teaspoonful to the cup of boiling water and stir it and drink while hot. Drink a small portion at a time, four or five times a day, or drink a cup as needed for griping and pain in the bowels. Use one-fourth teaspoon to a cup of other herbs to flavor them. Put it in with the herbs when you make the tea.

PRICKLEY ASH

The prickly ash is a beautiful little tree, growing from eight to twelve feet tall, full of thorns, and often just covered with berries about the size of the currant. I used to cut off a little of the bark and chew it. It will help sores in the mouth and toothache. Both the bark and the berries are used. This tree is a most wonderful remedy for many diseases. Look for Prickly Ash in Table of Contents under herbs.

CYPRESS

The cypress tree, the cones and nuts of this tree are an astringent and will stop bleeding of all kinds. For internal use, make a tea by taking a few of the cones in some water and simmering slowly for ten minutes. Take in small doses, two tablespoonfuls may be taken every two hours. In bad cases of diarrhea this tea is very effective. It will stop the bleeding or hemorrhages of lungs and stomach. Is very useful in bleeding piles and bloody diarrhea, also dysentery. Inject a little for too profuse menstruation. Is good for pyorrhea and bleeding gums when teeth are loose. Rinse the mouth with the tea.

MAPLE

The maple tree is one of our most beautiful shade trees. In my childhood and youth I admired this tree very much for the syrup and the maple sugar which we made from it. Then we raised plenty of buckwheat and had the whole kernel ground into flour and made into a pancake, upon which we used some butter and plenty of maple syrup. But now we have something better. Look under "Kloss Soybean Pancakes," which are a real health food.

The inner bark of the maple tree and also the leaves are a splendid medicine for both liver and spleen, and are very soothing to these organs. In fact they are a good medicine for the whole body, as they are a tonic and soother of the nerves.

Take one heaping teaspoonful to the cup of boiling water. One to three cups a day may be taken on an empty stomach. Sometimes when there is a pain in the liver or spleen, taking a wine glass full every hour or two has a splendid effect.

QUINCE

The quince tree grows to the size of an ordinary apple tree. The fruit has an acid taste, and the juice is a good stomach medicinne. It is a little astringent. It is quite a sedative. It will allay gas and vomiting. It checks the running off of the bowels, and in children nausea, vomiting, and running off of the bowels. Take two tablespoonfuls of the juice, and one-fourth tablespoonful of cinnamon, and one-fourth teaspoonful of powdered ginger. Add this to the two tablespoonfuls of juice, put in a cup, and fill with boiling water. Take a tablespoonful every hour. More may be taken, if needed. Children less according to age.

The juice of a quince is really a prevention against sickness. To rid the system of poison. The juice makes an excellent gargle. For gargling, is very effective if a little honey and lemon juice are added. Is also good to apply to sores on the outside. The juice of this fruit, rubbed with the tips of the fingers on the scalp, will keep hair from falling out, and make it grow where the roots of the hair are not entirely dead.

BAY

Of the bay tree, the bark, leaves, and berries are used. The bark is slightly astringent, is highly recommended for liver, stones in kidneys and bladder, and is a splendid remedy for the pancreas and spleen and various liver troubles. A tea made from the berries is very effectual for all poisonous insect bites and snack bites. A strong tea, both taken internally and applied to the wounds, is good for the stings of wasps and the bites of snakes, mad dogs, and poisonous insects. An excellent tea to be taken when contagious diseases are in the lands, such as smallpox, typhoid fever, measles, diphtheria, both taken internally and used as a gargle. Very efficient in tonsillitis, throat and nose troubles, and the various lung troubles. The berries are also very helpful in suppressed menstruation, womb troubles. The berries are very helpful in child-birth to be taken when the time of delivery is at hand. It is very useful to expel the after-birth. The tea of the berries is an excellent remedy in colds, la grippe, and fever. It helps to clear up the brain, the eyes, and the lungs, or any other part of the body. It is a regular cleanser, very good remedy for old coughs, consumption, and asthma troubles when there is shortness of breath. It will destroy the worms in the body. It helps to increase the flow of urine. Is an excellent tea for those troubled with fermentation and gas in the stomach and bowels. Make a tea of the leaves, bark, or berries for a sitz bath; is very excellent for any bladder or uterus troubles, or a pain in the bowels. When the soft palate hangs down and is inflamed, a gargle made into a tea of the berries, leaves, or bark will make it go back into place. A strong tea made of the berries or the oil of the berries is most excellent to apply to rheumatic joints, arthritis, and other nerve troubles, or pain in the bowels or womb. Good for any kind of cramps or pain in the chest or numbness in any part of the body. The oil is an excellent remedy for itch, or eczema, or for bruises after receiving a blow when the flesh becomes black; it will help to congeal the black blood and bring the color back to normal. It is also good for other black spots or brown spots on the flesh. Is excellent for sunburn. The berries, bark, and leaves are a most wonderful remedy for many troubles. Take a heaping teaspoonful of the granulated bark from the roots in a cup of boiling water. Let it steep for one-half hour and drink from one to three cups a day. The berries are also very useful in cough syrup.

WALNUT

The walnut is a well-known tree. It is only too bad that there are not more of them on every farm in the sections where they will grow, for the walnut is an excellent nut, and the leaves and bark are an effective medicine for a number of ailments. Will expel all kinds of worms from the intestinal tract, and is an excellent remedy for poisonous snake bites, or other poisonous bites, as mad dog bites. To be taken internally and also applied externally.

To boil the bark or leaves in honey makes an excellent throat and stomach remedy and for other lung troubles and any sores in the mouth. Both the leaves and the bark are astringent and are good in diarrhea and are excellent for women to take for profuse menstruation taken as a tea and used as a douche. To wet the tips of the fingers in the tea and massage the scalp once a day will keep the hair from falling out and give it a beautiful lustre. The tea is also very helpful for running sores. Bathe them with the tea three or four times a day.

DOSE: Take a heaping teaspoonful of the granulated leaves or bark. Steep in a cup of boiling water for thirty minutes and drink from one to three cups a day.

FIR TREE OR NORWAY SPRUCE

Fir tree or Norway spruce is a well-known tree. Both the leaves and the tops are used. A tea made from the leaves is very healing to wounds and ulcers, good for bladder, gonorrhea and leucorrhea. It is good to use an an enema and also a douche, as well as to take internally. Good for stones in the kidney and gravel in the bladder. It is also good for lung trouble. It will cut the phlegm in the throat and lungs and is very healing. When the breath is short, it helps to open up the air pipes. When the tree is tapped, there is a pitch that makes a very excellent turpentine and has very powerful healing properties. A tea made of the leaves and the young tops makes an excellent tea for scurvy and cleansing the system. It can be steeped or simmered for just a few minutes. This tea is an excellent remedy for those who have not access to plenty of fruits and greens.

The leaves and the branches of this tree have been used in that well-known spruce beer and have formerly been used in non-alcoholic beer, for its wonderful medical properties. For a tea, take a heaping teaspoonful to a cup of boiling water, steep for thirty minutes, and drink from one to three cups a day. This tea is excellent used both internally and externally.

JUNIPER

The juniper tree yields berries which are a most wonderful medicine. I used to gather these berries when just a young lad. For kidney and urinary troubles take one heaping teaspoonful of juniper berries, granulated or chopped up, or the whole berry, and one teaspoonful peach leaves, granulated, and one teaspoonful of the marshmallow. Mix together.

Take one heaping teaspoonful to the cup of boiling water and let steep. Take from one to three cups a day, more or less, as needed. Children according to age.

The tea of the juniper is very cleansing to the system, and combined as above makes a most excellent medicine. The juniper berries alone, made into a strong tea by taking two teaspoonfuls to cup of boiling water, make an excellent wash for the bites of poisonous insects, snake bites, dog bites, and bee stings. The tea of the berries alone, one teaspoonful to the cup of water, is an excellent stomach medicine, expelling the wind from the stomach and bowels..Can safely be called a good colic remedy. It is a very effective remedy for coughs, shortness of breath, consumption, pain in the bowels, cramps, convulsions. It is wonderful for women when their time of delivery has come, and it is a good brain medicine. Combining equal parts with rue makes an excellent remedy for any kind of head trouble. It is soothing and strengthening to the nerves and it also helps the vision of the eyes. In fact it strengthens the nerves in the whole body. It is a food for gout and sciatica rheumatism, or pain in any part of the body. It is very good combined with gentian and calamus. The juniper is excellent as a remedy for the gums and to gargle with. It also checks bleeding in hemorrhoids and piles. Good for worms in children, as well as adults.

The ashes of the wood, a teaspoonful to the pint of boiling water, is a splendid remedy for itch, scabs on any part of the body, also leper sores. The berries are also good for fits. They make a good medicine for the palsy. Take equal parts of prickly ash, juniper berries and calamus root; if constipated, add buckthorn bark.

FIG

The fig tree is one of our most wonderful trees. It has many valuable medical properties. Both the leaves and the fruit are used. Split open the fresh, ripe fruit and lay on a boil or carbuncle; will give great relief. The fruit is mildly laxative and one of the most delicious fruits. When the fruit is broken off the tree before it is ripe, a milk escapes which has wonderful healing properties. It may be put on sores and boils. If this milk is put freely on warts, it removes them. A tea made of the leaves will take the spots off the face or body. The tea is also excellent to wash old sores. The leaves boiled in Crisco make an excellent ointment. Where the flesh has turned black from bruises or blows, bathing with the warm tea brings about the circulation and carries away the discoloration. Snuff the tea up the nose when there are difficulties in the nostrils and pain. The tea is also good dropped in the ear for pain in the ear, but it must be lukewarm. It is also very excellent when there have been bites of poisonous insects. Good for a mouth wash and to gargle with, for hoarseness, sore throat, and bad breath. It is good for any kind of lung trouble, as asthma and bronchitis. A splendid medicine for dropsy, spasms, and fits. A syrup made of figs makes a very excellent cough medicine. It can be used alone or with a little lemon added. Take a pound of figs, cut them up, put them in a quart of water, simmer for a few minutes, then put them in a cheese cloth and squeeze out all the juices possible, add the juice of two lemons and a little honey if desired. This makes an excellent cough remedy. Of the leaves take one heaping teaspoonful (cut fine) to a cup of boiling water. Drink three or four cups a day one hour before meals. Sometimes the results are better if taken five or six times a day in wineglassful doses.

BALM OF GILEAD
(Buds)

Botanical Name: Populus condicans. Common Names: balsam poplar, American balm of Gilead, balm of Gilead buds. Medicinal Properties: Bark: Stimulant, tonic, diuretic, anti-scorbutic. Buds: Balsamic, vulnerary.

An excellent application for cuts, bruises, fresh wounds. Effective for coughs, dry asthma, and as an ointment for bedsores. The bark is useful in gout and rheumatism.

BIRCH
(Inner bark and small twigs)

Botanical Name: Betula lenta. Common Names: Black birch, cherry birch, sweet birch, mahogany birch, mountain mahogany, spice birch. Medicinal Properties. Aromatic, stimulant, diaphoretic.

This is the common birch tree. The tea makes a good wash for sore or cankered mouth. It is excellent for use in diarrhea, dysentery, and cholera infantum, given as an injection and taken internally. Splendid remedy for all kinds of bowel troubles, rheumatism, gout, stones in the kidneys and bladder and to expel worms. It will purify the blood, and excellent results will be obtained by drinking freely when afflicted with boils. The tea has a very pleasant taste, and makes an excellent drink in place of water for a time. It is much used in root beer.

BLACK WILLOW
(Bark and Buds)

Botanical Name: Salix nigra. Common Names: Catkin's willow, pussy willow. Medicinal properties: Bark: Astringent, antiseptic, antiperiodic, tonic. Buds: Antiaphrodisiac.

Exerts a good influence on the sex organs, as in cases of incontinence, excessive sexual desire, and acute gonorrhea. Combined with palmetto berries or scullcap is good for noctural emissions.

ELDER
(Flowers, leaves, bark, roots, berries)

Botanical Name: Sambucus, canadensis. Common Names: Sweet elder, American elder, rob elder, elder flowers, elder (juice or the berries). Medicinal Properties: Bark: Emetic, cathartic. Flowers: Diaphoretic, diuretic, exanthematous, alterative, emollient, discutient, rubrifacient.

Elder is an old-fashioned home remedy, and is found in nearly all old people's gardens. The whole tree has marvelous medicinal properties. Of some shrubs, trees, or plants there is only one part which is useful, but all parts of the elder—the flowers, berries, leaves, bark, and roots are useful.

The tea of the flowers is an excellent remedy for twitching eyelids and inflammation of the eyes. Made into an ointment, elder is valuable in burns, scalds, and all skin diseases. The tea is stimulating, a good tonic and a good blood purifier. Increases the flow of urine, is cooling, and good for building up the system. Very useful in liver and kidney diseases. A splendid remedy for children's diseases, such as liver derangements, erysipelas, etc. In skin diseases the sores should be washed with the tea, and the tea taken internally, also. Very useful for headache due to colds, palsy, rheumatism, scrofula, syphilis, and epilepsy. It is somewhat laxative and a wonderful remedy for dropsy as well as being useful in constipation. Very good in fever and many chronic diseases. Makes an excellent poultice for tumors and various swellings. The dry berries made into a tea are an excellent remedy for cholera, diarrhea, and summer complaint. It can be taken freely without harm. It is good for influenza combined with peppermint.

FRINGE TREE

Botanical Name: Chionanthus virginica. Common Names: Old man's beard, graybeard tree, poison ash, snowflower, white fringe. Medicinal properties: Blood purifier and general tonic. Abates fever. Acts as a gentle cathartic. Is good for the kidneys.

Fringe tree is very good for the liver, and all liver troubles, bilious fevers, jaundice, bilious colic, and gallstones.

GUM ARABIC
(Gum)

Botanical Name: Acacia arabica. Common Names: India gum tree, Egyptian gum, Arabic tree, gum Arabic Tree, bablah pods, acacia bambolah. Medicinal Properties: Mucilaginous, demulcent.

Used in poultices or applied externally, it retains warmth and moisture, thus proving relaxing. It absorbs discharges, and is excellent to use with the powdered herbs for poultices. Taken internally it lubricates mucous membranes, is soothing in inflamed conditions such as inflammation of stomach, bowels, uterus, and vagina.

(189)

HEMLOCK
(Inner bark and leaves)

Botanical Name: Abies canadensis. Common Names: Canada pitch tree, hemlock tree, hemlock, gum tree, hemlock pitch tree, weeping spruce, pine tops, tanner's bark, hemlock bark, hemlock leaves. Medicinal Properties: Diaphoretic, astringent.

This is the common hemlock, one of the old home remedies. The leaves can also be used, but should not be taken during pregnancy. This is the same kind of bark that tanners use in making shoe leather, but it is a very valuable remedy for a number of ailments. It is a wonderful astringent and can be used internally and externally. An ideal remedy for canker in mouth. Can be used in dropsy with splendid success, as it increases the flow of urine. Has a healing effect on the kidneys and bladder, and is good for gravel in urinary passages, uteritis, and other uterus troubles. Can be used as a douche for leucorrhea. A splendid remedy used as an enema for colon trouble and diarrhea. Good applied externally for gangrene, old sores, and ulcers, as a wash. The powder is excellent used in shoes or stockings for sore, tender or sweaty feet. For external use, simmer a teaspoonful in a cup of water for ten minutes. For internal use, a teaspoonful in a cup of boiling water. It is better to take smaller doses more often.

POPLAR
(Bark and leaves)

Botanical Name: Populus tremuloides. Common Names: Aspen, American aspen, quaking aspen, quaking asp, quiver leaf, trembling tree, trembling poplar, white poplar, aspen poplar, abele tree. Medicinal Properties: Stomachic, febrifuge, tonic, antiperiodic.

Poplar is better than quinine for all purposes for which quinine is used. Very useful for diseases of urinary organs, especially if weak. Excellent to aid digestion and to tone up run-down condition, either in disease or old age. Very good in all cases of diarrhea. Excellent for acute rheumatism. Good in all fevers, such as intermittent fever, influenza, etc. Good for neuralgia, la grippe, jaundice, liver and kidney trouble, diabetes, hay fever, cholera infantum. Will expel worms. Is splendid used externally as a wash for cancer, bad ulcers, gangrenous wounds, eczema, strong perspiration, burns, and sores caused by gonorrhea and syphilis. It is more effective than quinine in fever and la grippe.

PRICKLY ASH

(Bark and berries, the berries being most effective)

Botanical Name: Xanthoxylum fraxineum. Common Names: Northern prickly ash, toothache bush, toothache tree, suter berry, toothache bark, yellow wood, yellow wood berries, pellitory bark, suterberry bark, prickly ash berries. Medicinal Properties: Pungent, deobstruent, alterative, tonic, stimulant, sialagogue, nervine.

Is a most wonderful tonic and stimulant. Extremely useful in chronic rheumatism, syphilis, colic, derangement of the liver, scrofula, chronic female troubles. The berries are stimulant, anti-spasmodic, carminative, acting mostly in the mucous tissues. Removes obstructions in every part of the body. It will relieve asthma and colds generally. Is very beneficial in paralysis of the tongue and mouth, as it increases the flow of saliva. The berries are very fine in bad cases of cholera. A splendid blood purifier. The powder is excellent sprinkled on old wounds and indolent ulcers.

SLIPPERY ELM
(Inner bark)

Botanical Name: Ulmus fulva. Common Names: Slippery elm, red elm, Indian elm, sweet elm. American elm, British tea (the leaves). Medicinal Properties: Mucilaginous, demulcent, emollient, nutritive.

Slippery elm is an old-fashioned remedy which has many wonderful uses. It is highly nourishing and very soothing to the stomach as a tea. I have used it for many years with wonderful results. It is very effective in diarrhea, bowel, stomach, bladder, and kidney troubles. It is soothing and healing wherever it is used. Slippery elm will stay on an ulcerated and cancerous stomach when nothing else will. It is very nourishing, and in case of famine a person could live for some time on the inner slippery elm bark.

An excellent treatment in female troubles is the following: Make a thick paste with powdered slippery elm with pure, cold water. Shape into pieces about one inch long and one inch thick. Place in warm water for a few minutes. These are called vaginal suppositories. Insert three, afterwards inserting a sponge with string attached. Let it remain two days, then remove the sponge, and give douche which will remove the slippery elm. This is an excellent treatment for cancers and tumors of the womb, all growths in the female organs, fallen womb, leucorrhea, or inflammation and congestion of any part of the vagina or womb.

Slippery elm is one of the most effective ingredients known for a poultice. If the slippery elm powder is mixed with some cornmeal mush and powdered lobelia, it is wonderfully soothing as a poultice. For excellent poultices, take two parts of powdered slippery elm with one part of any one or all the following powdered herbs: Corn meal, bloodroot, blue flag, comfrey, ragweed, chickweed. Mix well together, add warm water to make required consistency, and use in cases of abscesses, dirty wounds, inflammations, congestions, or eruptions. The face of the poultice should be smeared with olive oil if it is to be applied to a hairy surface, such as the eye or head. This poultice is also good for enlarged prostate, swollen glands of the neck, groin, etc.

Slippery elm will roll up the mucous material troubling the patient and pass it down through the intestines. It cleans, heals, and strengthens.

As a diet, take a teaspoonful of the powdered slippery elm bark, and pour upon it a cupful of boiling milk (soybean). Sweeten to taste. This is useful in cases of consumption and inflammation of the stomach and intestines.

It makes a good food for children when mixed with soybean milk.

To make slippery elm tea, use a heaping tablespoonful to a pint of boiling water. Let soak one hour, then simmer a few minutes. Strain and use. It is well to soak and simmer twice as the full virtue does not usually come out the first time.

WHITE ASH
(Inner bark)

Botanical Name: Fraxinus Americana. Common Names: American white ash. Medicinal Properties: Diuretic, tonic, laxative.

Useful in dropsy, urinary troubles and constipation. Excellent for reducing. This is one of the old-fashioned, well-known remedies. Steep a heaping teaspoonful in a cup of boiling water for thirty minutes, drink one or more cupfuls a day, a half a glass at a time.

WHITE PINE
(Inner bark and Sprigs)

Botanical Name: Pincus strobus: Common Names: Deal pine, soft pine. Medicinal Properties: Expectorant.

A very old, reliable remedy for bronchial and catarrhal troubles, rheumatism, kidney troubles, and scurvy. For use in all chest affections such as tonsillitis, coughs, colds, laryngitis, croup, influenza, and sore throat. It is better combined with wild cherry bark or spikenard. Combined with uva ursi, marshmallow and poplar bark, it is excellent for diabetes. Will stop coughing and expel phlegm from the throat and lungs.

Chapter XXVIII

TONICS

A tonic is an agent that is used to give strength to the system. The remedies that are given in this book all work toward the strengthening of the system and are not like any of the patent medicines or drugs generally given to tone up the system. One of the best things to do to tone up the body is to accustom the system to cold showers in the morning, or cold towel rubs, which are better, followed by a vigorous, dry towel rub. Also at the beginning it is absolutely necessary to rid the system of poisons, by taking the high enemas, and taking laxative herbs so that the bowels move at least three times a day. A fruit diet for a time is advisable, as this makes it easier to rid the system of poisons at first. These tonics may be taken with great benefit by anyone who is not overflowing with health and vitality. But it is always good to take tonic herbs when convalescing from any disease or ailment. If the millions working in offices and those having taxing brain work knew what these things would do for them, with no harmful after effects, the herb business would increase a hundredfold. To overtaxed mothers and overtaxed nurses, with too many household duties and peevish, sick children, it would prove an untold blessing which no pen could fully portray. No pen could overdraw the benefit to be derived from the simple treatments given in this book for that purpose.

Be sure to study the herbs given under this article. You will be surprised to find out all the different properties the herbs have. The following are all tonic herbs:

White pond lily, boneset, ginger root, capsicum, bitter root, balmony, poplar bark, golden seal, white willow, black horehound, broom, centaury, comfrey, cudweed, ground ivy, elecampane, dandelion, valerian, meadow sweet, mistletoe, mugwort, wood betony, self heal, agrimony, sanicle, scullcap, red raspberry leaves, yarrow, sage, and vervain.

SPECIFIC NERVE TONICS: golden seal is a pure tonic to nervous systems and mucous membranes. It acts as a powerful cleanser to all the mucous membrane in the system. In my estimation there is no other herb that can take the place of golden seal.

White willow is a very effective tonic.

Scullcap is one of the finest nerve tonics; used alone it gives very successful results.

Valerian, taken cold, frequently during the day, acts powerfully on the nerves.

Mistletoe is good for nerves.

Equal parts of wood betony, agrimony, and self heal are good for nervous tremors.

TONIC FOR LUNGS: One teaspoonful equal parts of the following: comfrey, black horehound, cudweed, ground ivy, elecampane, ginger root, and one-half teaspoon of cayenne. Take as directed for use of herbs.

TONICS FOR GENERAL DEBILITY AND LOSS OF APPETITE: Centaury, dandelion, ground ivy, meadow sweet, mugwort, wood betony, self heal, agrimony, capsicum, balmony, poplar bark, black horehound, broom sanicle, yarrow, and sage. Boneset is a specific tonic in itself whenever a tonic is needed. Take as directed for use of herbs.

CHAPTER XXIX

USE OF HERBS IN DISEASE
(Their description and use in disease)

In reading the description of the herbs it may seem that many of the herbs have the same qualities. This is true. I give the description so if you should not be able to get a certain one, you can get some other having the desired qualities. Also different herbs grow in different parts of the earth. Knowing their qualities enables one to obtain one having the desired elements.

ALOES
(Leaves)

Botanical Name: Aloe socotrina. Common Names: Bombay aloes, Turkey aloes, Mocha aloes, Zanzibar aloes. Medicinal Properties: Cathartic, stomachic, aromatic, emmenagogue, drastic.

Promotes menstruation when suppressed. Will expel pinworms after several doses.

Aloes is one of the most healing agencies we have among the herbs. It is used in many cathartics. Aloes is one of the best to clean out the colon. The writer is personally acquainted with a lady who could not find anything that would move the bowels. This lady has used the aloes alone for many years with most splendid results. I have used it for many years in connection with other herbs as follows:

1 oz. powdered buckthorn bark
1 oz. powdered rhubarb root

1 oz. powdered mandrake root
¼ oz. Socotrina aloes powdered
1 oz. powdered calamus root

Dose; Each person should take the amount he needs to move bowels freely two or three times a day, starting, for instance, with one fourth teaspoonful, then increasing or decreasing the dose as needed. Some need so much more than others, so everyone must take the amount needed in his own case. Some who have very slow digestion do well if they take the full amount needed the first thing in the morning an hour or more before breakfast. Others prefer to take it just before retiring in the evening.

This is one of the finest body cleansers and brings most gratifying results. It cleans the morbid matter from the stomach, liver, kidneys, spleen, bladder, and is the finest colon cleanser known. It should be used in any case where a laxative is needed, does not gripe, and is very healing and soothing to the stomach—in fact, wherever it goes.

I also use aloes in my cancer liniment. (Look in Table of Contents for Cancer Liniment.)

Aloes may be used alone for any kind of sore on the outside of the body, and is a very excellent remedy for piles and hemorrhoids. Take a heaping teaspoonful to a pint of water, strain, and use. Two teaspoonfuls of boracic acid may also be added, which, besides being healing, will keep the mixture from souring.

ANGELICA
(Root and Seed)

Botanical Name: Angelica atropurpurea. Common Names: Dead nettle, purple angelica, masterwort, high angelica, archangel, American angelica. Medicinal Properties: Stimulant, carminative, emmenagogue, tonic.

Angelica is a good tonic, and remedy for stomach troubles, sour stomach, heartburn, gas; also for colic, la grippe, colds, and fevers. Tea made from this herb dropped into the eyes helps dimness of sight, and into the ears helps deafness. It should be taken hot to break up a cold quickly. For general tonic, one to three cupfuls should be taken every day. Angelica is a most effective remedy in epidemics and to strengthen the heart. Such wonderful results have been obtained from this plant that it has been given the name "archangel." Christ is an archangel and the results of this agent are compared with the mighty working power of God, Himself. Excellent in diseases of the lungs and chest, eases pains in colic, stoppage of urine, suppressed menstruation, expels afterbirth. Good in sluggish liver, and spleen. A tea made of angelica dropped into old ulcers will cleanse and heal them. The powder of the root may also be used for this purpose.

ANISE
(Seed or root)

Botanical Names: Pimpinella anisum. Common Names: Anise seed, common anise. Medicinal Properties: Aromatic, diaphoretic, relaxant, stimulant, tonic, carminative, stomachic.

Anise is one of the old-fashioned herbs, and has many valuable properties. It will prevent fermentation and gas in the stomach and bowels, and check griping in the bowels when taken as a hot tea. Anise is a very good stomach remedy to overcome nausea and colic. It is useful to mix with or take with other herbs to give them a palatable flavor.

APPLE TREE BARK
(Bark)

Botanical Name: Pyrus malus. Common Name: Apple tree. Medicinal Properties: Fruit: Diuretic, laxative. Bark: Tonic, febrifuge.

Tea made from apple tree bark is an old-fashioned remedy, which is excellent in intermittent fever, biliousness and for gravel in the bladder, to induce perspiration, good for suppressed menstruation, digestion, nausea, vomiting, low fever, liver, spleen, kidneys, bladder, griping in bowels, dysentery, boils, insect stings, mad dog bites, toothache.

BALM
(Herbs and flowers)

Botanical Name: Melissa officianlis. Common Names: Garden balm, sweet balm, lemon balm. Medicinal Properties: Diaphoretic, carminative, febrifuge, tonic.

A warm tea of balm will produce perspiration. It is very helpful in painful or suppressed menstruation, aids digestion, and is valuable in cases of nausea and vomiting. Useful in low fever, liver, spleen, kidney and bladder troubles, griping in bowels, and dysentery. A warm poultice of balm will bring a boil to a head, and it will break. For insect stings and mad dog bites, take the tea internally, and make a poultice to be applied to the bite or sting. Toothache remedy.

BALOMY
(Leaves)

Botanical Name: Chelone glabra. Common Names: Snake head, turtleloom, turtle head, salt rheum weed, fishmouth, shell flower, bitter herb. Medicinal Properties: Tonic, antibilious, stimulant, detergent, authelmintic.

Specific tonic for enfeebled stomach and indigestion, general debility and biliousness, jaundice, constipation, dyspepsia, and torpid liver. Almost a certain remedy for worms. Increases the gastric and salivary secretions, and stimulates the appetite. Good for sores and eczema.

BASIL SWEET
(Leaves)

Botanical Name: Ocimum basilicum. Common Names: Common basil, sweet basil. Medicinal Properties: Stimulant, condiment, nervine, aromatic. The tea taken hot is good in suppressed menses. Allays excessive vomiting. Effective when applied to snake bites and insect stings.

BAYBERRY
(Bark, leaves and flowers)

Botanical Name: Myrica Cerifera. Common Names: Bayberry Bush, American Bayberries, American vegetable tallow tree, Bayberry wax tree, Myrtle, wax myrtle, candleberry, candleberry myrtle, tallow shrub, American vegetable wax, vegetable tallow. Medicinal Properties: Astringent, tonic, stimulant. Leaves: Aromatic, stimulant.

One of the most valuable and useful herbs. The tea is a most excellent gargle for sore throat. It will thoroughly cleanse the throat of all putrid matter. Steep a teaspoonful in a pint of boiling water for thirty minutes, gargle the throat thoroughly until it is clean, then drink a pint luke-warm to thoroughly cleanse the stomach. If it does not come back easily, tickle the back of the throat. This restores the mucous secretions to normal activity. For chills make as above, adding a pinch of Cayenne, and take a half cup warm every hour. This is very effective.

Bayberry is excellent to take as an emetic after narcotic poisoning of any kind, and it is good to follow with a lobelia emetic.

Bayberry is valuable taken in the usual manner for all kinds of hemorrhages, whether from the stomach, lungs, uterus, or bowels. Bayberry is reliable to check profuse menstruation, and when combined with Capsicum is an unfailing remedy for this. Very good in leucorrhea. Has an excellent general effect on the female organs, also has an excellent influence on the uterus in pregnancy, and makes a good douche. Excellent results will be obtained from its use in goitre. In diarrhea and dysentery, use an injection of the tea as an enema.

In case of gangrenous sores, boils, carbuncles, use as a wash and poultice, or apply the powdered bayberry to the infection. The tea is an excellent wash for spongy and bleeding gums.

Bayberry is an excellent treatment in adenoids by snuffing the powder or tea up the nose, or using a straw through which to blow the powdered bayberry. This is also good for catarrh.

The tea taken internally is useful in jaundice, scrofula, canker in the throat and mouth. The tea taken warm promotes perspiration, and improves the whole circulation, and tones up the tissues. Taken in combination with yarrow, catnip, sage or peppermint, is unexcelled for colds.

An excellent formula used by the famous Dominion Herbal College made with bayberry for colds, fevers, flu, colic, cramps, and pains in the stomach, is as follows:

Bayberry	4 oz.
Ginger	2 oz.
White Pine	1 oz.

Cloves	1 dram
Capsicum	1 dram

This is prepared by mixing the herbs (in powdered form) and passing through a fine sieve several times. Use one teaspoonful, more or less as the case may require, in a cup of hot water. Allow the herbs to stand so they will settle and drink off the clear liquid, leaving the settlings. Anyone knowing the benefit of this wonderful composition would not be without it.

BAY LEAVES
(Bark, berries, and leaves)

Botanical Name: Laurus Nobilis. Common Names: Bay tree, Indian bay, bay laurel, laurel, European bay laurel. Medicinal Properties: Carminative, aromatic, stomachic, astringent.

A pleasant tonic, which gives tone and strength to the digestive organs. Expels wind from the stomach and bowels and is good for cramps.

BEECH
(Bark and leaves)

Botanical Name: Fagus ferruginea. Common Names: American beech, beech tree, beech nut tree. Medicinal Properties: Tonic, astringent, antiseptic.

This is the common beech tree that almost everyone is acquainted with. A good tonic, improves appetite. Very softening and healing to wounds and ulcers. Excellent in diabetes, internal ulcers, skin diseases, dyspepsia. Good for the liver, kidneys, and bladder. It is good to take once in a while to clean and tone up the system.

BETHROOT
(Root)

Botanical Name: Trillium Pendulum. Common Names: Birth-root, milk ipecac, three-leaved nightshade, trillium, Indian shamrock, cought root, nodding, wakerobin, lamb's-quarters, ground lily, snake bite, rattlesnake's root, Jew's harp plant. Medicinal Properties: Astringent, tonic, antiseptic, emmenagogue, diaphoretic, alterative, female complaints.

Useful in coughs, bronchial troubles, pulmonary consumption, hemorrhages from the lungs, excessive menstruation, leucorrhea, lax conditions of the vagina, and fallen womb. Remedy for diarrhea and dysentery.

BISTORT ROOT
(Root)

Botanical Name: Polygonum bistorta. Common Name: Patience dock, snake weed, sweet dock, dragonworth, red legs, Easter giant. Medicinal Properties: Astringent, diuretic, styptic, and alterative.

It is one of the strongest herb astringents, excellent for gargles, injections, and astringents used for cholera, diarrhea, dysentery, and leucorrhea. Excellent wash for sore mouth or gums and running sores. Combined with equal parts of red raspberries, it will cleanse internal cankers. Makes a good wash for the nose. Useful in smallpox, measles, pimples, jaundice, ruptures, insect stings, snake bites, expels worms. Combined with plantain is useful in gonorrhea. The powdered bistort will stop bleeding of a cut or wound when applied directly to the injury. Used in douche to decrease or regulate the menstrual flow.

BITTERROOT
(Root)

Botanical Name: Apocynum androsaemifolium. Common Names: Dogsbane, milkweed, honey bloom, milk ipecac, flytrap, wandering milkweed, catchfly, bitter dogsbanes, western wallflower. Medicinal Properties: Emetic, diuretic, sudorific, cathartic, stimulant, expectorant.

This is a very good remedy for intermittent fever, typhoid fever, and other fevers. Has an excellent effect on the liver, kidneys, and bowels. Increases the secretion of bile. Excellent for poor digestion. Bitterroot has been known to cure dropsy when everything else has failed. Expels worms. Is very useful in syphilis, and to rid the system of other impurities. Especially valuable in gallstones. Good in rheumatism, neuralgia, diseases of the joints and mucous membranes. Wonderful for diabetes.

BITTERSWEET
(Root and twig)

Botanical Name: Solanum dulcamara. Common Names: Woody nightshade, wolfe grape, bittersweet, nightshade, violet bloom, scarlet berry, bittersweet herb, bittersweet twigs, nightshade vine, garden nightshade, fever twig, felenworth, bittersweet stems, staff vine, woody nightshade. Medicinal Properties: Emetic, anodyne, deobstruent, herpatic, resolvent, depurative, aperient, laxative.

Has a splendid effect on the liver, pancreas, spleen, and other glandular organs of the body. Excellent in all skin troubles, and will purify the blood. It is very soothing and allays general irritability. Good in piles, jaundice, syphilis, gonorrhea, and rheumatism. It makes the skin and kidneys active, increases the menstrual flow, is helpful in leprosy, and is an important part in many salves. The tea is very healing to internal sores when bathed in it, especially burns and scalds. A salve made of equal parts of bittersweet and yellow dock forms an excellent ointment for various skin diseases and sores. A poultice made of the bruised berries will remove felons. Bittersweet may be combined with camomile as an ointment for bruises, sprains, swellings, and corns.

BLACK COHOSH

Botanical Name: Cimicifuga Racemosa. Common Names: Black snake root, bugwort, bugbane, squaw root, rattleroot, rattleweed, rattlesnake's root, rich weed. Medicinal Properties: Emmenagogue, nervine, alterative, expectorant, diaphoretic, astringent, antispasmodic.

A powerful remedy in hysteria, St. Vitus dance (or chorea), epilepsy, fits, convulsions, and all spasmodic affections. Good for pelvic disturbances, female complaint, all uterine troubles, and relieves pain in childbirth. Dependable herb to bring on menstrual flow that has been retarded by cold or exposure. Splendid for dropsy, rheumatism, spinal meningitis, asthma, delirium tremens, poisonous snakebites, and poisonous insect bites. A wonderful remedy for high blood pressure and for equalizing the circulation. By making into a syrup, black cohosh is effective in coughs, whooping cough, and in liver and kidney troubles.

BLUE COHOSH

Botanical Name: Caulophyllum thalictroides. Common Name: Blue berry, squaw root, papoose root, blue ginseng, yellow ginseng. Medicinal Properties: Stimulant, sudorific, parturient, emmenagogue.

Used to regulate mentrual flow and for suppressed menstruation. Is a most common remedy among the Indians to make childbirth easy and to bring on labor pains when the proper time arrives. Good for chronic uterine trouble, leucorrhea, rheumatism, neuralgia, vaginitis (inflammation of vagina), dropsy, cramps, colic, hysteria, palpitation of the heart, high blood pressure, and diabetes. Good for hiccough, whooping cough, spasms, fits, and epilepsy. Blue cohosh contains the following vital mineral elements: Potassium, magnesium, calcium, iron, silicon, phosphorous, helping to alkalinize the blood and urine.

BLUE FLAG

Botanical Name: Iris versicolor. Common Names: Poison flag, water flay, water lily, flay lily, fleur-de-lis, liver lily, snake lily, flowed-de-luce. Medicinal Properties: Alterative, resolvent, sialagogue, laxative, diuretic, vermifuge. The root is the part used.

Useful in cancer, rheumatism, dropsy, impurity of blood, constipation, syphilis, skin diseases, liver troubles, and as a laxative. It is very relaxing and stimulating.

BLUE VIOLET
(Whole plant)

Botanical Name: Viola cuculata. Common Names: Violet, common blue violet. Medicinal Properties: Mucilaginous, laxative, emetic, alterative.

Violet leaves are very effective in healing and give prompt relief in internal ulcers. For cancer they are a proven remedy. Use externally for this purose as a poultice, and take the tea internally. For cancer and cancerous growth and other skin diseases, violet is especially beneficial when combined with red clover and vervaine. Violet is a successful remedy in tumors, gout, coughs, colds, sore throat, sores, ulcers, scrofula, syphilis, bronchitis, and difficult breathing due to gases and morbid matter in the stomach and bowels. Violet is wonderful for nervousness or general debility when combined with nerveroot, scullcap, or black cohosh. Relieves severe headache and congestion in the head. Very effective for whooping cough.

BLOODROOT
(Root)

Botanical Name: Sanguinaria canadensis. Common Names: Red puccoon, Indiana plant, pauson, red paint root, red root. Medicinal Properties: Emmenagogue, tonic, diuretic. Stimulant, febrifuge, emetic, sedative, and rubefacient.

It is an excellent agency in adenoids, nasal polypus, sore throat, and syphilitic troubles. When the condition is not easily overcome, combine with equal parts of golden seal. It is also excellent for piles by using an injection of strong tea made from bloodroot. Effective remedy in coughs, colds, laryngitis, bronchitis, typhoid, fever, pneumonia, catarrh, scarletina, jaundice, dyspepsia and ringworm, liver, lungs, kidneys, whooping cough, running sores, eczema, skin diseases. Small doses stimulate digestive organs and heart. Large doses act as a sedative.

BORAGE

Botanical Name: Borago officinalis. Common Names: Burroge, bugloss, common bugloss. Medicinal Properties: Pectoral, cordial, aperient.

It is excellent to bathe sore inflamed eyes with the tea. Taken internally, the tea cleanses the blood and is effective for fevers, yellow jaundice, to expel poisons of all kinds due to snake bites, insect stings, etc., strengthens the heart, is good for cough, itch, ringworms, tetters, scabs, sores, ulcers. Use as a gargle for ulcers in mouth and throat, and to loosen phlegm.

BROOM

Botanical Name: Cytisus scoparius. Common Name: Common broom, broom flowers, Irish broom. Medicinal Properties: Top: Cathartic, diuretic. Seed: Cathartic, emetic. Contains forty-two parts potash. The stomach readily receives the nutritive salts in the plant, as they are naural.

Excellent for dropsy, toothache, ague, gout, sciatica, swelling of spleen, jaundice, kidney, and bladder troubles, especially in cases of gravel in the bladder. Makes an excellent remedy in connection with uva ursi, cleavers, and dandelion for cleansing the kidneys and bladders, and to increase the flow of urine. Broom is of great service in dropsy caused by a weak heart, also for hydrocephalus or water on the brain. Makes a good ointment for lice or vermin.

BUCHU
(Leaves)

Botanical Name: Barosma betulina. Common Names: Bookoo, bucku, short-leaved buchu, buku. Medicinal Properties: Diuretic, tonic, stimulant, diaphoretic. Use the short-leaved buchu.

One of the best remedies for urinary organs. It is very soothing and is a most excellent remedy when there is pain while urinating, catarrh of bladder, and dropsy. Excellent in stoppage of urine. When used specifically for this purpose, give a strong tea, cold. When given warm, it produces perspiration and soothes the enlargement of prostate gland, and irritation of the membrane of the urethra. Useful in diabetes in the first stages. Use for leucorrhea. DO NOT BOIL BUCHU LEAVES.

BUCKBEAN

Botanical Name: Menyanthes trifoliata. Common Names: Marsh trefoil, water shamrock, bog bean, bitter trefoil, marsh clover, bog myrtle, bitterworm, brook bean. Medicinal Properties: Tonic, bitter, cathartic, diuretic, anthelmintic.

Expels worms. Taken in large doses it is emetic. Promotes digestion by increasing the gastric juices. Excellent remedy in stomach catarrh, rheumatism, scrofula, scruvy, intermittent fevers, jaundice, dyspepsia, liver and kidney troubles.

BUCKTHORN BARK
(Bark and Fruit)

Botanical Name: Rhamnus frangula. Common Names: European buckthorn, black alder dogwood, black alder tree, alder buckthorn, black dogwood, vermifuge, Persian berries, European black alder. Medicinal Properties: Bitter, purgative, diuretic, emetic. Fruit: Purgative.

Buckthorn bark is a very effective remedy for appendicitis. Very beneficial for constipation, keeps the bowels regular. Not habit forming. Good in rheumatism, gout, dropsy, and skin diseases. Will produce profuse perspiration when taken hot. Take both internally and apply externally as a wash. The ointment made of buckthorn is very effective in curing itch. Expels worms. Will remove warts. Good used as fomentation or poultice.

BURDOCK
(Roots, leaves, and seeds)

Botanical Name: Arctium lappa. Common Names: Grass burdock, clotbur, bardana, burr seed, hardock, harebur, hurr-burr, turkey burr seed. Medicinal Properties: Root: Diuretic, depilatory, alterative. Leaves: Maturating. Seed: Alterative, diuretic.

The root is one of the best blood purifiers for syphilitic and other diseases of the blood. It cleanses and eliminates impurities from the blood very rapidly. Burdock tea taken freely will clear all kinds of skin diseases, boils, and carbuncles. Increases flow of urine. Excellent for gout, rheumatism, scrofula, canker sores, syphilis, sciatica, gonorrhea, leprosy. Wring a hot fomentation out of the tea for swellings. It is good to make a salve and apply externally for skin eruptions, burns, wounds, swellings, and hemorrhoids. Excellent to reduce flesh.

BURNET
(Root)

Botanical Name: Pimpinella saxifraga. Common Names: Burnet saxifrage, small saxifrage, pimpernel, small pimpernel, European burnet saxifrage, small saxifrage, small burnet saxifrage. Medicinal Properties: Aromatic, stimulant, stomachic, pungent.

It is very useful to cleanse the chest, lungs, and stomach. Will expel stones from the bladder. Good for cuts, wounds, running sores, toothache, earache, piles. Steep a teaspoonful of the root in a cup of boiling water, let cool, strain, and drink one or two cups a day cold, a large swallow at a time. Best remedy known for sour stomach.

BUTTERNUT BARK
(Bark)

Botanical Name: Juglans cinerea. Common Names: Oilnut, oilnut bark, white walnut, lemon walnut, Kisky Thomas nut. Medicinal Properties: Tonic, astringent, cholagogue, anthelmintic, alterative, cathartic.

Will expel worms from intestines. Excellent, slow remedy for chronic constipation, sluggish liver, fevers, colds, and la grippe. It is an old-fashioned remedy.

CALAMUS
(Root)

Botanical Name: Acorus calamus. Common Names: Sweet flag, grass myrtle, sweet grass, sweet root, sweet cane, sweet rush, sweet sedge, myrtle flag, sweet myrtle, sea serge. Medicinal Properties: Carminative, aromatic, tonic, vulnerary.

Excellent for use in intermittent fevers, fever in marshy regions. It is a valuable stomach remedy, and is good to mix with other herbs for that purpose, and is useful to prevent griping of other herbs. It improves gastric juices, is good for dyspepsia, wind colic, prevents acids, gases, and fermentation in the stomach, keeps the stomach fluids sweet, increases appetite. Will destroy taste for tobacco. The tea is excellent applied externally to sores, burns, and ulcers. Valuable in the treatment of scrofula.

CAMOMILE

Botanical Name: Anthemis nobilis. Common Names: Roman camomile, camomile, garden camomile, low camomile, ground apple, Whig plant. Medicinal Properties: Stimulant, bitter, tonic, aromatic.

An old, well-known home remedy, grows freely everywhere. Everyone should gather a bagful of camomile blossoms, as they are good for many ailments. Excellent general tonic, produces appetite, good for dyspepsia and weak stomach. Used in various parts of the world as a table tea. Good to regulate monthly periods. Splendid for kidneys, spleen, colds, bronchitis, bladder troubles, to expel worms, for ague, dropsy, jaundice. The tea is an excellent wash for sore and weak eyes, also for other open sores and wounds. As a poultice for pains and swellings. Intermittent and typhoid fever can be broken up in the early stages with the herb. Good in hysteria and nervous diseases. Made and used as a poultice, it will prevent gangrene. Combine with bittersweet as ointment for bruises, sprains, callous swellings, or corns.

CARAWAY
(Seed)

Botanical Name: Carum carui. Common Name: Caraway seed. Medicinal Properties: Carminative, aromatic, fragrant, stomachic.

Caraway seed is usually used to flavor baked and other food products.

It is very useful for colic in infants, taken in hot water or milk, also taken hot for colds and female trouble. It is very good to prevent fermentation in the stomach and aids digestion. Strengthens and gives tone to the stomach, also expels wind from the bowels. It is often used to flavor other herbs and to prevent griping. Used as a poultice for bruises.

CARROT
(Root and seed)

Botanical Name: Daucus carota. Common Names: Garden carrot, bee's nest plant, bird's nest root, wild carrot.

If carrots were used more extensively as a vegetable, they would prove of great benefit to mankind. Patients are often put on the carrot diet for a short period for cancer, liver, kidney and bladder troubles. They are very useful in dropsy, gravel, painful urination, to increase the menstrual flow, and in expelling worms from the bowels. Grated carrots make an excellent poultice for ulcers, abscesses, carbuncles, scrofulous and cancerous sores, and bad wounds. The seeds of carrots ground to powder, and taken as a tea relieves colic and increases the flow of urine. Carrot blossoms, used as a tea are most effective as a remedy for dropsy. It will very often effect a cure when all other means have failed.

CASCARA SAGRADA

Botanical Name: Rhamnus purschiana. Common Name: Purschiana bark, Persian bark, sacred bark, chittam bark, bearberry. Medicinal Properties: Bitter tonic.

It is one of the best remedies for chronic constipation. It does not form the drug habit. It is a good intestinal tonic. An excellent remedy for gallstones, increases secretion of bile, good for liver complaints, especially enlarged liver. Mix four teaspoonfuls of this in a quart of boiling water, let steep for one hour, and drink one or two cupfuls a day one hour before meals or on an empty stomach. It is well sometimes to drink a cupful on retiring. Cascara sagrada is a wonderful remedy. Among the Indians it was known as "sacred bark." It was called sacred by them because of the excellent results they obtained from its use. The writer has used this remedy for over thirty years, and is getting gratifying results. The bark is very bitter and disagreeable to the taste of many people. In recent years it can be procured from drugstores in three and five grain chocolate-coated tablets, called abstract cascara sagrada. Do not mistake this for Cascarets, as they are an entirely different product. Have them on hand when needed. When there is a bad taste in the mouth, or the bowels do not move as they should, take one or more of these tablets according to your needs. Take them immediately after meals, or upon retiring. An excellent remedy for children when constipated.

CATNIP

Botanical Name: Nepeta cataria. Common Names: Catmint, catrup, cat's-wort, field balm, catnip. Medicinal Properties: Anodyne, antispasmodic, carminative, aromatic, diaphoretic, nervine.

Catnip is one of the oldest household remedies. It is wonderful for very small children and infants. Use the tea as an injection for children in convulsions. Very useful in pain of any kind, spasms, wind colic, excellent to allay gas, acids, in stomach and bowels, prevent griping. A tablespoonful steeped in a pint of water used as an enema is soothing and quieting, and very effective in insanity, fevers, expelling worms in children; also fits. A high enema of catnip will relieve hysterical headaches. It is good to restore menstrual secretions. Catnip, sweet balm, marshmallow and sweet weed make an excellent baby remedy. If mothers would have this on hand and use it properly, it would save them many sleepless nights and doctor's bills, and also save the baby much suffering. It is a harmless remedy and should take the place of the various soothing syrups on the market, many of which are very harmful. This wonderful remedy should be in every home. A little honey or malt honey may be added to make it palatable. Steep, never boil, catnip. Take internally freely. An enema of catnip will cause urination when it has stopped.

CAYENNE
(Fruit)

Botanical Name: Capsicum annuum. Common Names: Cayenne pepper, red pepper, capsicum, Spanish pepper, bird pepper, pod pepper, chillies, African pepper, chili pepper, African red pepper, cockspur pepper, American red pepper, garden pepper. Medicinal Properties: Pungent, stimulant, tonic, sialagogue, alterative.

Red pepper is one of the most wonderful herb medicines we have. We do wonderful things with it that we are not able to do with any other known herb. It should never be classed with black pepper, vinegar, or mustard. These are irritating, while red pepper is very soothing. While red pepper smarts a little, it can be put in an open wound, either in a fresh wound or an old ulcer, and it is very healing instead of irritating; but black pepper, mustard, and vinegar are irritating to an open wound and do not heal. Red pepper is one of the most stimulating herbs known to man with no harm or reaction.

It is effective as a poultice for rheumatism, inflammation, pleurisy, and helpful also if taken internally for these. For sores and wounds it makes a good poultice. It is a stimulant when taken internally as well as being antispasmodic. Good for kidneys, spleen, and pancreas. Wonderful for lockjaw. Will heal a sore, ulcerated stomach, while black pepper, mustard, or vinegar will irritate it. Red pepper is a specific and very effective remedy in yellow fever, as well as other fevers and may be taken in capsules followed by a glass of water.

It is one part of a most wonderful liniment, which may be made as follows:

> 2 oz. gum myrrh
> 1 oz. golden seal
> ½ oz. African red pepper

Put this into a quart of rubbing alcohol, or take a pint of raspberry vinegar and a pint of water. Add the alcohol or vinegar to the powder. Let it stand for a week or ten days, shaking every day. This can be used wherever liniment is used or needed. It is very healing to wounds, bruises, sprains, scalds, burns, and sunburns, and should be applied freely. Wonderful results are obtained in pyorrhea by rinsing the mouth with the liniment or applying the liniment on both sides of the gums with a little cotton or gauze.

CAPSICUM-CAYENNE, RED PEPPER

"From the Greek kapto, I bite—a biting plant. The best Capsicum is obtained from Africa and South America, one province of the latter, Cayenne, giving its name to the article. It can be produced in good quality in the Southern States, especially those that lie beyond the southern line of Tennessee. It grows abundantly and of excellent quality in the West Indies, where the negroes count it almost a certain remedy for nearly all their maladies. They have no fears of fatal effects from fevers, even the terrible and devastating yellow fever, if they can get plenty of Capsicum. They not only drink a tea of it, but they chew and swallow the pods one after another, as we should so many doughtnuts, and never dream of it doing them any injury. Dr. Thomas, of London, who practised a long time in the West Indies, found cayenne pepper an almost certain remedy for yellow fever, and almost every other form of human malady. There is, perhaps, no other article which produces so powerful an impression on the animal frame that is so destitute of all injurious properties. It seems almost incapable of abuse, for however great the excitement produced by it, this stimulant prevents that excitement subsiding so suddenly as to induce any great derangement of the equilibrium of the circulation. It produces the most powerful impression on the surface, yet never draws a blister; on the stomach, yet never weakens its tone. It is so diffusive in its character that it never produces any local lesion, or induces permanent inflammation.

"Yet its counter excitation is the most salutary kind, and ample in degree. A plaster of cayenne is more efficient in relieving internal inflammation than a fly blister ever was, yet I never knew it to produce the slightest vesication, though I have often bound it thick as a poultice on the tenderest flesh to relieve rheumatism, pleurisy, etc., which, by the aid of an emetic, an enema, and sudorifics, it is sure to do. I have thus cured with it, in a single night, cases of rheumatism that had been for years most distressing. Though severe on the tissue to which applied, it is so diffusive that it does not long derange the circulation, but, on the contrary, equalizes it. Thus it is not only stimulant, but antispasmodic, sudorific, febrile, anti-inflammatory, depurating, and restorative. It is powerful to arrest hemorrhage from the mucous membranes. When the stomach is foul, a strong dose of the powder will excite vomiting and an enema of it and lobelia and slippery elm will relieve the most obstinate constipation. Taken in powder in cold water it is sure to move not only the internal canal, but all the splanchnic viscera, as the liver, the kidneys, the spleen, and the pancreas, the mesentery, etc. This article, along with lobelia, some good astringent, such as bayberry or sumach leaves, a good bitter, a mucilage, a good sudorific and the vapor bath, must ever constitute the basis of the most effective medication." *Standard Guide to Non-Poisonous Herbal Medicine,* pp. 52, 53.

"There are several species of Capsicum, but the most prominent are the Capsicum Annuum and the Capsicum Fastigiatum-Guinea or African Bird's Eye Pepper. The last named is the official article, and is possessed of greater medicinal virtue; yet the small American species are nearly its equal. The fruit of the Fastigiatum is quite small, while that of the American species is very much larger and is heart-shaped. The African species is quite a shrub, while the American is more like an herb in appearance. Capsicum, strange though it may seem, is not a true pepper. The popular but erroneous idea is that anything that is hot is a pepper, and that therefore Capsicum must belong to the pepper family. The African or small varieties are the most pungent—I should say nearly twice as much so as the others, but owing, I suppose to the American species being cheaper, it is used as a substitute for the African. They both contain a resin and an oil, each of which is very acrid, sharp, and biting. Its properties are completely extracted by 98% alcohol, and to a considerable extent by vinegar or boiling water.

"One of the best *LINIMENTS* in use is prepared as follows: Boil gently for ten minutes one tablespoonful of cayenne pepper in one pint of cider vinegar. Bottle that hot, unstrained. This makes a powerfully stimulating external application for deep-seated congestions, sprains, etc.

"Capsicum is a pure stimulant, permanent in its action, and ultimately reaching every organ in the body. It creates at first a sensation of warmth, which afterwards becomes intense, and in large doses strongly excites the stomach, which influence can be utilized in the administration of emetics, when the emesis is delayed and needs to be accelerated. For this purpose give a quarter of a teaspoonful in syrup. Capsicum, by its sudden and intense stimulation of the stomach, will produce hiccoughs. It acts mainly upon the circulation, but also on the nervous structures. Its influence, which is immediate on the heart, finally extends to the capillaries, giving tone to the circulation, but not increasing the frequency of the pulse so much as giving power to it. In prostrating fevers and putrescent tendencies it may be used in full quantities combined with other suitable agents. It is a good addition to relaxant cathartics, to prevent griping and facilitates their operation when the tissues are in a sluggish condition. In cases of constipation, capsicum is efficacious in stimulating the peristaltic motion of the bowels. For this effect, give small doses daily. Of course, constipation never can be cured by physic alone. Temporary relief may be obtained from carthartics, but any medicinal efforts must be combined with proper diet in order to effect a permanent cure.

"Capsicum is valuable in all forms of ague by sustaining the portal circulation. In cases of chill, give large doses of cayenne. By a large dose is meant 10 to 15 grains, or a No. 0 to a No. 00 capsule. Of course some patients require more than others. (A No. 0 capsule should contain about ten grains, and No. 00 about 15 grains.) In coughs where there is an abundant secretion of mucus in the respiratory passages, capsicum increases the power of expectoration, and thus facilitates its removal. In connection with capsicum may be mentioned the *slippery elm compound,* which is excellent for coughs. Cut obliquely into small pieces about the thickness of a match, one ounce or more of slippery elm bark: add a pinch of cayenne, flavour with a slice of lemon, sweeten with sugar, and infuse one pint of boiling water. Take this in small doses, frequently repeated. Let a consumptive patient drink a pint of this each day. It is one of the grandest remedies that can be given, as it combines both stimulating and demulcent properties. As slippery elm is mucilaginous it will roll up the mucus material troubling the patient, and pass it down through the intestines. It is also very nourishing, and possesses wonderful healing properties. For an infant's food mix with an equal quantity of milk, and leave out the lemond and cayenne.

"Cayenne is good in coughs, torpor of the kidneys, and to arrest mortification. A peculiar effect of capsicum is worth mentioning. In Mexico the people are very fond of it; and their bodies get thoroughly saturated with it, and if one of them happens to die on the prairie the vultures will not touch the body on account of its being so impregnated with the capsicum.

"It is good in all forms of low diseases. The key to success in medicine is stimulation, and capsicum is the great stimulant. There are many languid people who need something to make the fire of life burn more brightly. Capsicum, not whiskey, is the thing to do it. It can be given without stint or measure. It is excellent in yellow fever, black vomit, putrefaction or decay, given frequently in small doses. It is good, also, in asthmatical asphyxia (i.e., when a person cannot get his breath) combined with lobelia in what would be called the lobelia compound. It is good in profound shock. For local application it is, or should be, the base of all stimulating liniments. It is not injurious to the skin, as is turpentine or acetic acid. It is an agent that is seldom used alone. A *capsicum tincture* may be made as follows:

"Take two ounces of cayenne and macerate for ten to fourteen days in one quart of alcohol. Then strain and bottle. Keep in a warm place while macerating during cold weather.

"A splendid *stimulating liniment* is made as follows:

Tinct. Cayenne	1 qt.
Castille Soap	2 oz.
Oil of Hemlock Spruce	½ oz.
Oil of Origanum	½ oz.
Oil of Cedar	½ oz.
Oil of Peppermint	½ oz.

Shave or scrape the soap very fine, and dissolve in one pint of water. Stir the oils into the tincture and mix with the soapy solution. A little additional oil of peppermint will greatly increase its efficacy. In a four-ounce bottle put one ounce of lobelia compound (without gum myrrh) and fill the bottle up with the stimulating liniment. Shake this well, and after application cover the affected part with a piece of warmed flannel.

"The oil of capsicum represents the stimulating property of the plant in highly concentrated form. It is exceedingly strong, and the dose must be not more than one drop given on sugar. For the relief of toothache, first clean out the cavity of the tooth, then make a small plug of cotton wool saturated with oil of capsicum, which press into the cavity, and it will, in most cases, cure the toothache by its stimulating and antiseptic qualities. The beneficial effect will last for months.

"Having considered the various ingredients in the myrica compound ('composition powder'), we will now pass it under review. The bayberry bark is astringent and stimulant, the ginger root is a diffusive stimulant and antispasmodic, prompt but kindly in its action; the Canada snake root has an influence similar to that of ginger, but is more aromatic, and corrects the acridness of the other ingredients; the prickly ash berry constitutes the peripheral stimulant; and the capsicum is the great arterial stimulant, and imparts energy to the action of the whole compound." *Standard Guide to Non-Poisonous Herbal Medicine,* pp. 95, 96, 97, 98.

MYRICA COMPOUND

Bayberry Bark .... 8 oz.
African Ginger .... 4 oz.
Prickly Ash Berries .... 1 oz.

Canada Snake Root .... 3 oz.
African Cayenne .... 2 drachms

Pass these powders twice through a sifter, and they will be mixed to perfection. For emetic teas, make three pints of composition, two pints of lobelia infusion, and three pints of catnip or peppermint infusion.

"Capsicum (red pepper) is the most pronounced, natural and ideal stimulant known in the entire materia medica. It cannot be equaled by any known agent when a powerful and prolonged stimulant is needed, as in congestive chills, heart failure and other conditions calling for quick action. The entire circulation is affected by this agent and there is no reaction. In this it stands alone as ideal.

"In congested, ulcerated or infectious sore throat it is an excellent agent, but should be combined with myrrh to relieve and remove the morbidity.

"Capsicum is antiseptic and therefore a most valuable agent as a gargle in ordinary sore throat or in diphtheria.

"In uterine hemorrhages it is ideal combined with bayberry and will do more than any other remedy could. Capsicum has the power to arouse the action of the secreting organs and always follows the use of lobelia.

"When there is inactivity of the entire system, as in 'spring fever,' capsicum is indicated. In fact, whenever there is disinclination to activity it is an ideal stimulant, arousing the sluggish organism to action.

"In indigestion where gas is present, it should be given in conjunction with small doses (1 to 5 grains) of lobelia, as capsicum increases the glandular activity of both stomach and intestines.

"In all so-called 'low' fevers, where the temperature is subnormal capsicum is indicated and should be prescribed consistently.

"On the inset of a cold, when there are chills, cold and clammy feelings, the feet damp and cold, capsicum should be taken in full dose (5 to 10 grains). In these cases capsicum is more efficient than quinine and there is no reaction—no undesirable after effects.

"Even in cholera morbus and atonic diarrhea, where stimulants are usually contra-indicated, capsicum is valuable in that it 'tones' up the organs and establishes natural activity.

"In all diseases prostrating in their nature, whether pneumonia, pleurisy or typhoid fever, capsicum is invaluable in the prescription as the toning agent which helps the system to throw off the disease and reestablish equilibrium.

"In all acute conditions where capsicum is indicated, the call is for the maximum dose—from three to ten grains, preferably in tablet form, followed by a large drink of hot water. In chronic and sluggish conditions, the small dose frequently given, is 1 to 3 grains with either hot or cold water.

Capsicum plasters are valuable in pneumonia, pleurisy and other acute congestions. Combine with lobelia and bran or hops. One hour is the maximum time to keep them applied."—*The Medicines of Nature,* by R. Swinburne Clymer, pp. 69, 70, 71.

"As the common red pepper of table use, capsicum is well known to almost all people. None know better its virtue than the habitual drinker who considers it his best friend and never fails to use plenty of it in his hot soups when sobering up and soothing his cold and sore stomach after a prolonged spree. Common red pepper may be given safely in capsules and take the place of tablets. In the onset of chills and colds it is the sovereign remedy." *The Medicines of Nature,* by R. Swinburne Clymer, pp. 79, 80.

"Whenever a stimulant is necessary Capsicum should have first consideration. It is indicated in low fevers and prostrating diseases. Capsicum is non-poisonous and there is no reaction to its use. It is the only natural stimulant worth while considering in diarrhea and dysentery with bloody mucus, stools and offensive breath."—*The Medicines of Nature,* by R. Swinburne Clymer, p. 143.

"The stimulant. There is no other stimulant known to medical science so natural, so certain and with less reaction following its constant use. Capsicum is indicated in all low fevers and prostrating diseases. Capsicum increases the power of all other agents, helps the digestion when taken with meals, and arouses all the secreting organs. Whenever a stimulant is indicated, capsicum may be given with the utmost safety." *The Medicines of Nature,* by R. Swinburne Clymer, p. 150. Capsicum, cayenne (red pepper) is not a pepper, no more than water pepper or peppermint. Water pepper is also called smart weed, is very hot but a wonderful medicine.

"Peppermint well known all over the civilized world is very heating, will stimulate like a drink of whiskey, but there is no reaction from it, no bad after effects. It permanently strengthens the whole system. Red pepper does the same. There are a number of other herbs that are very hot which are God-given medicines.

"Capsicum, cayenne, red pepper: This plant is indigenous to the warmer climates, Asia, Africa, and the Southern States. The kind bearing the larger berries grows in the more northern places and is frequently used for culinary purposes.

"The African bird pepper is the purest and best stimulant known. It has a pungent taste, and is the most persistent heart stimulant ever known. It is exceedingly prompt in its effects. Through the circulation, its influence is manifest through the whole body. The heart first, next the arteries, then the capillaries, and the nerves. We have known in cases of apoplexy a bath of hot water and mustard with half a teaspoon of cayenne added and the feet thrust in to give good results, the pressure being removed from the brain by equalizing of the circulation.

"The negroes of the West Indies soak the pods in water, add sugar and the juice of sour oranges, and drink freely in fevers. Capsicum has a wonderful place in inflammation. We have often been told that it would burn the lining of the stomach, and our medical, as well as lay friends, have at times shown fear at its use. We assure the student that the fear of Capsicum is unfounded. We have used it freely for over a quarter of a century, and therefore feel that our experience is worth more than the opinions of those who know nothing about it experimentally.

"Some twenty years ago we were asked to send something to a lady whom we were told was suffering from pleurisy. After getting what little information we could, we decided to send some African bird pepper, as it was in the early hours of the morning and we were on the prairie and could not get anything in the way of supplies. Being satisfied that there was inflammation, we ordered three number four capsules filled with cayenne to be given every hour until the pains ceased. We were surprised later to learn that the pains had ceased in two and a half hours and no other remedies of any kind had been used, the capsules having been taken in smaller dosage after the pain eased. We were asked what was the wonderful remedy we had sent and when we told the husband of the patient, he said, had they known what was in the capsules, he would not have given them.

"We do not, of course, refer to this case to indicate that capsicum is a cure for pleurisy. We should have used other means as well, had the circumstances permitted. We mention it to show its use in inflammatory conditions.

"It is useful in cramps, pains in the stomach and bowels, and sometimes in constipation will create a heat in the bowels, causing peristaltic action of parts previously contracted. In these later cases it would be well to give it in small doses in the form of warm infusion, from half to one teaspoonful to a cup of boiling water. In typhoid fever, in combination with hepatics and a little golden seal, it will sustain the portal circulation and give much more power to the hepatics used.

"In colds, relaxed throat, cold condition of the stomach, dyspepsia, spasms, palpitation, particularly in the acute stages, give a warm infusion of capsicum in small repeat doses, about two teaspoonfuls every half hour or more frequently if required.

"A little capsicum sprinkled in the shoes will greatly assist in cold feet. Some place a sprinkle in the socks. Don't place too much however; you may find it too warm.

"In hemorrhage from the lungs place your patient in the vapour bath and give an infusion of Capsicum. The pressure will be taken from the ruptured vessels and good results obtained.

"In quinsy and diptheria, apply the tincture of cayenne (red pepper) around the neck. Then place a flannel around

(227)

the neck wet with the infusion of cayenne and use the infusion internally at the same time freely.

"A good liniment for sprains, bruises, rheumatism, and neuralgia may be made as follows:

Tincture Capsicum (Red Pepper)	2 Fluid Ounces
Fluid Extract Lobelia	2 Fluid Ounces
Oil of Wormwood	1 Fluid Drachm
Oil of Rosemary	1 Fluid Drachm
Oil of Spearmint	1 Fluid Drachm

"In setting forth the above uses of this agent, we do not wish the student to consider it a cure-all. Such is not the case; but where a stimulant is needed of this type, it will not fail the physician. It is not used more because its value is not realized." *Dominion Herbal College, Ltd.* pp. 1, 2, Lesson 5.

"Capsicum is the botanical name of a large genus or family of plants which grow in various countries, as Africa, South America, and the East and West Indies. We use only the African bird pepper, as it retains its heat longer in the system than any other, and is the best stimulant known. It has a pungent taste, which continues for a considerable length of time; when taken into the stomach it produces a pleasant sensation of warmth, which soon diffuses itself throughout the whole system, equalizing the circulation. Hence it is so useful in inflammation and all diseases which depend upon a morbid increase of blood in any particular part of the body. According to analysis, cayenne consists of albumen, pectin, (a peculiar gum), starch, carbonate of lime, sesquioxide of iron, phosphate of potass, alum, magnesia, and a reddish kind of oil. In apoplexy we have found it beneficial to put the feet in hot water and mustard, and at the same time give half a teaspoonful of cayenne pepper in a little water. This treatment has caused a reaction, taking the pressure of the blood from the brain, and by this means saved the patients. Some may ask, 'Will it produce an inflammatory action?' We say decidedly not, for there is nothing that will take away inflammation so soon. We have used it in every stage of inflammation and never without beneficial results. Mr. Price, the well-known traveler, lays it down as a positive rule of health that the warmest dishes the natives delight in are the most wholesome that strangers can use in the putrid climates of lower Arabia, Abyssinia, Syria, and Egypt. Marsden, in his history of Sumatra, remarks that cayenne pepper is one of the ingredients of the dishes of the natives. The natives of the tropical climates make free use of cayenne, and do not find it injurious. Dr. Watkins, who visited the West Indies, says the negroes of those islands steep the pods of the cayenne in hot water, adding sugar and the juice of sour oranges, and drink the tea when sick or attacked with fever. It is very amusing to see the medical men prohibiting the use of cayenne in inflammatory diseases as pernicious, if not fatal, and yet find them recommending it in their standard works for the same diseases. Dr. Thatcher, in his dispensatory, says: 'There can be but little doubt that cayenne furnishes us with the purest stimulant that can be introduced in the stomach.' Dr. Wright remarks that cayenne has been given for putrid sore throats in the West Indies with the most signal benefit. Paris, in his *Pharmacologia,* says that the surgeons of the French army have been in the habit of giving cayenne to the soldiers who were exhausted by fatigue. Dr. Fuller, in his prize essay on the treatment of scarlet fever, says: 'Powdered cayenne made into pills with crumbs of bread and given four times a day, three or four each time, is a most valuable stimulant in the last stages of the disease, and is also good in all cases of debility, from whatever cause it may arise.' Cayenne given in half teaspoonful doses, mixed with treacle and slippery elm, at night, is a valuable remedy for a cough. Bleeding of the lungs is easily checked by the use of cayenne and the vapor bath. By this means circulation is promoted in every part of the body, and consequently the pressure upon the lungs is diminished, thus affording an opportunity for a coagulum to form around the ruptured vessel. In advocating the use of cayenne we do not wish to be understood that it will cure everything, nor de we recommend it to be taken regularly, whether a stimulant is required or not. Medicines ought to be taken only in sickness. If persons take a cold a dose of cayenne tea will generally remove it, and by this means prevent a large amount of disease. It is an invaluable remedy in the botanic practice." *The Model Botanic Guide to Health*, pp. 33-34-35.

The above quotations on capsicum are from some of the world's foremost herbalists, therefore are very valuable. I quote these herbalists because I know them to be Christian men and they verify my own practical experience with capsicum.

CEDRON
(Seed)

Botanical Name: Simaba cedron. Common Names: Cedron, rattlesnakes' beans. Medicinal Properties: Antispasmodic, nervine, stomachic.

Cedron permanently strengthens and invigorates the entire system. It is excellent for the stomach, prevents gas and fermentation. A good remedy in intermittent fevers, spasms, fits, and nervous troubles. Make a strong tea of it, apply to a snake bite or poisonous insect bite, moisten a cloth in the tea, and keep it over the bite; keep it well saturated with the tea. Take plenty of the tea internally.

CELANDINE (WILD)
(Plant)

Botanical Name: Impatiens pallida. Common Names: Jewel weed, quick-in-hand, slippers, snap weed, pale touch-me-not, slipper weed, balsam weed, weathercock, touch-me-not. Medicinal Properties: Plant: Diuretic, alterative, emetic.

Effective for bladder and kidneys, jaundice, dropsy, liver, ulcers.

CELERY
(Root and Seed)

Botanical Name: Apium graveolens. Common Names: Smallage, garden celery. Medicinal Properties: Diuretic, stimulant, aromatic.

Excellent for use in incontinence of urine, dropsical and liver troubles. Produces perspiration, is a splendid tonic. Good in rheumatism and neuralgia, also nervousness. Is much used as a table relish, and the ground seed for flavoring soups.

CHICKWEED

Botanical Name: Stellaria media. Common Names: Stitchwort, scarwort, satin flower, adder's mouth. Medicinal Properties: Alterative, demulcent, refrigerant, mucilaginous, pectoral resolvent, discutient.

Chickweed can be used in many ways. It is considered a great nuisance by gardeners, but it can be used as a food as spinach. It may be used fresh, dried, powdered, in poultices, fomentations, or made into a salve. Excellent in all cases of bronchitis, pleurisy, coughs, colds, hoarseness, rheumatism, inflammation, or weakness of the bowels and stomach, lungs, bronchial tubes—in fact, any form of internal inflammation. It heals and soothes anything it comes in contact with. It is one of the best remedies for external applications to inflamed surfaces, skin diseases, boils, scalds, burns, inflamed or sore eyes, erysipelas, tumors, piles, cancer, swollen testes, ulcerated throat and mouth, deafness, and all kinds of wounds.

Bathe the surface with the decoction, and the swelling and inflammation will go down. In blood poisoning it should be taken internally, and a poultice applied externally. For constipation when the bowels are completely obstructed, take three heaping tablespoonfuls of the fresh herb, boil in one quart of water down to one pint. Take a cupful warm every three hours or oftener until the desired results are obtained.

Chickweed salve should be applied after bathing any external part with tea and left on as long as possible. Apply at night and leave on. Give several applications during the day if possible. It will cure burning and itching genitals. Anyone who is covered with any kind of sores should take a chickweed herb bath, and then apply the chickweed salve. Good for scurvy and blood disorders. For tea to be taken internally, steep a heaping teaspoonful for half an hour to a cup of boiling water, take three or four cups a day between meals, taking a swallow at a time. Take a cup warm upon retiring.

CHICORY

Botanical Name: Cichorium endiva. Common Names: Garden endiva, garden chicory, endive, garden endive. Medicinal Properties: Root: Tonic, laxative, diuretic.

While chicory is a very well-known herb for its combination with coffee, its value for various remedies is not well known. Chicory is effective in disorders of the kidneys, liver, urinary canal, stomach, and spleen. It is good for jaundice. Is good to settle an upset condition in the stomach, expelling the morbid matter and toning up the system.

CINCHONA BARK (See Peruvian Bark)

CLEAVERS
(Whole herb)

Botanical Name: Galium aparine. Common Names: Goose grass, gravel grass, grip grass, goose's hair, clabber grass, catchweed, savoyan, milk sweet, poor robin, clivers, bedstraw, scratchweed, cleaverwort, cheese rent herb. Medicinal Properties: Refrigerant, diuretic, aperient, alterative, tonic.

One of the best remedies for kidney and bladder troubles, scalding urine, and in suppressed urine, especially when used with broom, uva ursi, buchu and marshmallow. Makes an excellent wash for the face to clear complexion. Due to its refrigerant properties it is excellent in all cases of fever, scarlet fever, measles, and all acute diseases. Good in many skin diseases, such as cancer, scrofula, and severe cases of eczema. Also good for inflammatory stages of gonorrhea. Excellent for stone in the bladder, scurvy, and dropsy. This herb may be used freely. Is excellent in jaundice. Can be used as spinach. Is excellent to cleanse the blood and strengthen the liver used in this way.

CLOVER (See Red Clover, White Clover)

COHOSH (See Blue Cohosh, Black Cohosh)

COLOMBO

Botanical Name: Cocculus palmatus. Common Names: Colombo, colombo root, columba, foreign colombo kalumb, calumba root. Medicinal Properties: Anti-emetic, tonic, febrifuge.

One of the best and purest tonics to strengthen and tone up the entire system. Useful in intermittent and remittent fevers. Will keep the system pure and toned up in debilitating and hot swampy climates. Excellent to allay vomiting in pregnancy, can be used with good effect before and after pregnancy, can be used for colon trouble, no matter of how long standing, cholera, chronic diarrhea, and dysentery. A splendid stomach remedy, useful in dyspepsia and improves the appetite. Good for rheumatism and pulmonary consumption.

COLTSFOOT
(Root and leaves)

Botanical Name: Tussilago farfara. Common Names: Bullsfoot, horsehoof, butter, British tobacco, folesfoot, flower velure, coughwort, ginger root. Medicinal Properties: Emolient, demulcent, expectorant, pectoral, diaphoretic, tonic.

Is an excellent remedy for catarrh, consumption, and all lung troubles. It is very soothing to the mucous membranes. Good results are obtained when a tea is made by steeping a heaping tablespoonful in a quart of water, and using as a fomentation, or just moisten a cloth in the tea and apply to the lung and throat. Is excellent to relieve the chest of phlegm in all coughs, asthma, bronchitis, whooping cough, and spasmodic cough. Is good for inflammations and swellings, piles, stomach troubles, and ague or fever. The powdered leaves snuffed up the nostrils are excellent for nasal obstruction and headache. For scrofula or scrofulous tumors, take internally or make a poultice and apply externally. Coltsfoot has been much used in cough and lung medicines. It is excellent made into a cough syrup combined with other herbs.

COMFREY
(Root)

Botanical Name: Symphytum officinale. Common Names: Gum plant, healing herb, knitback, slippery root. Medicinal Properties: Demulcent, astringent, pectoral, vulnerary, mucilaginous, styptic, nutritive.

Powerful remedy in coughs, catarrh, ulcerated or inflammation of the lungs, consumption, hemorrhage, excessive expectoration in asthma, and tuberculosis. Very valuable in ulceration of the kidneys, stomach or bowels, or when sore. The best remedy for bloody urine.

Give fomentations wrung out of the strong hot tea in bad bruises, swellings, sprains, fractures, and it will greatly reduce the swelling and relieve the pain. Also give as fomentation in boils.

A poultice of the fresh leaves is excellent for ruptures, sore breasts, fresh wounds, ulcers, white swellings, burns, bruises, and sores. The tea taken internally is useful in scrofula, anemia, dysentery, diarrhea, leucorrhea, and female debility. Has an excellent effect on inward bruises and pains. A poultice of the fresh leaves is excellent for gangrenous sores, gangrene, mortifications, and moist ulcers.

CORAL
(Root)

Botanical Name: Corallorhiza odontorhiza. Common Names: Crawley, chicken's toes, turkey claw, Crawley root, coral root, fever root, scaly dragon's claw, dragon's claw. Medicinal Properties: Febrifuge, sudorific, sedative, diaphoretic.

A most powerful and effective remedy in skin diseases of all kinds, scrofula, scurvy, boils, tumors, fevers, acute erysipelas, cramps, pleurisy, night sweats, and is highly recommended for cancer. Very useful for enlarged veins. Dip a cloth in the tea and apply to boils and tumors. Will produce profuse perspiration, without exciting the system. Especially good in the low stages of fever. Valuable in typhus, and inflammatory diseases. Excellent combined with blue cohosh for scanty or painful menstruation.

CORIANDER
(Seed)

Botanical Name: Coriandrum satium. Common Names: Coliander, coriander seed herb. Medicinal Properties: Aromatic, stomachic, cordial, pungent, carminative.

Coriander is a good stomach tonic, and very strengthening to the heart. Will allay griping caused by other laxatives, and expel wind from the bowels. Good to flavor other unpleasant tasting herbs.

CORN SILK
(Use fresh or dried)

Botanical Name: Zea mays. Common Name: Corn, Indian corn, maize jagnog, Turkish corn. Medicinal Properties: Anodyne, diuretic, demulcent, alterative, lithontryptic.

Corn silk is one of the best remedies for kidney and bladder troubles. Where there is trouble with the prostate gland in urinating, also for painful urination. Useful to prevent bedwetting.

CUBEB BERRIES
(Berries)

Botanical Name: Piper cubeba. Common Names: Java pepper, cubebs, tailed cubebs, tailed pepper. Medicinal Properties: Aromatic, purgative, stimulant, diuretic, antisyphilitic, carminative, stomachic.

Is excellent in chronic bladder troubles, scalding urine, water passage, leucorrhea, gonorrhea, gleet, bronchial troubles, cough, wind colic, gives tone to the stomach and bowels. Heretofore has been used largely for seasoning soups. Increases flow of urine.

DANDELION
(Leaves and root)

Botanical Name: Taraxicum dens-leonis. Common Names: Lion's tooth, swine snout, puff ball, wild endive, priest's crown, white endive. Medicinal Properties: Hepatic, aperient, diuretic, depurative, tonic, stomachic.

Dandelion green has been much used in the same way as spinach or fresh green salad. Dandelion has twenty-eight parts sodium. The natural nutritive salts purify the blood and destroy the acids in the blood. Anemia is caused by the deficiency of nutritive salts in the blood, and really has nothing to do with the quantity of the good blood. Dandelion contains these nutritive salts. It is one of the old well-known remedies. The root is used to increase the flow of urine, and is slightly laxative. It is a splendid remedy for jaundice and skin diseases, scurvy, scrofula, and eczema. Useful in all kinds of kidney trouble, diabetes, dropsy, inflammation of bowels, and fever. Has a beneficial effect on the female organs. Increases the activity of the liver, pancreas, and spleen, especially in enlargement of the liver and spleen. The ground roots make an excellent substitute for coffee.

DILL
(Seed)

Botanical Name: Anethum graveolens. Common Name: Garden dill, dilly. Medicinal Properties: Stomachic, aromatic, stimulant, carminative, diaphoretic.

The leaves and seed have been used in putting up pickles, but pickles should never be introduced into the stomach. Dill has been used to flavor other foods also. Dill is an old-fashioned stomach remedy. It prevents gas and fermentation. It is a splendid remedy for colic in children and can be used in hot milk. Very quieting to the nerves, useful in swellings and pains, and stops hiccoughs.

ECHINACEA

Botanical Name: Brauneria angustifolia. Common Names: Purple cove flower, Sampson root, Kansas niggerhead.

Excellent blood cleanser. For blood poisoning, fevers, carbuncles, boils, peritonitis, syphilitic conditions, bites and stings of poisonous insects or snakes, erysipelas, gangrenous conditions, diphtheria, tonsillitis, pus formations, sores, infections, wounds, gargle for sore throat. An excellent remedy to combine for all these purposes with myrrh. This is powerful to cleanse the morbid matter from the stomach and to expel poisons, toxins, and pus or abscessed formations.

ELECAMPANE

Botanical Name: Inula helenium. Common Name: Scabwort. The root contains the medicinal virtues. Medicinal Properties: Diaphoretic, diuretic, expectorant, aromatic, stimulant, stomachic, astringent, and tonic.

Useful in coughs, asthma, bronchitis. An excellent remedy in tuberculosis, combined with echinacea. It is a stimulant, relaxant, and tonic to the mucous membranes. Warming and strengthening to the lungs, promoting expectoration. A tea of elecampane is useful in whooping cough. It strengthens, cleanses, and tones up the pulmonary and gastric membranes. It can also be used in retention of urine, delayed menstruation, kidney and bladder stones.

FENNEL
(Seed and leaves)

Botanical Name: Foeniculum officinale. Common Names: Large fennel, wild fennel, sweet fennel. Medicinal Properties: Stomachic, carminative, pectoral, diuretic, diaphoretic, aromatic.

Fennel is an old household remedy, also used as a culinary herb. Good for flavoring foods and other medicines. The tea makes an excellent eye wash. Fennel is one of the thoroughly tried remedies for gas, acid stomach, gout, cramps, colic, and spasms. Sprinkled or ground fennel on food will prevent gas in the stomach and bowels. An excellent remedy for small children. For colic, the herb should be steeped and given in small doses every half-hour until the infant or child is relieved. Fennel seed ground and made into a tea is good for snake bites, insect bites, or poison from food. Good for obstruction of liver, spleen and gall, and for yellow jaundice. Excellent for obesity. Increases the flow of urine. Increases the menstrual flow.

FENUGREEK
(Seed)

Botanical Name: Trigonella foenum graecum. Common Name: Foenugreek seed. Medicinal Properties: Mucilaginous, farinaceous.

Excellent made into a poultice for wounds and inflammations. Grind the seed, make into a thick paste, mix with powdered charcoal. The charcoal makes the poultice more effective. Treating ulcers and swellings in this manner will prevent blood poisoning. The tea is an excellent gargle for sore throat. The seed is jelly-like when moistened and has a very cooling effect on the bowels, lubricates the intestines, and is very healing. The tea is excellent taken in fevers. The seed boiled in soybean or nut milk is very nourishing.

FIRE WEED
(Whole plant)

Botanical Name: Eretchites hieracifolius. Common Names: Pilewort, various leaved fleabane. Medicinal Properties: Astringent, tonic, emetic, alterative.

Is strongly astringent; therefore, most excellent in diseases of the mucous membranes, colon troubles, cholera, and dysentery, and will quickly relieve pain in these conditions. Is almost a specific for piles. Very effective for children for summer complaints. It gives prompt relief when taken very hot. Excellent remedy for fevers, as a tonic, and will purify blood.

FIT ROOT
(Root)

Botanical Name: Monotropa uniflora. Common Names: Ice plant, Indian pipe, fit root plant, pipe plant, Dutchman's-pipe, bird's nest plant, ova ova, bird's nest, corpse plant, nest root, convulsion weed. Medicinal Properties: Antispasmodic, nervine, tonic, sedative.

Is splendid in all kinds of fevers. Takes the place of quinine and opium perfectly. An excellent remedy for restlessness, faints, nervous irritability, spasms, and convulsions. Should be used in place of opium and quinine. It will cure intermittent and remittent fevers. Oh, why will not people use this wonderful remedy in place of poisonous drugs? It is efficient and harmless. A teaspoonful of fit root and fennel seed, steeped in a pint of boiling water for twenty minutes is an excellent douche for inflammation of the vagina and uterus, also good used as a wash for sore eyes. A valuable remedy for epilepsy and lockjaw in children, and for spasmodic affections.

FLAXSEED
(Seed)

Botanical Name: Linum usitatissimum. Common Names: Linseed, common flax, winterlien. Medicinal Properties: Demulcent, pectoral, maturating, mucilaginous, emollient.

This is the common flaxseed with which almost everyone is familiar. The ground seed, when mixed with boiling water, makes a thick mush which is excellent for use in poultices. Any herb may be added for this purpose, such as smart-weed, alum bark, granulated hops, mullein, or any of the other herbs recommended for use in poultices. These herbs mixed and used as a poultice with flaxseed make one of the best poultices for all kinds of old sores, boils, carbuncles, inflammations, and tumors. The oil from flaxseed is good for coughs, asthma, and pleurisy.

FLEABANE

Botanical Name: Erigeron canadense: Common Names: Canada fleabane, horse tail, cow's tail, horse weed, pride weed, colt's tail, fire weed, mare's tail, scabious, blood staunch, butter weed. Medicinal Properties: Styptic, astringent, diuretic, tonic.

Excellent for cholera, dysentery, and summer complaint, especially for children, when all other remedies fail. In these affections, use as an enema. Steep a teaspoonful in a quart of boiling water for twenty minutes, use hot, about 112° to 115° F. See Enema in Table on Contents. This is an excellent remedy for all colon troubles. Can be improved by taking equal parts of white oak bark, wild alum root, and catnip. Taken internally it is very reliable for bladder troubles, scalding urine, and hemorrhages from the bowels and uterus. Good for consumption.

GIANT SOLOMON SEAL
(Root)

Botanical Name: Convallaria multiflora. Common Names: Drop berry, sealwort, seal root. Medicinal Properties: Tonic, mucilaginous, astringent, emetic, pectoral.

Useful in chest affections, female debility, inflammation of the stomach and intestine, erysipelas, neuralgia. Will allay vomiting. Helpful in ruptures, taken internally and applied externally as a poultice. Helpful in broken bones. Will disperse congealed blood caused from blows and bruises. Removes black and blue marks, and eases pain caused from blows. Apply by poultice.

GENTIAN ROOT

Botanical Name: Gentiana lutea. Common Names: Bitterroot, bitterwort, gentian, yellow gentian, pale gentian, felwort, gentian root. Medicinal Properties: Stomachic, tonic, anthelmintic, antibilious.

A most effective and reliable tonic. Purifies the blood. Good for liver complaints and dysentery. Most effective for jaundice. Excellent for the spleen. Gentian root will improve the appetite, strengthen the digestive organs, increase the circulation, is beneficial to the female organs, and invigorates the entire system. Useful in fevers, colds, gout, convulsions, scrofula, and dyspepsia. It will expel worms. Excellent in suppressed menstruation and scanty urine. Because of its bitterness, it is better to combine gentian root with some aromatic herb. It is more effective than quinine. Allays poison from mad dog, insect, and snake bites.

GINGER

Botanical Name: Zingiber officinale. Common Names: Black ginger, race ginger, African ginger. Medicinal Properties: Stimulant, pungent, carminative, aromatic, sialagogue, condiment. When taken hot, is diaphoretic.

Taken hot, ginger is excellent for suppressed menstruation. A little of the root chewed stimulates the salivary glands and is very useful in paralysis of the tongue, also good for sore throat. Prevents griping, good for diarrhea, colds, la grippe, chronic bronchitis, dyspepsia, gas, and fermentation, cholera, gout, and nausea when combined with stronger laxative herbs.

GINSENG

Botanical Name: Panax quinquefolia. Common Names: Five fingers' root, American ginseng, ninsin, red berry, garantogen, sang. Medicinal Properties: Demulcent, stomachic, slightly stimulant.

Ginseng is very much used in hot, moist climates as a preventive against all manner of illnesses, and is also used in severe diseases of all types. Promotes appetite, and is useful in digestive disturbances. Flavored with any flavoring you like makes an agreeable and very effective drink for colds, chest troubles, and coughs. If taken when hot, will produce perspiration. It is also good for stomach troubles and constipation. Has been much used in lung troubles and inflammation of the urinary tract.

GOLD THREAD
(Root)

Botanical Name: Coptis trifolia. Common Names: Yellow root, mouth root, canker root. Medicinal Properties: Tonic.

Excellent for digestion. A well-tried remedy for canker in the mouth and stomach, ulcers of both stomach and throat, and inflammation of the stomach in dyspepsia.

Effective to destroy the desire for strong drinks. Especially beneficial and effective when used in combination with golden seal in ulcers and cancerous affections of the stomach.

GOLDEN SEAL
(Root)

Botanical Name: Hydrastis canadensis. Common Names: Yellow paint root, orange root, yellow puccoon, ground raspberry, eye root, yellow Indian paint, Indian plant, tumeric root, Ohio curcuma, eye balm, yellow eye, jaundice root. Medicinal Properties: Laxative, tonic, alterative, detergent, opthalmicum, antiperiodic, aperient, diuretic, antiseptic, deobstruent.

This is one of the most wonderful remedies in the entire herb kingdom. When it is considered all that can be accomplished by its use, and what it actually will do, it does seem like a real cure-all.

It is one of the best substitutes for quinine, is a most excellent remedy for colds, la grippe, and all kinds of stomach and liver troubles. It exerts a special influence on all the mucous membranes and tissues with which it comes in contact. For open sores, inflammations, eczema, ringworm, erysipelas, or any skin disease, golden seal excels. Golden seal tea is made by steeping one teaspoonful in a pint of boiling water for twenty minutes and used as a wash, then after the place is thoroughly clean (It is well to use peroxide of hydrogen also for cleansing.) sprinkle some of the powdered root and cover. Taken in small but frequent doses, it will allay nausea during pregnancy. Steep a teaspoonful in a pint of boiling water for twenty minutes, stir well, let settle, and pour off the liquid. Take six tablespoonfuls a day. It equalizes the circulation and combined with scullcap and red pepper (cayenne) will greatly relieve and strengthen the heart. It has no superior when combined with myrrh, one part golden seal to one-fourth myrrh for ulcerated stomach, duodenum, dyspepsia, and is especially good for enlarged tonsils and sores in the mouth. Smoker's sores, caused by holding a pipe in the mouth, will heal after just a few applications of the powder to the sore. I have used it in a number of cases that were called "skin cancers" with excellent results.

It is an excellent remedy for diphtheria, tonsillitis, and other serious throat troubles, and has a good effect combined with a little myrrh and cayenne. Excellent for chronic catarrh of the intestines and all catarrhal conditions. Will improve appetite and aid digestion. Combined with scullcap and hops, it is a very fine tonic for spinal nerves; is very good in spinal meningitis. Very useful in all skin eruptions, scarlet fever, and smallpox.

To cure pyorrhea or sore gums, put a little of the tea in a cup, dip the toothbrush in it, and thoroughly brush the teeth and gums. The results will be most satisfactory. In any nose trouble, pour some tea in the hollow of the hand and snuff up the nose. Very useful in typhoid fever, gonorrhea, leucorrea and syphilis. For bladder troubles, it should be injected into the bladder immediately after the bladder had been emptied, and retained as long as possible, repeating two or three times a day. I do not recommend that individuals do this for themselves unless experienced. Have a physician or nurse inject it for you with a rubber catheter.

Golden seal combined with alum root, taken internally, is an excellent remedy for bowel and bladder troubles. Use two parts of golden seal and one part wild alum. This is a laxative. Good for piles, hemorrhoids, and prostate gland. When combined with equal parts of red clover blossoms, yellow dock, and dandelion it has a wonderful effect on the gall bladder, liver, pancreas, spleen, and kidneys. Combined with peach leaves, queen of the meadow, cleavers and corn silk, it is a reliable remedy for Bright's disease and diabetes. Golden seal is excellent for the eyes. The following is the way the writer uses it for the eyes: Steep a small teaspoonful of golden seal and one of boric acid in a pint of boiling water, stir thoroughly, let cool, and pour liquid off. Put a tablespoonful of this liquid in a half cup of water. Bathe the eyes with this, using an eye cup, or drop it in with an eye dropper. If the eyelids are granulated or there is film over the eyes, add one teaspoonful burnt alum powder. If you use it a little too strong, there is no harm done; it will only smart a little. Golden seal may be taken in different ways, and may be used alone in all cases given above where it is suggested to combine with others. Take one-fourth teaspoonful of golden seal dissolved in a glass of hot water immediately upon arising, a glass one hour before noon and evening meal. Or you may steep a teaspoonful in a pint of boiling water, stir thoroughly, let cool, pour liquid off and take a tablespoonful four to six times a day. Children should take less of all doses according to age.

There are many remedies much advertised as containing golden seal, but the fact is, there is so little golden seal in the preparations, that it does very little good, as it is very expensive.

Chronic catarrh of the intestines, even to the extent of ulceration, is greatly benefited by golden seal. Golden seal produced healing in ulceration of the mucous lining of the rectum, effectual in hemorrhage of the rectum. Is a remedy for chronic and intermittent malarial poisoning or enlarged spleen of malarial origin. From above it will be seen how applicable golden seal is in all catarrhal conditions, whether of the throat, nasal passages, bronchial tubes, intestines, stomach, bladder, or wherever there is a lining of mucous membrane. It kills poisons.

HEMP (See Indian Hemp)

HENNA LEAVES
(Root and leaves)

Botanical Name: Lawsonia inermis. Common Names: Jamaica mignonette, Egyptian privet, alcanna, henna plant. Medicinal Properties: Root: Astringent; Bark: Dyeing.

The leaves can be used internally or externally for jaundice, leprosy, and other infections of the skin.

HOLY THISTLE
(Plant)

Botanical Name: 'Centaura benedicta. Common Names: Bitter thistle, blessed cardus, spotted thistle. Medicinal Properties: Diaphoretic, emetic, tonic, stimulant, febrifuge.

This plant has very great power in the purification and circulation of the blood. It is very effective for dropsy, strengthens the heart, and is good for the liver, lungs, and kidneys. It is soothing to the brain, strengthens the memory, and clears the system of bad humors, and is effective for insanity. It is a good tonic for girls entering womanhood. It is claimed that the warm tea given to mothers will produce a free supply of milk.

It is such a good blood purifier that by drinking a cup of tea twice a day it will cure chronic headaches. Some have called it "blessed thistle" on account of its excellent qualities. About two ounces of the dried plant simmered in a quart of water for two hours makes a tea satisfactory for most purposes. This tea is best taken at bed time as a preventive of disease and it will cause profuse perspiration. Holy thistle is a plant which has been used for centuries. It is very good combined with any of the dock roots (red dock, yellow dock or burdock).

HOPS
(Flowered)

Botanical Name: Humulus lupulus. Medicinal Properties: Febrifuge, tonic, nervine, diuretic, anodyne, hypnotic, anthelmintic, sedative.

Hops is an old-fashioned and very useful remedy. An excellent nervine. Will produce sleep when nothing else will. Two or three cups should be taken hot. Valuable in delirium tremens. Is a good remedy for toothache, earache, neuralgia, and like ailments. Will tone up the liver, increase the flow of urine, and increase the flow of bile, and is good for excessive sexual desires and gonorrhea. Put a tablespoonful in a pint of water, simmer for ten minutes. Drink a half pint morning and evening. A pillow stuffed with hops has long been used to produce sleep and is very effective. Good in diseases of the chest and throat. Hop poultices are very effective for inflammation, boils, tumors, painful swellings, and old ulcers.

HOREHOUND
(Plant)

Botanical Name: Marrubium vulgare: Common Names: Horehound, white horehound. Medicinal Properties: Pectoral, aromatic, diaphoretic, tonic, expectorant, diuretic, hepatic stimulant.

Horehound will produce profuse perspiration when taken hot. Taken in large doses, it is a laxative. When taken cold, is good for dyspepsia, jaundice, asthma, hysteria, and will expel worms. Very useful in chronic sore throat, coughs, consumption, and all pulmonary infections. If the menses stop abnormally, it will bring them back. Horehound is one of the old-fashioned remedies and should be in every home ready for immediate use. Horehound syrup is excellent for asthma and difficult breathing. For children in coughs or croup, steep a heaping tablespoonful in a pint of boiling water for twenty minutes, strain, add honey, and let them take freely.

HYDRANGEA
(Root and leaves)

Botanical Name: Hydrangea aborescens. Common Names: Wild hydrangea, seven barks. Medicinal Properties: Root: Diuretic, lithrontryptic. Leaves: Tonic, diuretic, sialagogue, cathartic.

An old remedy. Valuable in bladder troubles. Will remove bladder stones and will remove the pains caused by the stones, brick, and dust in the bladder. Will relieve backache caused by kidney troubles. Good for chronic rheumatism, paralysis, scurvy, and dropsy.

HYSSOP
(Whole plant)

Botanical Name: Hyssopus officinalis. Medicinal Properties: Aromatic, sudorific, pectoral, expectorant, febrifuge, anthelmintic, aperient.

Hyssop is an old Bible remedy. David knew the benefits to be derived from its use. He drew the most wonderful lessons from it, which he used in showing the cleansing of the body from sin, for he said "Purge me with hyssop, and I shall be clean; wash me, and I shall be whiter than snow." (Psalms 51:7) Hyssop, in connection with the proper use of water and deep breathing, is a most wonderful body cleanser.

Valuable in quinsy, asthma, colds, la grippe, and all chest affections. Loosens phlegm in the lungs and throat. Is excellent for children and infant's diseases, such as sore throat and quinsy. Can be applied as a compress and used as a gargle. In fevers, give a glassful every hour of a tea made by simmering a tablespoonful of the herb in a pint of boiling water for ten minutes. It will start perspiration, relieve the kidneys and bladder, and is slightly laxative. Hyssop increases the circulation of the blood and will reduce blood pressure. Excellent blood regulator and is a fine tonic when the system is in a weakened condition. It is excellent for scrofula, gravel, and various stomach troubles, jaundice, dropsy, and for the spleen. It has a splendid effect on the mucous lining of the stomach and bowels. It is good for cough and shortness of breath. A fine remedy for epilepsy and fits in connection with other hygienic measures. It will expel worms. The leaves applied to inflammations and bruises remove the pain and discoloration. Effective for insect stings and bites. Kills body lice.

Soak the herb fifteen minutes in boiling water and place in a cloth for use as a poultice.

Hyssop is good for intermittent fever and other fevers. Hyssop tea is an excellent remedy for eye trouble. It should be used in an eye cup.

For general use, steep a heaping teaspoonful to a cup of boiling water for twenty minutes. Take from one to three cups a day, a large swallow at a time. Children less according to age.

INDIAN HEMP
(Root)

Botanical Name: Pilocorpus selloanus. Common Name: Brazilian jaborandi root. Medicinal Properties: Stimulant, expectorant, sialagogue, antivenomous.

This is excellent for breaking up colds, for rheumatism, influenza, Bright's disease. It causes profuse perspiration. Effective in various fevers, in diabetes, dropsy, pleurisy, catarrh, and jaundice. An excellent remedy for mumps, taken internally as a tea, and applied externally as a fomentation or poultice to reduce the swelling. Fold the cloth three or four thicknesses and dip in the hot tea and apply. Very effective in asthma and diphtheria. It will stop hiccoughs. Excellent to stimulate the growth of the hair. Dip the fingers in tea made of the leaves several times a day and massage the scalp thoroughly.

JUNIPER BERRIES
(Bark and berries)

Botanical Name: Juniperus communis. Common Names: Juniper bush, juniper bark. Medicinal Properties: Diuretic.

This is very effective as a tea for kidney, urinary, and bladder trouble, and catarrh of the bladder, gleet, leucorrhea, gonorrhea, scorbutic diseases, and dropsy. For leucorrhea, it may be combined with the other herbs as a douche. For most purposes, Juniper berries are most effective used in combination with such herbs as broom, uva ursi, cleavers, and buchu.

Juniper berries are excellent as a spray or fumigation of a room in which there has been a patient with an infectious disease, as it thoroughly destroys all fungi.

They are excellent as a preventive of disease, and the berries should be chewed or a strong tea used to gargle the throat when exposed to contagious diseases.

LAVENDER
(Plant)

Botanical Name: Lavandula vera. Common Names: Garden lavender, spike lavender, common lavender. Medicinal Properties: Stimulant, aromatic, and fragrant.

A tea steeped from the flowers is tonic, prevents fainting, and allays nausea. Excellent combined with other herbs to overcome their taste. The flowers are also used in making perfumes. The dried flowers and leaves are used to put in drawers and linen closets. Sometimes used to keep moths from clothing and fur. Leaves are used as a culinary herb for seasoning.

LILY OF THE VALLEY
(Root)

Botanical Name: Convallaria majalis. Common Name: May lily. Medicinal Properties: Sweet and mucilaginous.

Very quieting to the heart, good for the heart generally. Useful in epilepsy, vertigo, and convulsions of all kinds. Good for palsy and apoplexy. Strengthens the brain, makes the thoughts clearer.

Removes dizziness from the head. Extremely useful in dropsy.

Dose: Take same as other herbs. (See Herbs in Table of Contents.)

LOBELIA
(Plant and seed)

Botanical Name: Lobelia inflata. Common Names: Bladder podded lobelia, wild tobacco, emetic herb, emetic weed, lobelia herb, puke weed, asthma weed, gag root, eye-bright, vomit wort. Medicinal Properties: Emetic, expectorant, diuretic, nervine, diaphoretic, antispasmodic.

Lobelia is the most powerful relaxant known among herbs that have no harmful effects. Lobelia acts differently upon different people, but it will not hurt anyone. It makes the pulse fuller and softer in cases of inflammation and fever. Lobelia reduces palpitation of the heart. It is fine in the treatment of all fevers and in pneumonia, meningitis, pleurisy, hepasitis, peritonitis, phrenitis, nephritis, and perositis. Lobelia alone cannot cure, but it is very beneficial if given in connection with other measures, as an enema of catnip infusion morning and evening. The enema should be given even if the patient is delirious. It will relieve the brain. Pleurisy root is a specific remedy for pleurisy, but it is excellent if combined with lobelia for its relaxing properties. The use of lobelia in fevers is beyond any other remedy. It is excellent for very nervous patients. Poultices of hot fomentation of lobelia are good in external inflammations such as rheumatism, etc. It is excellent to add lobelia to poultices for abcesses, boils, and carbuncles. Use one-third lobelia to two-thirds slippery elm bark or the same proportion to any other herb you are using.

While lobelia is an excellent emetic, it is a strange fact that given in small doses for irritable stomach, it will stop spasmodic vomiting. In cases of asthma, give a lobelia pack, followed the next morning by an emetic. The pack will loosen the waste material, and it will be cast out with the emetic. In bad cases, where the liver is affected and the skin yellow, combine equal parts of pleurisy root, catnip, and bitter root. Steep a teaspoonful in a cup of boiling water. Give two tablespoonfuls every two hours, hot. For hydrophobia, steep a tablespoonful of lobelia in a pint of boiling water, drinking as much as possible to induce vomiting. This will clean the stomach out; then give a high enema. This treatment should be given immediately after the person is attacked. Lobelia is excellent for whooping cough. (For this purpose look in the Table of Contents under "Whooping Cough.") There is nothing that will as quickly clear the air passages of the lungs as lobelia. A tincture made as follows will stop difficult breathing and clear the air passages of the lungs, if taken a tablespoonful at a time:

Lobelia herb	2 ounces
Crushed lobelia seed	2 ounces
Apple vinegar	1 pint

Soak for two weeks in a well-stoppered bottle, shaking every day. Strain and it is ready for use. This is also good to use as an external application, rubbing between the shoulders and chest in asthma. Lobelia poultice is excellent for sprains, felons, bruises, ringworm, erysipelas, stings of insects, and poison ivy.

LOBELIA (Lobelia inflata)

"This plant is also called emetic weed, and India tobacco. Do not suppose, however, that tobacco and lobelia are one and the same thing. All species of this plant are common in North America, and several are to be found in England. It is a very pretty little plant, having blue, or it may be, red, flowers. When ripe, the flowers change into small pods containing numerous black or dark brown seeds. The plant grows to from six to twenty inches high. It is an annual in warm latitudes, but bi-annual in moderate and northern latitudes. It blooms from July to September. It prefers meadows, pastures, and other grassy places.

"There has been a great deal of opposition to this herb, mainly by the allopaths. These people say that it is a poison. We are reminded of a challenge which was once given to an allopath, the conditions of which were, that the challenger was to take all the lobelia that the allopath was inclined to give him, if the allopath, on his part, was inclined to take as much strychnine. The challenge was never accepted. Lobelia is not a poison.

"Lobelia acts differently upon different people, causing in some cases alarming symptoms. It will, however, never hurt anyone, but it should not be given before a stimulant has been administered. A big, strong man may take lobelia without a stimulant, but in ninety-nine cases out of a hundred a stimulant should be first administered. To Dr. Samuel Thompson is due the credit of first clearly defining the action of this remedy. He learned its value solely from personal observation and experiment. It is the most powerful relaxant known of those that have no bad or harmful effects. The seeds are twice as relaxing as the herb: but do not use the seed in preference to the herb, as splendid results may be obtained from the use of the herb. It may be given in either small or large doses, at shorter or longer intervals, without any fear whatever of harm being done. The blood vessels are relieved from undue tension, and the circulation thereby materially equalized. It makes the pulse fuller and softer, whether the case be one of inflammation or fever. We note that the difference between these two terms is just simply that the former is local and the latter systemic. (The word 'inflammation' is this: an increased flow of blood in and through a part.) Lobelia reduces the excitability of the heart. In cases of angina pectoris or when the heart is in an excitable condition, lobelia compound is the one thing required. Allopathy has nothing like it.

"Lobelia is fitted for the treatment of all fevers, such as phrenitis, meningitis, pneumonia, pleurisy, hepatitis, peritonitis, nephritis, periostitis. Let us consider these conditions separately: The terminal 'itis' in all these names means fever-inflammation. Phrenitis: In this case lobelia must not be given with the idea of curing by that alone. Give first of all, morning, noon, and night, an infusion of catnip to the bowels, which of itself will do wonders to relieve the brain. This may be administered even when the patient is delirious. Give lobelia in small quantities as the case may require, but clean out the waste material and relieve the locked-up condition of the body which is causing the trouble. The thought is this—clean out, clean up, and keep clean. Meningitis (or spotted fever): The main treatment is lobelia with catnip injection, for relieving the congested condition of the vertebral arteries. The allopath does nothing to clean out this waste material. He merely gives morphine and other opiates to relieve the pain. Pneumonia: This system of medicine has done wonders in the treatment and cure of pneumonia. Allopaths lose 50 per cent of their cases, many of whom would recover were it not for their maltreatment. Use the following treatment: First, give a large injection of catnip—there may be a temperature of from 103° to 105° F., and the patient hardly able to bear the weight of the bedclothes—and as soon as the patient is quieted down by this injection, give a stomach treatment, if he can stand it. With several cupfuls of the warm, stimulating tea in the stomach, the blood, instead of going to the lungs and staying there, will be kept circulating, and the treatment will thus prevent the dreaded stage of congestion. After this stomach treatment, put a wet pack (cold and sopping wet) on the back and chest, and wrap the patient up in a heavy woolen blanket. Do it quickly. In about ten or fifteen minutes' time, give him a small dose of medicine appropriate to the condition, or a small dose of hot lemonade, and repeat this dose every ten or fifteen minutes. In about an hour and a half or two hours time, there will be a profuse perspiration. When the towels are taken off, they will be so hot and steaming as to give the idea that they have just been taken out of the hot water. When the pack is removed, rub the patient dry; have a bowl of cold water ready, and with this, wash the body quickly with the bare hands; dry thoroughly, and put on a clean bed-dress. It will then be seen that the temperature has been materially reduced. Pleurisy: Pleurisy root is a specific for this condition; combine lobelia with it for its relaxing effect. Use pleurisy root, catnip, and some of the myrica compound, as a mixture, in conjunction with the use of the pack as mentioned when dealing with pneumonia, and the pleurisy will be cured in grand style. Hepatitis (inflammation of the liver): Pack the patient in the region of the liver; the condition calls for water. Put on cold packs, which are the things to relieve the inflammation. Then give something to act on the liver. The same principles of treatment apply in cases of peritonitis, nephritis, etc. They all come under the same head, and the same treatment is applicable in every case.

"The use of lobelia in fever is beyond any other remedy that has ever been introduced to the notice of the profession, and that without reference to its emetic action. For a very nervous patient, take some of this lobelia seed, mix it up with a little syrup into a hard mass, and give a small pill of it two or three times a day, and that nervous condition will be wonderfully relieved, providing that relaxation is needed.

"Local applications of lobelia are good in external inflammation, such as rheumatism; give the injection of catnip with stomach treatment, and cold packs where needed, and a cure will result. Lobelia may be made into poultices for boils, abscesses, etc., combined with powdered slippery elm bark thus: One-third lobelia seed, two-thirds slippery elm bark.

"Notwithstanding what has been said of lobelia as an emetic, it is a striking fact that when it is given in small doses in cases of irritable stomachs, it arrests spasmodic or sympathetic vomiting. It is emphatically the grandest remedy, with varied qualities, in the Botanic Pharmacopoeia. For asthmatic cases, put on a pack the first day, and the next morning, on an empty stomach, give the stomach treatment. The pack loosens up all the waste material, and by the emetic next morning it is cast out of the system. In a very bad case, where the liver is affected, and the skin is very sallow and yellow, then give on the first day, of equal parts of powdered lobelia, catnip, bitter root, and pleurisy root, one teaspoonful infused in a cupful of boiling water, one-fourth, of the cupful every two hours, but, after the first dose, fill up the cup so as to get five doses in all from the infusion.

"Lobelia is a good thing in hydrophobia. Don't have your patients pasteurized. Go to work at once and give the sufferer a thoroughly stimulating emetic and get the poison cleaned out. Don't attempt to compromise or temporise.

"Besides being a splendid agent for asthma, lobelia is also good for whooping cough. In the latter case, prohibit all starchy foods, and put the child exclusively upon fruits, nuts, and vegetables. Do not allow even brown bread, as that is too starchy. The fruit, nut, and vegetable diet, with lean lamb, mutton, and beef, is the best. The three best nuts are the walnut, the Brazil nut, and the pecan nut, because of the oil they contain. For this reason, also, they are very good for consumptive patients.

"The 'alarming stage' of lobelia, sometimes spoken of, need not alarm at all. Just simply go ahead, giving the patient more stimulation. Here is a compound which will prove very useful:

LOBELIA COMPOUND

Lobelia Seed	1 lb.
Ladies' Slipper	¾ lb.
Capsicum	¼ lb.

"Exhaust this mixture with 80 per cent alcohol, making half a gallon. The uses of this compound are many. For a cough, put two drachms into a 4-oz. bottle, and fill the bottle with syrup. Dose: One teaspoonful as needed. This compound may be put into liniment if it is desired. No gum myrrh is needed for this purpose. All that gum myrrh is needed for, because of its antiseptic qualities, is diptheria in the malignant condition.

"For angina pectoris, put one drachm (teaspoonful) of the compound into a cup of water, and give teaspoonful doses every minute. For a person who has sustained a profound shock, lobelia compound is the remedy to give.

"HOW TO GIVE A THOROUGH THOMPSONIAN EMETIC: Procure three enamelled pitchers, or jugs—

teapots or coffeepots are the best because they have covers to them and retain the heat—and put into the one on the right hand one ounce of peppermint (This is in case of an irritable stomach; but in the case of nervousness, employ catnip instead.), and call this 'No. 1'; put into the middle vessel one heaping teaspoonful of the myrica compound, and call this 'No. 2'; into the vessel on the left put one ounce of lobelia herb, and call this 'No. 3.' Pour onto these about three pints of boiling water for the myrica compound and the peppermint, and a good quart for the lobelia herb. Stir them, and cover up immediately; let them steep. If time is pressing, five or ten minutes will do, but fifteen, or twenty minutes will be so much the better. Besides a cup and saucer, and a very fine strainer, have a cold jug of water handy, for cooling the tea, if too hot; also a bowl of sugar, if the patient should prefer the tea sweetened. Provide the patient with a towel and large bowl. Now give a cupful of No. 1, then a cup of No. 2, then a cup of No. 1, and again a cup of No. 2, then a cup of No. 3. You have thus given four cups of stimulation to one of relaxation. (It frequently happens, in cases of irritated stomachs, that when the peppermint and the myrica have been received, vomiting occurs. Don't be alarmed, but if this should happen two or three times, give the lobelia, and that will stop it.) Then give a cup of No. 2, followed by a cup of No. 1, then a cup of No. 3. This makes eight cups—six of stimulation and two of relaxation. Usually vomiting ensues at this point; perhaps part, or it may be, the whole of the teas will return. Usually, however, about half the quantity taken is returned, which is best. Then give cups of Nos. 1, 2, 3 in turn. If a little vomit follows, all right. Repeat the last procedure, which will be followed by another vomit. The idea is to get the patient to vomit at least three times. Now, supposing that the patient when he vomits brings up blood. Don't get worried, but for subsequent teas use raspberry leaves instead of catnip or peppermint, and make the myrica compound a little stronger by adding more cayenne. Tell the patient that he may have a gastric ulcer, and when these remedies are taken they will cleanse the ulcer and, of course, it naturally bleeds. If it is not that, it means that the walls of the stomach are so relaxed as to bleed easily, and myrica compound will stimulate and astringe them.

"What is the emetic good for? Is it simply to clean out the stomach? No; it has an extensive physiological influence. It does not simply go into the stomach, stay there a while, and then be vomited out; but it cleans the mucus from the lining of the stomach, and, if there is bile brings it away, and so enables the stomach to perform its functions. This stomach treatment washes the blood, washes out the accumulations of unassimilated material from the entire system, and restores the tissues to a more normal condition.

"Note—There are many conditions under which this treatment ought not to be administered, and this part of the Lectures is given for information but not for domestic use. None but an experienced Botanic Practitioner, who is qualified to judge of the suitability of the conditions of the patient, should undertake the use of the treatment." —*Standard Guide to Non-poisonous Herbal Medicine,* pp. 102, 103, 104, 105, 106, 107.

NUMBER 1, THE EMETIC—LOBELIA

1. The powdered leaves and pods. This is the most common form of using it; and from half to a teaspoonful may be taken in warm water, sweetened: or the same quantity

may be added either of the other numbers when taken to cleanse the stomach, overpower a cold, and promote a free perspiration.

2. A tincture made from the green herb. This is used to counteract the effects of poison (taken either internally or applied externally) and for asthma and other complaints of the lungs. For a dose add a grain or two of capsicum in a half teacupful of warm water, sweetened, and in all cases of nerve affection add half a teaspoonful of nerve powder. For the external effects of poison, take the above dose with the tincture, and bathe the parts affected, repeating until relieved.

3. The seeds reduced to a fine powder and mixed with Nos. 2-6 is for the most violent attacks of spasms and other complaints, such as lockjaw, bite of dog with hydrophobia, fits, and in all cases of suspended animation, where the vital spark is nearly extinct. For a dose, give a teaspoonful, and repeat until relief is obtained; then follow with tea made of No. 3 for canker.

For children, the dose must be regulated according to their age. If very young, steep a dose of the powder in half a teacupful of warm water, or in a tea of raspberry leaves, and give a teaspoonful of the tea at a time. First strain through a cloth, and sweeten. Repeat the dose every fifteen minutes until it operates. Give pennyroyal or other herb tea, for a drink.

4. Tablets may be substituted for the herb. Use ten to fifteen grains in half a cup of warm water every fifteen minutes until the stomach has been completely relieved of all its contents.

Lobelia will do quickly all that the stomach pump can do, do it as efficiently, and with better results.

LOBELIA

According to Drs. Thompson, Scudder, Lyle, Greer, Stephens, and modern physicians.

"Lobelia is indicated when the pulse is full and oppressed, or small and feeble, oppression in the precordium, labored action of the heart, cardiac (heart) pain, oppression of the chest with difficult and labored respiration and the accumulation of mucus in the bronchial tubes.

"Lobelia is a specific in most cases of angina pectoris and neuralgia of the heart. It is the indicated remedy when the patient complains of oppressions in the chest and difficult breathing. It is the remedy in laryngitis in both children and adults. It is directly indicated in all conditions where there is a morbid congestion of the mucous membranes. Lobelia is one of the most direct and valuable stimulants to the sympathetic nervous system, and it favorably influences every organ and function supplied or controlled by these nerves.

"When there is lack of power, lobelia is always indicated.

"Lobelia is dual in its activity. It is a relaxant, and it is a stimulant. In small doses it stimulates. In large doses it relaxes and must be followed by a stimulant such as capsicum.

"In all conditions of congestions, wherever they may be, lobelia due to its influence on the blood vessels, lessens the depression through the vaso-motor and strengthens the muscular action of the vessel walls which propel the blood onward overcoming the condition.

"In asthma, from any cause, lobelia will be found invaluable, because the condition is due to vaso-motor inefficiency in all cases.

"For spasms in children, lobelia is the ideal remedy. It will give quick relief, after which the cause must be sought and relieved by the indicated remedies.

"In whooping cough, false heart spasms, spasmodic coughs, and many forms of asthma, it is the ideal remedy.

"Lobelia is a powerful antispasmodic, acting on the nerve centers and respiratory centers, thereby improving oxygenation of the blood.

"In the convulsions of childhood, as in all other forms of convulsion, it should be the first remedy given.

"In pneumonia and all other conditions of the congestions of the lungs, when breathing is difficult and painful, the pulse rapid, and the expression of the countenance drawn, lobelia is the first remedy to be given to induce relaxation and equalize the circulation of the blood, thereby removing the congestions.

"On the contrary, when the circulation is feeble, the extremities cold, face palid, and there is oppression, it is equally efficient to restore normalcy.

"In all cases of zymotic inner filth diseases such as scarlet fever, chickenpox, measles, and smallpox, it is of supreme importance. First in a large dose to cleanse the stomach of poisonous matter, then in conjunction with other remedies to cleanse the entire system of congestion and establish equilibrium.

"Lobelia acts directly upon the regulating centers of the system (thus its influence to establish equilibrium), those of heat, the circulation, nervous system, and digestive organism. It supports the heart, overcomes excessive blood pressure in any portion of the body, and restores interaction between the functions of the various organs.

"Lobelia is a restorative to the nerve force at the several centers, acts directly upon the heart and the lungs, restores the resisting potency of every center to the invasion of disease, and establishes harmony between the nervous and circulatory systems.

"When the heart is weak, lobelia is a restorative, and following its use the pulse becomes strong and natural.

"In the dreaded diphtheria, lobelia hypodermically given is of greater potency and in every sense far more valuable, not to mention being more natural, than any serum ever devised.

"In all bronchial difficulties, whether asthma, croup or pneumonia, lobelia should be given in a relaxant dose— sufficient to cause free vomiting and thus cleanse the stomach, and then be given as part of the after-treatment.

"In epilepsy and all other contractive ailments, Lobelia should be given in doses large enough to cleanse the stomach and relax the system and be followed by corrective treatment. Spasms, whether of the chest, spine, muscles or sex organisms should be treated in the same manner.

"In many forms of digestive disturbances, lobelia is an ideal remedy. This is especially true in nervous dyspepsia, where there is a feeling more of nausea than of pain, an oppressive feeling, like a dead weight, after eating. Also in those conditions where there is a feeling of coldness or a faintness at the pit of the stomach. In such conditions, a few grains of lobelia and an equal amount of capsicum (tablet form) may be taken directly after eating. In acute indigestion, a condition which has killed countless people, and where the verdict has nearly always been heart failure, lobelia, given in a dose sufficiently large to properly empty the stomach, will hardly, if ever, fail. It is the one agent that one may safely rely upon. It should always be followed by a stimulant and nervine.

"Lobelia is essential in labor. It will allay and regulate the violent pains in the loins during labor, which are due to rigidity of the passages, and is far safer and much to be preferred to ergot or other agents generally employed.

"In disorders of the menstrual period, it is, with the addition of such agents as pennyroyal, the ideal agent to relieve contraction and pain, and to establish normalcy.

"In hysteria, whether due to congested ovaries, swollen uterus or other cause, lobelia with nervines, may be safely relied upon to bring relief.

"IMPORTANT—Whether Lobelia is given in the powdered, tinctural or tablet form, it is always to be remembered that the full dose should be given at once. If emesis does not occur promptly, follow with slightly warm water every five minutes until there is free vomiting. This plan is followed in all cases where emptying of the stomach and relaxation is desired, as in spasms, congestions, fits, and infectious diseases. As soon as the vomiting ceases, stimulants and nervines must be given.

"When stimulation is desired, then the dose is always small—from one to five grains in conjunction with a stimulant such as capsicum.

"EXTERNAL APPLICATION—In all cases where an external compress or plaster is indicated, as in pneumonia, pleurisy, boils, and acute swellings, a compress may be made with hops and lobelia herb, or bran and lobelia herb, or a plaster with lard and lobelia herb. In each case these are to be applied as hot as the patient can comfortably bear and changed as they become cold."—*The Medicines of Nature,* pp. 65, 66, 67, 68, 69.

LOBELIA INFLATA: The herb and seeds of this plant are largely used by all herbal practitioners. It is employed in quite a number of cases and has won a richly deserved place in the annals of herbal writers. To Dr. Samuel Thompson is due the credit of first bringing this article into real use. It had, no doubt, been used to produce emesis in some localities previously, but its great uses were made known by him.

So successfully did he use it that the regulars of his day classed it a poison, as some writers said only a poison could bring about the speedy results that Thompson obtained by its use. If the student goes to buy an ounce package of the herb from the drugstore, he will find it labeled poison, and in practically all the official works such as the B.P. the C.P., and the U.S.P. and the American Dispensatory, etc., it is classed as a poison.

That it has no poisonous properties we very definitely affirm. Much has been said and written on this point, and it is because of this we devote a special lesson to this herb. Dr. H. Nowell has used it for nearly thirty years, in all manner of cases, and at all ages. We have friends who have likewise used it freely, and if half that is said against it by the medical world were true, thousands should have been dead from its use.

In cases of cough, asthma, bronchitis, etc., we have used it with remarkable success. We believe there is nothing known to man that will so effectively clear the air passages of the lungs of viscid matter. Its influence is rapidly manifested, and it is frequently felt throughout the system, even to the toes.

As stated above, the allopathic schools call lobelia a poison, and as the student may possibly have done some medical work to which reference may be made, we desire to make very clear something of the history as well as some of the uses of this most valuable herb.

Samuel Thompson employed lobelia quite extensively in Vermont, New York, New Hampshire, and Massachusetts as early as 1795. There are extant many allopathic works such as Thatcher's Dispensatory (1817), the U. S. Dispensatory, Griffith, Royle, Carson, etc; wherein the reader is informed that "Thompson himself was tried for murder for killing a man with this article." Did one know nothing outside the medical records, one would possibly accept the conclusion that Thompson was a careless empiric, who was called to account for using a deadly article.

We give the student a concise outline of the facts of the case. The trial took place in December, 1809, before the Supreme Court in Salem, Mass. Thompson was charged with the murder of one Ezra Lovett, Jr., by the administering of lobelia. The complaint was laid by a Dr. French, an allopathic physician, who had repeatedly persecuted Thompson. So bitterly had this Dr. French persecuted Thompson that the latter had been compelled to take steps to have Dr. French bound over to keep the peace, owing to the M.D.'s having publicly threatened to blow Thompson's brains out.

Following this, Dr. French, seeking an opportunity to injure this wonderful man, Thompson, finally procured his arrest on a charge of murder. (It is evidently the venom of French, and his charge against Thompson that is the basis of the allopathic claim that lobelia is a poison.) We quote a few lines from Dr. Thompson's report of the case: "Just before night, Dr. French arrived with the sheriff and ordered me to be delivered up by the constable to the sheriff. Dr. French again vented his spleen upon me by the most savage abuse that language could express, saying that I was a murderer, that I had murdered fifty and he could prove it, that I should be either hung, or sent to the State Prison for life, and he would do all in his power to have me convicted.

"I was then put in irons by the sheriff, and conveyed to the jail in Newburyport and confined in a dungeon with a man who had been convicted of an assault upon a girl six years of age. I was not allowed a chair or a table, nothing but a miserable straw bunk on the floor, with one poor blanket which had never been washed. I was put into this prison on the tenth day of November, 1889." He then tells of the cold, the filth, the vermin, that infested the place, etc.

As there was no session of the court until the fall of the next year, it was expected that he would have to lie in this unhealthy confinement for a year, which would most likely have killed him. There were, however, some eminent friends who had been benefitted by his work, who, through their influence, after making fifteen trips from Salem to Boston, secured a hearing before Judge Parsons in a special session on Dec. 10, 1809.

"Vol. VI Massachusetts Criminal Reports contains the report of the trial written by Judge Parsons himself. It is supposed that the Judge was favorably disposed to the prosecution, and gave only that which plain justice called for to Thompson. The report states, among other things, Thompson 'had administered the like medicines with those given to the deceased to several of his patients, who had died under his hands.' This charge was made by the Solicitor General; and to prove this statement he called several witnesses, of whom but one appeared. He testified that he had been the prisoner's patient for an oppression at his stomach, that he took the emetic powders several times in three or four days and was relieved from his complaint, which had not since returned, and there was no evidence in the case that the prisoner in the course of his very novel practice had experienced any fatal accident among his patients.

"As the Court were satisfied that the evidence produced by the commonwealth did not support the indictment, the prisoner was put upon his defense. The prisoner was acquitted."

Such is the report of the case (written by the Judge himself) that evidently gave rise to the blind repetition that lobelia is a poison. There were four justices on the bench at the trial, and only the blindness of allopathic prejudices continues to ban from general use one of our best remedies.

After this, laws were sought forbidding the prescribing, selling, or even the giving away of lobelia; meanwhile the same brand of allopathic knave went on prescribing arsenic, antimony, strychnine, prussic acid, etc. During the following years many of the reformatory physicians were prosecuted and allopathic regulars swore on oath that ten, eight, or even four grains of lobelia were sufficient to cause death. Yet no proof was ever found that any life had ever been lost or injured by it, while some physicians and many patients testified that they had taken from half an ounce upwards in the space of a few hours, always to their benefit.

There was no single instance in all the prosecutions of any harm ever resulting from the use of lobelia. For the further information of the student, we quote from the late Prof. W. Tully, of Yale College, in a letter written to Dr. H. Lee, of Middletown, Conn. dated March 22, 1838. "Lobelia inflata is entirely destitute of any narcotic powers. I have been in the habit of employing this article for twenty-seven years, in large quantities and for a long period, without the least trace of any narcotic effect. I have used the very best official tincture in the quantity of three fluid ounces in twenty-four hours and for four to seven days in succession, and I have likewise given three large tablespoonfuls of it within half an hour, without the least indication of any narcotic operation.

"I have known four and five tobacco pipes full of it smoked in immediate succession and without any narcosis, and I have also known it given by enema and with the same result—Dr. Bigelow, of Boston, was the first person who ascribed narcotic powers to this agent, and he did this in 1817, but not from his own observation. I am confident (the old women's stories in the books to the contrary notwithstanding) that lobelia inflata is a valuable, a safe, and a sufficiently gentle article of medicine, and I think the time will come when it will be much better appreciated."—William Tully.

Now for the uses of this plant. The herb and seed have similar properties, the seed, however, being much the stronger. In infusing the seed, it is best to crush them. Both herb and seed contain a volatile oil, and if the seed is kept in paper, some of the oil will be absorbed by the paper.

Lobelia is a most efficient relaxant, influencing mucous, serous, nervous, and muscular structures. It is a good rule to always give a stimulant before administering lobelia, or to combine a stimulant with it. It is used in coughs, bronchitis, asthma, whooping cough, pneumonia, hysteria, convulsions, suspended animation, tetanus, febrile troubles, etc. It may be used in substance, i.e. the powdered herb or seed, in fluid extract, acid tincture, infusion, decoction, pills or capsules, in syrup, by enema, and in poultices.

We have used the acid tincture of lobelia for nearly thirty years and have had splendid results. Dr. H. Nowell tells how that twenty-five years ago he was asked to try to help a case of asthma in a patient where the regulars, after consultation, had declared the patient's cough could not be stopped. To stop the cough, they declared, would stop the patient. The case was a woman forty years of age, and at the time was seven months pregnant with her first baby. The asthmatic spasms were most trying, the patient being unable to lie in bed, and she would tear at the throat, fighting for breath, and both she and her husband begged of their doctor to stop the cough.

They were told that nothing could be done until after the child was born. The husband was given a one-ounce bottle of the acid tincture of lobelia and instructed that a teaspoonful be given when the spasm came on, with instructions to give a second teaspoonful ten minutes later if necessary.

The next morning, upon inquiry as to the patient, he was told that almost immediately after taking the first dose the patient brought up long, thick masses of phlegm from the lungs the size of a man's fist. No further dose was taken and the patient has never had a trace of asthma or any chest trouble since—and she is living today.

We quote here the statement of Dr. Butler: "It has been my misfortune to be an asthmatic for about ten years, and I have made a trial of a variety of the usual remedies with very little benefit. The last time I had an attack it was the worst I ever experienced. It continued for eight weeks. My breathing was so difficult that I took a tablespoonful of the acid tincture of lobelia, and in about three or four minutes my breathing was as free as it ever was. I took another in ten minutes, after which I took a third, which I felt through every part of my body, even to the ends of my toes, and since that time I have enjoyed as good health as before the first attack."

We have also used the acid tincture as an external application, rubbing it between the shoulders and on the chest in asthma and have found it most helpful. Dr. H. Nowell uses this regularly in this manner and has had some surprising results in cases where the breathing has been most difficult. Dr. Nowell's method of making the acid tincture is as follows:

Lobelia herb ....2 ounces
Lobelia seed (crushed) ....2 ounces
Best malt vinegar ....1 pint

Macerate in a closely stoppered bottle for ten days to two weeks, shaking every day. Strain off and bottle for use. This is the formula he has used for nearly thirty years.

Another formula for the acid tincture of lobelia:

Lobelia seed (crushed) ....2 ounces
Lobelia herb ....½ ounce
Cayenne ....1 teaspoonful

Macerate ten days in one pint of malt vinegar, shaking well daily. Strain and bottle for use.

Another extremely useful acid tincture of lobelia is made by using raspberry vinegar instead of the plain malt vinegar. For the benefit of those who may not know, we give herewith a formula for raspberry vinegar, which we always use ourselves. We strongly advise the student to make his own; he is then sure of having a pure article.

Bruise two quarts of raspberries. Add two quarts of best malt vinegar, stand for two days, then strain off the liquor, and to each quart of liquid add twelve ounces of good sugar (loaf sugar, if obtainable). Bring to a boil and remove the scum as it rises. The longer it boils the thicker the syrup becomes.

Allow to cool and bottle for use. Keep in a dry place. This makes an excellent raspberry vinegar and is useful to add to some cough syrups and makes a pleasant drink with water added.

The acid tincture can be added to horehound, hyssop, sage or other teas, or may be added to the composition tea in doses of a teaspoonful to a cupful of the herb tea for cough, asthma, colds, etc. It is also extremely useful as an emetic when one feels that the stomach should be thoroughly cleansed.

ANTISPASMODIC TINCTURE OR THIRD PREPARATION

What is known among the herbal practitioners as spasmodic tincture of the third preparation of lobelia is a most effective compound. It is useful in many violent cases such as epilepsy, convulsions, lockjaw, delirium tremens, fainting, hysteria, cramps, suspended animation, etc. We give below what we believe to be two of the best compounds that can be made.

ANTISPASMODIC TINCTURE

Lobelia seed, crushed scullcap, skunk cabbage, gum myrrh, black cohosh, of each one ounce, cayenne, one-half ounce.

Infuse for one week in one pint of rectified spirits of wine (alcohol) in a closely corked vessel. Shake well once daily. It is well if possible to have a somewhat wide neck on the bottle. After one week strain and press out the clear liquid when it is ready for use. We assure the student that we have used this very formula with remarkable results. We have given just a drop or two on the tip of the finger, thrusting the finger into the mouth of a baby in convulsions, and in less time than it takes to write this statement the convulsions have ceased.

We have seen a man rolling in agony and moaning with pain and have given one teaspoonful of antispasmodic tincture in half a cup of warm water sweetened and had the patient drink the whole, warm, and we affirm that within fifteen seconds all traces of cramps and spasm had gone.

Dr. H. Nowell has poured a teaspoonful of the antispasmodic tincture, full strength, between the clenched teeth of a case of lockjaw and before a second teaspoonful could be poured from the bottle the locked jaws have relaxed and the patient asked, "My God! What have you done?" It traverses the system with most remarkable rapidity, and we verily believe that in cases of suspended animation, locked jaws, spasms, and cramps it stands unequalled in the whole realm of therapeutic agents.

The formula of the late Mr. Hool, of Lancashire, in making his antispasmodic tincture, is as follows: Powdered lobelia herb, lobelia seed, scullcap, valerian, skunk cabbage, gum myrrh, cayenne; of each one-half ounce.

Place in a bottle with one and a half pints of rectified spirits of wine (pure alcohol, called also spirit vini rect, and written S.V.R.), cork well and shake once daily for fourteen days. Filter through white blotting paper and bottle for use.

We quote from Mr. Hool's latest writings, knowing his wonderful work and integrity of character. He says, "The above tincture will be found superior to any other single agent, as its purely innocuous character renders it a safe and reliable remedy for patients of all ages. In mucous and spasmodic croup the tincture must be administered promptly and in full teaspoonful doses in warm water and repeated at intervals of every ten or fifteen minutes until free vomiting ensues, as it is necessary in all such cases to induce complete relaxation of the system, by means of full emetic doses repeated at suitable intervals."

"Where the case is very severe or the tincture is difficult to administer, as in the case of infants, it should be rubbed well into the neck, chest, and between the shoulders at the same time. Two or three drops of the tincture in a raw state should be placed in the mouth and washed down with teaspoonful doses of warm water and the patient kept warm in bed. In all such cases relief will be experienced in a few minutes, and by repeating the same treatment every one or two hours a cure will soon be effected and the patient brought to a state of convalescence.

"But how is this result brought about? The properties of the lobelia, by immediate action on the muscular and mucous parts of the esophagus, glottis, larynx, windpipe and bronchial tubes, cause immediate relaxation, the parts previously contracted are made to expand and breathing is made easier. The properties of the cayenne pepper warm and stimulate the blood, allay inflammation of the parts, cause better secretions and action of the mucous membranes.

"The scullcap and valerian, being nervines, allay the irritation of the nerves and prevent too much straining and excitement and by that means prevent rupture of the small vessels, while the action of the properties of the skunk cabbage and gum myrrh is to keep canker away and to brace up the system."

As we feel the above writer, Mr. Hool, is absolutely reliable, we quote further from him as to his method of treating:

SCARLET FEVER AND OTHER FEBRILE CONDITIONS

"In typhoid, typus, spotted black or slow fever, and especially malignant scarlet fever, its (antispasmodic tincture) value cannot be half told. I have seen in my time some of the worst cases of scarlet fever cured by the following simple treatment, even when death seemed to have set in and there has been no apparent hope of recovery. I have gone into such cases and caused to be administered one teaspoonful of the antispasmodic tincture of lobelia in a little water made warm, and given every half hour until the patient seemed easier. Then make up a good fire in the room, have clean underclothing warm and ready to put on.

"Then get two quarts of hot water and one quart of the best malt vinegar. Mix the water and vinegar together, bring the patient near the fire and wash the body all over with the vinegar and water and wipe dry. Put the clean clothing on and clean sheets on the bed. Put the patient back in bed and give a teaspoonful of the preparation in warm tea (herbal tea) or warm water every two hours afterwards, taking care to wash with vinegar and warm water every day and Hey Preste, the patient will be on the highway to recovery. I have treated some scores of cases of scarlet fever in the above way, and never lost a single case by death.

"We have thus quoted extensively because we personally know of the long life work, the labor of love, and the remarkable success of this noble-hearted man. We have used the acid tincture and the antispasmodic tincture in our parctice and commend all that has been said to the careful study of the nature cure physician.

"In rheumatic fever, the antispasmodic tincture will generally work wonders with the patient. Proceed as follows: Rub the whole body from neck to toes with the tincture, and if the case is bad, such as cannot sit up or move arms or legs, give a teaspoonful of the tincture in a little hot water, every half hour until free perspiration ensues. Keep patient in bed and allow to cool down, then wash the whole body down with vinegar and hot water. After this give the tincture in teaspoonful doses in hot water every two hours for one day, then every three hours for a few days. If the case demands it, use a little for rubbing as needed also. Sponge down daily with the hot water and vinegar. If this course is followed, the practitioner will find both himself and his patient surprised at the speedy recovery the case will make.

"Finally, we believe that lobelia is one of the finest remedies a kind Providence has blessed mankind with." Dominion Herbal College, Ltd. Lesson 26.

"Lobelia inflata is one of the most valuable herbs used in the botanic practice. Much has been written as to whether this herb is a poison or not. Practical experience—which is far better than theory—has proved that it is as harmless as milk, and instead of being a poison, it is an antidote to poison. The analysis of its chemical constituents show it to contain an alkaloid lobelina and an acid lobelic acid, resin, wax, and gum; the seeds contain in addition about 30 percent of fixed oil. We have attended cases where poison had been given in mistake, and lobelia has had the desired effect of discharging the contents of the stomach. Medical men are often deluded by giving heed to mere opinions instead of noticing facts; but men who have divested themselves of that which has been taught them in medical schools have discovered truth from error.

"Dr. Butler, who wrote about lobelia in 1810, says: 'It has been my misfortune to be an asthmatic for about ten years, and I have made a trial of a variety of the usual remedies with very little benefit. The last time I had an attack it was the severest I ever experienced; it continued for eight weeks. My breathing was so difficult that I took a tablespoonful of the acid tincture of lobelia, and in about three or four minutes my breathing was as free as it ever was. I took another in ten minutes, after which I took a third, which I felt through every part of my body, even to the ends of my toes; and since that time I have enjoyed as good health as before the first attack.'

"We have prescribed the acid tincture of lobelia inflata for whooping cough with striking success. There is no other medicine that so effectually frees the air passages of the lungs of their viscid secretions. As an emetic, we are satisfied that it is as kind and destitute of all hazard as ipecacuanha, though it is more efficient; and we consider it one of the best remedies in the whole materia medica: and are confident—the old women's stories in the books (meaning the medical school books) to the contrary nothwithstanding —that lobelia is a valuable, a safe, and sufficiently gentle article of medicine; and we think the time will come when it will be much better appreciated. Little, however, of its value, can be specified within the compass of a single sheet of paper. We not only give it to our patients, but take it ourselves whenever we have occasion for an emetic. We can assure the public that it can be used without apprehension of danger; we have given it to infants a few months old. It tends to remove obstructions from every part of the system, and is felt even to the ends of the toes; it not only cleanses the stomach, but exercises a beneficial influence over every part of the body; it is very diffusable, however, and requires to be used with cayenne or some other permanent stimulant. The effects of lobelia may be compared to a fire made of shavings, which will soon go out unless other fuel be added; cayenne therefore, may be said to keep alive the blaze which the lobelia has kindled. We can bear testimony that it is harmless when given in a proper manner; we never saw any evil effect, and our experience should be worth something when we say that we have sold in our practice upwards of one hundred pounds weight per year for seventy years past, which, according to the notions of some medical men, would have been sufficient to poison one-half of the population of England. There is no other medicine that is half so effective as lobelia in removing the tough, hard, and ropy phlegm from asthmatic and consumptive persons. It is an indispensable medicine in fevers, bilious, and longstanding chronic complaints. We have used it for deafness with good results. It is also useful in poultices to assist supperation. There are some writers who state that it will cure hydrophobia, if taken inwardly and applied externally as well. The medical qualities of this invaluable herb are so multifarious that a large treatise might well be written on its curative powers. Suffice it, however, to say that it is a general corrector of the whole system, innocent in its nature, and moving with the general spirits. In healthy systems it will be silent and harmless. It is fully as well calculated to remove the cause of disease as food is to remove hunger; and it clears away all obstructions in the circulation regardless of the nature of the disease." *The Model Botanic Guide to Health*, pp. 35, 36, 37.

There are untold mysteries hid in the nonpoisonous herbs, that are not yet all uncovered.

I do thank God for the good herbal colleges we have today, which we did not have when I was a young man.

There is a number of herbs which you can do miracles. Will mention some of them: Scullcap, golden seal, myrrh, yarrow, milkweed, fennel, cubeb berries, chickweed, aloes, mandrake, calamus root, dandelion root, blueberry leaves, tansy, yellow dock, burdock root, lobelia, coltsfoot, palmetto berries, hyssop, cayenne, sage, catnip, peppermint, echinacea, and witch hazel.

Lobelia possesses most wonderful properties; it is a perfectly harmless relaxant. It loosens disease and opens the way for its elimination from the body. Its action is quick and more effective than radium, and lobelia leaves no bad after effects, while radium does. Shun radium as you would a rattlesnake.

Nonpoisonous herbs will do everything for which the allopath gives radium, mercury, antitoxin, serums, vaccines, insulin, strychnine, digitalis, and all the poisonous drug preparations, and nonpoisonous herbs do not leave any bad after effects.

LUNGWORT
(Whole plant)

Botanical Name: Pulmonaria officinalis. Common Names: Spotted lungwort, maple lungwort, Jerusalem cowslip, Jerusalem sage, spotted comfrey. Medicinal Properties: Expectorant, demulcent, pectoral, mucilaginous.

Lungwort is a most valuable remedy for coughs, influenza, catarrh, colds, la grippe, yellow jaundice, lung troubles, bleeding lungs, and all bronchial troubles. It decreases the flow of the menses when excessive. Used to wash ulcers in the private parts.

MAGNOLIA
(Bark)

Botanical Name: Magnolia glauca. Common Names: Swamp laurel, red laurel, sweet magnolia, red bay, white bay, beaver tree, Indian bark, sweet bay, swamp sassafras, holly bay. Medicinal Properties: Astringent, stimulant, febrifuge, tonic, aromatic, anti-periodic.

This is an excellent tonic, very valuable in intermittent fever, dyspepsia, dysentery, and erysipelas. Use as a douche for leucorrhea. A wash made by simmering a tablespoonful of magnolia bark in a pint of water for ten minutes is fine for salt rheum and other skin diseases. Magnolia is excellent to use in place of quinine, and will do the work when quinine fails. Effective to cure tobacco habit. This herb can be taken a long time without any bad effects.

MANDRAKE

Botanical Name: Podophyllum peltatum. Common Names: Hog apple, May apple, American mandrake, wild lemon, raccoon berry, yellow berry, wild mandrake, Indian apple, duck's foot, ground lemon. Medicinal Properties: Antibilious, cathartic, emetic, diaphoretic, cholagogue, alterative, resolvent, vermifuge, deobstruent.

Excellent regulator for liver and bowels. Good physic. It is often combined with senna leaves. In chronic liver diseases it has no equal. It is very beneficial in uterine diseases. It acts thoroughly upon all the tissues of the system. Valuable in jaundice, bilious, or intermittent fever. Use wherever a powerful cathartic is required. Steep a teaspoonful in a pint of boiling water and take a teaspoonful of this tea as often as required. Children less according to age.

MARJORAM
(Plant)

Botanical Name: Origanum marjorana. Common Names: Sweet marjoram, knotted marjoram. Medicinal Properties: Aromatic, tonic, condiment, emmenagogue.

This is a good tonic. Very effective in combination with camomile and gentian. Excellent for sour stomach, loss of appetite, cough, consumption, spleen, eruptive diseases, suppressed menstruation, to increase the flow of urine, for poisonous insect bites and snake bites, dropsy, scabs, scurvy, itch, jaundice, deafness, toothache, headache, and indigestion. Taken hot, it produces perspiration.

MASTERWORT
(Root and seed)

Botanical Name: Heracleum lanatum. Common Names: Madnep, cow parsnip, youthwort, madness. Medicinal Properties: Carminative, stimulant, antispasmodic.

A useful remedy for colds, fevers, increasing flow of urine, gravel in kidneys, colic, suppressed menstration when scanty and painful cramps, dyspepsia, dropsy, epilepsy, spasms, asthma, palsy, and apoplexy. Will expel wind from the bowels. Good as a wash for sores and ulcers.

MARSHMALLOW
(Root and leaves)

Botanical Name: Althaea officinalis. Common Names: Althaea, sweat weed, wymote, mortification root. Medicinal Properties: Diuretic, demulcent, mucilaginous, emollient.

As a poultice it is excellent for sore or inflamed parts; is very soothing and lubricating. For lung troubles, hoarseness, catarrh, diarrhea, dysentery, put a teaspoonful in a cup of water, simmer for ten minutes, let stand until cool. Drink one to two cupfuls a day, a large mouthful at a time. For irritation of the vagina, use as a douche, also take internally. The tea is also good to bathe sore, inflamed eyes. Very soothing and healing to an inflamed condition of the bowels. Valuable in pneumonia, strangury, gravel, and all kidney diseases.

MILKWEED
(Root)

Botanical Name: Asclepias syriaca. Common Names: Milkweed, milkweed root, silkweed, silky swallow wort.

Medicinal Properties: Emetic, purgative, alterative, diuretic, tonic.

This is the common milkweed with which almost everyone is familiar. A splendid remedy for female complaints, bowel and kidney troubles. It increases the flow of urine; therefore is good for dropsy, also good for asthma, stomach troubles, and scrofulous conditions of the blood.

It is a very effective remedy for gallstones. Is much used in place of lobelia. Take equal parts of milkweed and marshmallow, steep a teaspoonful in a cup of boiling water, take three cups daily, and one hot upon retiring. It will expel gallstones in a few days, when combined with this. Fomentations applied to the liver and the liver thoroughly massaged at the same time is very effective. Children less according to age. The boiled roots taste similar to asparagus.

MINT
(Whole plant)

Botanical Name: Monarda punctata. Common Names: Horsemint, American horsemint, origanum, monarda. Medicinal Properties: Stimulant, carminative, sudorific, diuretic, emmenagogue.

Very quieting and soothing. Eases pain. Excellent for suppression of urine, suppressed menstruation, nausea, vomiting, and gas in the stomach and intestines.

MISTLETOE

Botanical Name: Viscum flavescens. Common Names: Birdlime, mistletoe, golden bough. Medicinal Properties: Narcotic, antispasmodic, emetic, tonic, nervine.

Excellent specific remedy for cholera or St. Vitus's dance. Is a fine nervine, effective in epilepsy, convulsions, hysteria, delirium, nervous debility, and heart troubles.

MOTHERWORT
(Whole plant)

Botanical Name: Leonurus cardiaca. Common Names: Lion's tail, lion's ear, throwwort. Medicinal Properties: Antispasmodic, nervine, emmenagogue, laxative, hepatic.

Very well known and used with excellent results in suppressed menstruation and other female troubles. Take warm. Very useful in nervous complaints, fainting, heart flutters, cramps, convulsions, hysteria, delirium, sleeplessness, also liver affections. Good for suppressed urine. Increases the menstrual flow. A hot fomentation wrung out of the strong tea will relieve cramps and pain in painful menstruation. A remedy for colds, particularly chest colds. Kills worms. Has an excellent effect if taken during pregnancy.

MUGWORT
(Whole plant)

Botanical Name: Artemisia vulgaris. Medicinal Properties: Emmenagogue, anti-epileptic.

Splendid for female complaints when combined with marigold flower, cramp bark, and black haw. Mix together. Take a heaping teaspoonful to a cup of boiling water. Steep twenty minutes, and drink one to three cups a day as needed. The leaves and flowers are full of virtue. It is a most safe and excellent medicine for female complaints. It is safe and certain for young girls and others in suppressed menstruation. Steep a tablespoonful in a pint of water twenty minutes and drink two or three cups a day a few days before the monthlies are expected. Mugwort is very useful to overcome inflammatory swellings, gravel and stones in kidneys and bladder, to increase flow of urine, for fevers and gout. After using a poultice of chickweed or slippery elm, thoroughly bathe the affected part for some time with the hot tea, made by steeping a tablespoonful of mugwort to a pint of boiling water for twenty minutes. Bruises, whitlows, abscesses, carbuncles, and sometimes even tumors will yield to this treatment if persevered with. Good for rheumatism and gout. Acute pain in the bowels and stomach can quickly be relieved by drinking the warm infusion and applying hot fomentations wrung out of the boiling infusion.

MULLEIN
(Leaves and root)

Botanical Name: Verbascum thapsus. Common Names: Velvet plant, white mullein, verbascum flowers, woolen, blanket herb, bullock's, lungwort, flannel flower, shepherd's club, hare's beard, pig taper, cow's lungwort. Medicinal Properties: Anodyne, diuretic, demulcent, anti-spasmodic, vulnerary, astringent, emolient, pectoral.

This is one of the old household herbs we have used from childhood. The root has been successfully used for many years in asthma. For this purpose, burn the root and inhale the fumes. A tea of the leaves is very valuable in asthma, croup, bronchitis, all lung affections, bleeding from the lungs, difficult breathing, and hay fever. The tea is good as a throat gargle, for toothache, and for washing open sores. A tea made from the flowers will induce sleep, relieve pain, and in large doses act as a physic. The fresh flowers, crushed, will remove warts. Fomentations wrung from hot tea made from the leaves are helpful for inflamed piles, ulcers, tumors, mumps, acute inflammation of the tonsils, and malignant sore throat. Fomentations are excellent in any glandular swelling. This is a splendid remedy taken internally for dropsy, catarrh, swollen joints. Boil for a few minutes one ounce of mullein in a pint of boiling water or milk (soybean preferred) and take a half teacupful after each bowel movement, for dysentery, diarrhea, and bleeding of the bowels. For swollen testicles or scrotum apply fomentations for one hour three or four times a day wrung out of the tea, made by simmering one ounce of mullein and one ounce of sanicle herb in two quarts of water for fifteen minutes. These fomentations are good for any kind of swelling or bad sores.

MUSTARD
(Ground seed)

Botanical Name: Sinapis aĺba. Common Names: White mustard seed, yellow mustard, kedlock, yellow mustard seed, white mustard. Medicinal Properties: Pungent, laxative, stimulant, condiment, emetic.

A tablespoonful steeped in a quart of boiling water and taken lukewarm acts as an emetic. This is the common yellow ground mustard which is used so much in food, but it is harmful to use mustard in food. It is excellent to put in a foot bath to draw the blood to the lower part of the body in congestion of the lungs, also to draw the blood from the head when congested. An old fashioned remedy to produce vomiting. Steep a teaspoonful of mustard in a large cup of boiling water. Stir well. Let cool to lukewarm. Drink all at one time. If this does not produce vomiting, tickle the back of the throat with the finger. A good mustard plaster is made as follows: One part mustard and four parts whole wheat flour. Make into a paste by mixing with warm water. Have it thick enough to nicely spread on a piece of cloth. Mustard plaster is excellent applied over the kidneys in irritation of the kidneys. If the mustard is very strong, be careful not to draw a blister. Do not leave it on too long. If you wish to keep it on a long time, make it weaker. If you mix the mustard and flour with the whites of eggs in place of water, it will not blister.

MYRRH
(Powdered gum)

Botanical Name: Balsamodendron myrrh. Common Name: Gum myrrh tree. Medicinal Properties: Antiseptic, stimulant, tonic, expectorant, vulnerary, emmenagogue.

An ancient Bible remedy which is still in use today, and one of the best remedies. It is valuable as a tonic and stimulant for bronchial and lung diseases. Excellent for pyorrhea, as it is antiseptic and very healing. Brush the teeth with the powder, thoroughly rinse the mouth with the tea, and bathe the gums. Removes halitosis or bad breath, when taken internally. Take a small teaspoonful of powdered myrrh and one of golden seal to a pint of boiling water. Steep a few minutes, pour off the clear liquid, and take teaspoonful doses five or six times a day. It is also an excellent remedy for ulcers, piles, hemorrhoids, and for bathing bedsores or any sores on the body. Made into an ointment with equal parts of golden seal, it is an excellent injection for piles and hemorrhoids; or the tea can be used for this purpose as a wash. After thoroughly washing sores, ulcers, etc., with the tea, sprinkle a little of the powder on the sore. Charcoal moistened with this tea and applied to old ulcers and sores is healing. Is also effective for gangrene. For use as a gargle and mouth wash, steep a teaspoonful of myrrh and one of boracic acid to a pint of boiling water. Let stand one-half hour, pour off clear liquid and use. This is also an excellent remedy for diphtheria, ulcerated throat, and sores in the mouth. Use for cough, asthma, tuberculosis, and all chest affections, as it diminishes the mucus discharges.

NETTLE
(Whole plant)

Botanical Name: Urtica dioica. Common Names: Common stinging nettle, great stinging nettle, stinging nettle, common nettle, nettle. Medicinal Properties: Pectoral diuretic, astringent, tonic, styptic, rubifacient.

This herb will prevent scrofula. It is an excellent remedy for kidney trouble. It will expel gravel from the bladder and increase the flow of urine. Splendid for neuralgia. A poultice of the green steeped leaves will relieve pain. Such a poultice will raise blisters if kept on too long. The tea increases the menstrual flow. It will kill and expel worms. For diarrhea, dysentery, piles, hemorrhages, hemorrhoids, gravel, inflammation of the kidneys, make a decoction using a teaspoonful to a cup of water and simmer for ten minutes. For chronic rheumatism, take the bruised leaves and rub on the skin. Excellent for reducing in combination with seawrack. Tea made from the root will cure dropsy in the first stages and will stop hemorrhages from the urinary organs, lungs, intestines, nose, and stomach. The boiled leaves applied externally will stop bleeding almost immediately. Nettle tea is good for fever, colds, and la grippe. It is an old-fashioned remedy for backache. Very fine for eczema. Tea made from the leaves of the nettle will expel phlegm from the lungs and stomach and will clean out the urinary canal.

Nettle tea is an excellent hair tonic and will bring back the natural color of the hair. Use as the last rinse when shampooing. Make a cup of the tea by steeping a teaspoonful in a cup of boiling water for thirty minutes. Dip the fingers in and thoroughly massage the scalp. This will cure dandruff. It is well to boil the leaves in vinegar for this purpose.

In the summer when you get the green leaves, cook them like spinach. They are a splendid blood purifier. Nettle is a weed people generally dislike, as when they touch it, it burns the hands, but they do not know the wonderful medicinal properties it contains.

NUTMEG

Botanical Name: Nigella sativa. Common Names: Nutmeg flower, black caraway, nutmeg, flower seed, black cummin, nigella seed, bishop's wort, small fennel flower. Medicinal Properties: Expectorant, deobstruent, sialagogue, emmenagogue, antigas.

Much used for seasoning food. Prevents gas and fermentation.

ORIGANUM
(Whole plant)

Botanical Name: Origanum vulgare. Common Names: Wild marjoram, origanum, winter marjoram, mountain mint, winter sweet. Medicinal Properties: Aromatic, pungent, stomachic, tonic, stimulant, emmenagogue, carminative, diaphoretic.

Very strengthening to the stomach, excellent for relieving sour stomach, promotes appetite. Excellent in consumption and extreme cough. Will expel poison from the body. Good in suppressed urine, suppressed menstruation, dropsy, yellow jaundice, scurvy, and itch. The extracted juice is excellent for deafness or pain and noise in the ears. Drop a few drops in the ear whenever necessary. The oil dropped in the hollow of an aching tooth will stop the pain. Will expel gas from the stomach and bowels. Very helpful in dyspepsia. Good for rheumatism, colic, nausea, and neuralgia. Poultice made from this herb is very beneficial for painful swellings, sprains, felons, boils, and carbuncles. Is an excellent medicine in nervous cases. Good to use in salves and liniments. Is excellent for sore throat when applied as a heating compress. Steep a heaping tablespoonful in a pint of boiling water for thirty minutes. Dip a cloth in this hot tea, apply, binding loosely with a dry cloth. It is well to cover the compress with oiled silk, which will keep it moist. For general use, steep a teaspoonful to a cup of boiling water twenty minutes; drink cold one or two cupfuls a day, one hour before meals. Children less according to age.

OREGON GRAPE
(See Wild Oregon Grape)

PARSLEY
(Leaves, root, and seed)

Botanical Name: Petroselinum sativum. Common Names: Garden parsley, rock parsley, common parsley, march. Medicinal Properties: Diuretic, aperient, expectorant. Juice: Antiperiodic. See: Febrifuge, emmenagogue.

The root or leaves is one of the most excellent remedies for difficult urination, dropsy, jaundice, fevers, stones in kidneys, gravel, obstructions of liver and spleen, strangury, syphilis, and gonorrhea. Also excellent for cancer, and should be classed among the preventive herbs. Simmer a tablespoonful to a pint of water for ten minutes, let stand, strain, and drink one to three cups a day, a large swallow at a time, more or less, as needed. For female troubles, it is well to combine the leaves with equal parts of buchu, black haw, and cramp bark. One of the most excellent remedies for gallbladder and expels gallstones. A hot fomentation wrung out of the tea and applied to insect bites and stings will cure them. Use a tablespoonful of the leaves to a cup of boiling water, and steep twenty minutes. Parsley is rich in potassium, and cancerous germs cannot live in potassium. A poultice of the bruised leaves is excellent for swollen glands, swollen breasts, or to dry up milk. A tea made of the crushed seed, a teaspoonful to the cup, steeped, strained, and applied to the hair, will kill vermin. Parsley should be used freely in salads, soups, and slaws for its beneficial results.

PEACH

(Bark, leaves, twigs, and kernels)

Botanical Name: Amygdalus persica. Common Names: Common peach tree, peach tree. Medicinal Properties: Relaxant, demulcent, sedative, aromatic, laxative.

The common peach tree leaves should be on hand in every home. They are laxative and exert an excellent influence over the nervous system. Used with good results in whooping cough. Good for dyspepsia, other stomach troubles, jaundice, inflammation of the abdomen, and will expel worms. Excellent for bladder and uterine troubles such as scalding urine, inflammation, tenderness and aching of those parts. When taken hot in small doses, a large swallow every hour or two, it will stop vomiting in cholera morbus. Is also a very effective remedy for morning sickness in pregnancy. The powdered bark or leaves heals sores or wounds. The kernels or buds, bruised and boiled in vinegar until they become thick, are excellent for baldness to grow hair. More effective than quinine as a substitute for the purposes for which quinine is used.

PENNYROYAL

(Whole plant)

Botanical Name: Hedeoma Pulegioides. Common Names: Tickweed, squaw mint, stinking balm, thickweed, American pennyroyal. Medicinal Properties: Sudorific, carminative, emmenagogue, stimulant, diaphoretic, aromatic, sedative.

Is excellent in burning fevers. Will promote perspiration. Take hot. Excellent remedy for toothache, gout, leprosy, colds, consumption, phlegm in chest and lungs, jaundice, dropsy, cramps, convulsions, headache, ulcers, sores in mouth, insect and snake bites, itch, intestinal pains, colic, and griping. If troubled with suppressed or scanty menstruation, take one or two cupfuls hot at bedtime along with a hot foot bath, several days before expected. It will relieve nausea, but should not be taken by a pregnant woman. Good as poultice and wash for bruises, black-eye. Good for nervousness and hysteria. Useful for skin diseases.

PEPPERMINT

Botanical Name: Mentha piperita. Medicinal Properties: Aromatic, stimulant, stomachic, carminative. Oil: Stimulant, rubfacient.

This is one of the oldest household remedies and should be in every garden, as it grow very prolifically. Excellent remedy for chills, colic, fevers, dizziness or, gas on stomach, nausea, vomiting, diarrhea, dysentery, cholera, heart trouble, palpitation of the heart, influenza, la grippe and hysteria. Applied externally is good for rheumatism, neuralgia and headache. Peppermint enemas are excellent for cholera and colon troubles. It is helpful in cases of insanity, and especially useful for convulsions and spasms in infants.

Peppermint is a general stimulant. A strong cup of peppermint tea will act more powerfully on the system than any liquor stimulant, quickly diffusing itself through the system and bringing back to the body its natural warmth in case of sudden fainting or dizzy spells, with extreme coldness and pale countenance.

Will bring back to the body its natural warmth and glow without the usual tendency to relapse. Good for griping pain caused by eating unripe fruit or irritating foods.

Do not drink coffee and tea, which are so harmful. Coffee weakens the heart muscles—peppermint tea is delicious and strengthens your heart muscles. Coffee hinders digestion, weakens the heart, is one cause of constipation, poisons the body. Peppermint tea cleanses and strengthens the entire body. Give it a fair trial and see how much better you feel when you leave off coffee and tea and drink peppermint tea.

In place of aspirin for the headache or any other harmful headache drug, take a cup of as-strong-as-you-like-it peppermint tea, lie down for a little while, and see what a good effect it will have. If need be, drink two or three cups, or enough so it gets into the system so it can help you, and it will not disappoint you. Strengthens the nerves instead of weakening them as aspirin and other drugs do.

If the tea is not at hand, take some of the leaves and chew them up fine until you can swallow them easily. This will start the food to digesting and assist the entire system to do its work more normally.

PERUVIAN BARK
(Bark)

Botanical Name: Cinchona calisaya. Common Names: Cinchona bark, calisaya bark, yellow Peruvian bark, yellow bark, jacket bark, yellow cinchona, Jesuits bark. Medicinal Properties: Antiperiodic, astringent, febrifuge, tonic, aperient.

It has an excellent effect upon the stomach in convalescence. Quinine is derived from this bark. As is well known, quinine often causes deafness, but this bark, used in its natural state, is harmless. It exerts an excellent influence on the entire nervous system. In fevers, drink the tea freely. It is excellent for dyspepsia, neuralgia, epilepsy, fevers, female debility, aids digestion, has healing influence on the lungs, and therefore is useful in cases of pneumonia.

PILEWORT
(Whole plant)

Botanical Name: Amaranthus hypochondriacus. Common Names: Amaranth, lovely bleeding, red cockscomb, pileworth, spleen amaranth, prince's feather. Medicinal Properties: Astringent, detergent in piles.

Excellent for excessive menstruation, leucorrhea, diarrhea, dysentery, hemorrhage from the bowels. Simmer a tablespoonful in a pint of water for ten minutes. Let cool, strain, and drink freely for the above diseases. An excellent gargle and wash for ulcers in the mouth and throat, also for an injection for leucorrhea, and as an external wash for old foul ulcers, piles, hemorrhoids, and wounds.

PIMPERNEL (See BURNET)

PLANTAIN
(Whole plant)

Botanical Name: Plantago major. Common Names: Way bread, roundleaved plantain, Englishman's foot, common plantain, ribworth. Medicinal Properties: Alterative, diuretic, antisyphilitic, antiseptic, astringent, deobstruent, styptic, vulnerary.

Plantain is an old-fashioned herb. The Indians used it to a great advantage. It grows practically all over the United States. Every family should gather some and have it ready for use. It has wonderful properties and many uses. There are two kinds of plantain—narrow and wide leaf. Both are good. The whole plant should be used.

Plantain has a soothing, cooling, and healing effect in cases of sores and ulcers. The fresh leaves pounded into a paste are good applied to wounds to check bleeding. It is extremely useful in erysipelas, eczema, burns, and scalds.

Make a strong tea and apply to the affected parts, using frequently in bad cases.

For piles and hemorrhoids, make a strong tea with an ounce of granulated plantain to a pint of boiling water. Let steep for twenty to thirty minutes. For hemorrhoids, use a glass syringe and inject one tablespoonful of this tea three or four times a day, at least, and especially after each stool, using more frequently in bad cases. For piles, apply externally with soft gauze or cotton. A saturated piece of gauze may be kept on the piles by using a belt or band around the body to which has been attached a narrow strip of cloth for holding the saturated gauze against the piles. An ointment for piles may be made by boiling slowly for about two hours two ounces of granulated plantain in one pint of soybean oil, peanut oil, or any other soluble oil.

For use in leucorrhea, make a strong tea and use as a douche with a whirling spray syringe.

For diarrhea, kidney and bladder trouble, and aching in the lumbar regions and bedwetting, plantain is wonderful. Make a tea by using one teaspoonful of granulated herbs in one cup of boiling water. Let steep for twenty or thirty minutes. If powdered herbs are used, take one small teaspoonful in a cup of hot water. Let stand about fifteen or twenty minutes, and drink a cupful of hot water. Let stand about fifteen or twenty minutes and drink a cupful of this tea four or five times a day until relief is obtained.

For use in scrofulous diseases and syphilis, use both internally and externally.

The green leaves give wonderful relief if mashed up and applied as a poultice to any part of the body stung by poisonous insects, snake bites, boils, carbuncles, and tumors.

Plantain tea will ease pains in the bowels. It will help clear the head of mucus, and stays all manner of flowings, even in women's courses, when too abundant. The plantain seed is good for dropsy, by making a tea of one teaspoonful to a cup of boiling water. The roots, beaten into powder, are good for toothache. A tea made with distilled water is good for inflamed eyes. The tea kills worms in the stomach and bowels. Equal parts of plantain and yellow dock make a very excellent wash for itch, ringworms, and all running sores. Plantain is excellent to heal fresh or old wounds or sores, either internal or external.

PLEURISY ROOT
(Root)

Botanical Name: Asclepias tuberosa. Common Names: Butterfly weed, wind root, Canada root, silkweed, orange swallow wort, tuber root, white root, flux root, asclepias. Medicinal Properties: Expectorant, carminative, tonic, diuretic, diaphoretic, relaxant, antispasmodic.

As the name suggests, it is very valuable in pleurisy. Excellent to break up colds, for la grippe, and all bronchial and pulmonary complaints. Very useful in scarlet fever, rheumatic fevers, lung fever, bilious fever, typhus, and all burning fevers, also measles. Good for suppressed menstruation and acute dysentery.

Treatment of pleurisy: Clean the stomach out first with an emetic. Steep a teaspoonful of powdered pleurisy root in a cup of boiling water for forty-five minutes, strain, and take two tablespoonfuls every two hours—oftener, if necessary. Apply to the affected part a cold compress, covering well with a flannel. Give a high enema of pleurisy root, using a tablespoonful to a quart of boiling water. Let steep and use about 112° F.

It is a tonic for the kidneys. Good for asthma.

POKE ROOT

Botanical Name: Phytolacca decandra. Common Names: Red weed, red ink plant, poke weed, garget, pigeon berry, scoke coakum, Virginia polk, pocan bush, cuncer jalap, American nightshade, red ink berries. Medicinal Properties: Alterative, resolvent, deobstruent, detergent, antisyphilitic, antiscorbutic.

The root is the part used as a medicine, but the tender leaves are excellent for greens for the dinner table. Especially in the early spring, they are eaten by many people for the purpose of toning up the whole system.

Poke root makes a good spring tonic. The green root of poke is a most useful agent. Very good in enlargements of the glands, spleen, and particularly the thyroid gland. Very good for hard liver, biliousness, inflammation of the kidneys, enlarged lymphatic glands. It is effective in goitre, taken internally, also applied as a poultice or liniment. It is effective for growths and for enlargements of bone from injury, if in a chronic state. Excellent in skin diseases, also syphilis, scrofula, and eczema. If a tea is made of the root applied to the skin, it will cure the itch.

It makes a good poultice for caked breasts. It has been used successfully for cancer of the breast as a poultice by grinding fine the fresh root. Roll this out so as to make a plaster to cover the breast completely, cutting out a hole for the nipple. Use a piece of cheese cloth or other thin material to put this on the breast, and once daily moisten the poultice with poke root tea made fresh each time. Do this for three days and put on a fresh poultice, continuing the treatment for fifteen days. The skin will be covered with little sores with pus. In about four to six weeks the hardness should then leave the breast. Then cleanse thoroughly and cover with boric acid powder, and allow the entire surface to become dry. In about ten days the sores will be completely healed and the trouble cured.

PSYLLA
(Seed)

Botanical Name: Plantago psyllium. Common Names: Branching plantain, flea seed, flea wort. Medicinal Properties: Demulcent, purgative, deturgent.

Psylla assists greatly in cases of colitis, ulcer, and hemorrhoids by relieving the stress occasioned during evacuation of the bowel. It relieves auto-intoxication, the cause of many diseases, by cleansing the intestines and removing the putrefactive toxins. Psylla being a purely vegetable product, no harmful effects, either physiological or chemical, can result from its use. It is superior to emulsions, oils, and agar compounds, which are widely known and used. For adults, take one or two teaspoonfuls with meals, preferably; or take an hour before meals in half a glass of water, hot water being preferred. For children the dose is one half to one teaspoonful. Vary the dose according to the individual needs. When soaked in water or any liquid, the seed gives out a substance like jelly which lubricates the intestines. Psylla could really be called a regular colon broom, as it cleans out the colon.

QUEEN OF THE MEADOW
(Root and whole herb)

Botanical Name: Eupatorium purpureum. Common Names: Gravel root, kidney root, Joe Pye, purple boneset, trumpet weed. Medicinal Properties: Diuretic, stimulant, tonic, astringent, relaxant.

This is a good remedy for gravel in the bladder, chronic urinary disorders, dropsy, neuralgia, lame back, and all such ailments. Excellent for rheumatism. Very soothing and will relax the nerves. Increases the flow of urine. Wonderful remedy when combined with uva ursi, marshmallow, blue cohosh, and lily root for female troubles, bladder and kidney affections, diabetes, and Bright's disease.

RAGWORT
(Plant)

Botanical Name: Senecio aureus. Common Names: Uncum root, waw weed, uncum, liferoot, liferoot plant, false valerian, golden sececio, cough weed, squaw weed, female regulator, cocash weed. Medicinal Properties: Expectorant, diaphoretic, febrifuge, emmenagogue, pectoral, tonic.

Has a very powerful influence upon the female organs. Combined with lily is one of the most certain and safe cures known for aggravated cases of leucorrhea, and also for suppressed menstruation. Good in all urinary diseases and gravel.

QUASSIA
(Wood and bark)

Botanical Name: Simarouba excelsa. Common Names: Quassia wood, quassia bark, bitter bark, bitter quassia, lofty quassia, bitter ash, bitter wood. Medicinal Properties: Tonic, febrifuge, anthelmintic.

The tea is an excellent tonic to tone up a run-down system. It will expel worms. Is a wonderful remedy to destroy the appetite for strong drink. In olden days cups were made of the wood and water and other liquids let to stand in them for a few minutes, thus receiving the virtue of the wood. Quassia is good in fevers, dyspepsia, and rheumatism.

RED CLOVER
(Flower)

Botanical Name: Trifolium pratense. Common Names: Cleaver grass, marl grass, cow grass. Medicinal Properties: Depurative, detergent, alterative, mild stimulant.

Red clover is one of God's greatest blessings to man. Very pleasant to take and a wonderful blood purifier. Combined with equal parts of blue violet, burdock, yellow dock, dandelion root, rock rose and golden seal, it is a most powerful remedy for cancerous growths and leprosy affections, also pellagra. Learn to use this God-given remedy effectively. Used alone it is excellent for cancer of the stomach, whooping cough, and various spasms. The warm tea is very soothing to the nerves. I have used red clover blossoms for many years with excellent results. When I was a boy, my parents had me gather it for their postmaster, who had a serious cancer. He lived to be an old man, without an operation.

Red clover blossoms were also one of Mrs. E. G. White's home remedies. Red clover is quieting to the nerves, effective in spasmodic, bronchial troubles, whooping cough, is healing to fresh wounds as well as old ulcers, and makes an excellent healing salve. Red clover is splendid for syphilis. A good prescription is the following:

> 1 oz. Red Clover
> 1 oz. Burdock Seed
> 2 oz. Oregon Grape
> ½ oz. Blood Root.

Use the granulated herbs. Mix well in one pint of hot water and one pint of hot apple cider. Cover and let stand for two hours. The dose is one wineglass four times a day.

Red clover is an exceedingly good remedy for cancer on any part of the body. If in the throat, make a strong tea and gargle four or five times a day, swallowing some of the tea. If in the stomach, drink four or more cups a day on an empty stomach. If there are sores on the outside of any part of the body, bathe freely with the tea. If in the rectum, inject with syringe, five or six times a day. If in the uterus, inject with bulb syringe, holding the vagina closed after the syringe is inserted so the tea will be forced well around the head of the womb. This should be held in for several minutes before expelling.

Every family should have a good supply of red clover blossoms. Gather them in the summer when in full bloom. Dry in the shade on papers. Put in paper bags when dry and hang in a dry place. Use this tea in place of tea and coffee and you will have splendid results. Use it freely. It can be taken in place of water.

RED PEPPER (See CAYENNE)

RED RASPBERRY
(Leaves and fruit)

Botanical Name: Rubus strigosus. Common Names: Wild red raspberry, raspberry. Medicinal Properties: Leaves: Anti-emetic, astringent, purgative, stomachic, parturient, tonic, stimulant, alterative. Fruit: Laxative, esculent, anti-acid, parturient.

Will remove cankers from mucous membrane. Excellent for dysentery and diarrhea, especially in infants. It decreases the menstrual flow without abruptly stopping it. Is very soothing and does not excite. Good to combine in such cases with prickly ash, blue cohosh, wild yam, and cinnamon. Will allay nausea. When the bowels are greatly relaxed, use in place of coffee and tea.

RED ROOT
(Root)

Botanical Name: Ceanothus Americana. Common Names: Walpole tea, bobea, New Jersey tea, wild snow ball, Jersey tea, mountain sweet, New Jersey tea tree. Medicinal Properties: Astringent, expectorant, sedative.

This is one of the most wonderful remedies for any spleen trouble. It has direct action on the spleen. It is good in dysentery, asthma, chronic bronchitis, whooping cough, and consumption, and is a splendid wash for the sore mouth of fevers and for canker in the mouth or throat. It will reduce sore, swollen tonsils by gargling with a strong tea every two hours. If tonsils are very sore and swollen, make a swab and work around good and gargle. It will reduce very badly enlarged tonsils, and the trouble will rarely ever recur. Excellent for piles or hemorrhoids. Inject the strong tea often.

It is effective in spasms, also is very effective in syphilis and gonorrhea. It is good for bilious sick headache, acute indigestion, and nausea due to inactivity of the liver, when combined with fringe tree and golden seal. Use one teaspoonful of the granulated red root to a pint of boiling water. Steep for twenty or thirty minutes. Drink one cupful of this tea before each meal and before going to bed. If the powdered herb is used, take half a teaspoonful in a cup of hot or cold water, using the same as directed for the granulated herb, that is, a cupful an hour before each meal and before going to bed.

Red root is also an excellent remedy used in diabetes.

RHUBARB
(Root)

Botanical Name: Rheum palmatum. Common Names: Turkey rhubarb, China rhubarb. Medicinal Properties: Vulnerary, tonic, stomachic, purgative, astringent, aperient.

Rhubarb is an old-time remedy, very useful for diarrhea and dysentery in adults and children. An excellent laxative for infants, as it is very mild and tonic. Excellent to increase the muscular action of the bowels. Excellent for use in stomach troubles. Will relieve headache. It stimulates the gall-ducts, thereby causing the ejection of bilious materials. Excellent for scrofulous children with distended abdomens. Good for the liver. Cleans and tones the bowels.

ROCK ROSE

Botanical Name: Helianthemum canadense. Common Names: Frostwort, frost weed, frost plant, sun rose, scrofula plant. Medicinal Properties: Aromatic, tonic, alterative, astringent. The oil from the plant is the valuable part.

Superior remedy for cancer. Valuable remedy for scrofula and has long been used for this purpose. Simmer a teaspoonful of the herb in a cup of water for ten minutes. Cool, strain, and take from four to six large swallows. A poultice made from the leaves is good for scrofulous tumors and ulcers. Excellent gargle for cankered sore throat and scarletina. Good for diarrhea, syphilis, and gonorrhea.

ROSEMARY
(Leaves and flower)

Botanical Name: Rosemarinus officinalis. Common Names: Garden rosemary, rosemary plant. Medicinal Properties: Stimulant, antispasmodic, emmenagogue, tonic, astringent, diaphoretic, carminative, nervine, aromatic, cephalic.

An old-fashioned remedy for colds, colic, and nervous conditions. Very good in headaches caused by nervousness. Shoud be taken warm for these complaints. Good as wash for mouth, gums, halitosis (foul breath), and sore throat. Is useful for female complaints. The leaves are used for flavoring. The oil is used as a perfume for ointments and liniments. This is an excellent ingredient for shampoos. Rosemary is helpful in cases of insanity. It aids digestion, cough, consumption, and strengthens the eyes.

RUE
(Whole plant)

Botanical Name: Ruta Graveolens. Common Names: Herb of grace, garden rue, countryman's treacle. Medicinal Properties: Aromatic, pungent, tonic, emmenagogue, stimulant, antispasmodic.

This is one of the herbs that have been used since time immemorial. It was anciently used by the priests, and even in Christ's time was a well-known herb and used by the people. It has been much used by Germans and other nationalities since then. This herb should be in every garden. Rue is very much like hyssop as a fine remedy for the many ills of humanity. Will relieve congestion of the uterus, lending a very stimulating and tonic effect. Excellent in suppressed menstruation. Steep a tablespoonful in a pint of boiling water for half an hour. Strain, drink warm, a cupful every two hours. Also good for painful menstruation. Excellent remedy for stomach trouble, cramps in the bowels, nervousness, hysteria, spasms, convulsions, will expel worms, relieve pain in the head, confused mind, dizziness, and insanity. Excellent for colic and convulsions in children. A poultice of rue is good for

sciatica, pain in the joints, and gout. It resists poison.
Steep a teaspoonful in a cup of boiling water for one-half
hour. Drink one to three cups a day, a large swallow at a
time. DO NOT BOIL RUE.

SAFFRON
(Flower and seed)

Botanical Name: Carthamus tinctorius. Common
Names: Dyers saffron, saffron seed, American saffron,
thistle saffron, false saffron, bastard saffron, parrot's corn,
safflower. Medicinal Properties: Laxative, emmenagogue,
condiment, carminative, sudorific, diuretic, diaphoretic.
Seed: Aromatic, laxative, diuretic.

Saffron is one of the old-fashioned remedies. One of
the most reliable in measles, all skin diseases, and scarlet
fever. Will produce profuse perspiration when taken hot;
therefore, very useful in colds and la grippe, also in regulating and increasing the menstrual flow, especially when
checked by cold. Very good in chlorosis hysteria.

As a culinary herb, it is used for dyeing.

SAGE
(Leaves)

Botanical Name: Saliva officinalis. Common Name:
Garden sage. Medicinal Properties: Sudorific, astringent, expectorant, tonic, aromatic, antispasmodic, nervine,
vermifuge.

Sage is a well-known seasoning for roasts, soups, etc.
The tea is an excellent gargle for ulcerated throat or mouth.
It can be mixed with a little lemon and honey. An excellent article for excessive sexual desire and sexual debility.
One of the best remedies for stomach troubles, dyspepsia,
gas in the stomach, and bowels. For quinsy, take the tea
externally and also gargle the throat. Will expel worms in

adults and children. Will stop bleeding of wounds, very cleansing to old ulcers and sores. Good for spermatorrhea. Also in liver and kidney troubles. Wounds of any kind will heal more rapidly when washed with sage tea. It is very soothing in nervous troubles and delirious fevers. A most effective hair tonic. Will make hair grow when roots are not destroyed, and remove dandruff. As a substitute for quinine, it is better than this drug.

For fever, la grippe, or pneumonia, first take a high enema; next take a big dose of body cleanser and laxative. Then go to bed and take three, four, or five cups of hot sage tea in short intervals—say a half hour apart. This will cause free perspiration, will make the whole body active, and will throw off the cold. It will relieve the pains in the head. It produces strong circulation. A strong tea is excellent to gargle for sore throat. This tea, drunk cold during the day, will prevent night sweats.

The American people would do well if they would use sage instead of tea and coffee. The Chinese make fun of the American people because they buy the expensive tea for their drink and pay a big price for it, while the Chinese buy sage from America for a small price and drink that for their tea, which is a most wonderful remedy. The Chinese know that the sage tea will keep them well, while the tea that we buy from the Chinese makes the American people sick, is a cause of great nervousness, and one of the causes of insanity. Sage tea is very soothing and quieting to the nerves, while the tea that we buy from China is a great cause of nervousness, headache, and delirium. In case of weaning a child, or when it is desired that the milk should cease in the breasts, in case of sickness or other reasons, the sage tea, drunk cold, will cause the flow of milk in the breasts to cease.

This tea should not be boiled, but just steeped. It should be kept covered while steeping. The ordinary dose is a heaping teaspoonful to a cup of hot water. Let it steep twenty or thirty minutes. Drink three or four cups a day. Never steep herbs in aluminum.

RED SAGE
(The whole herb)

Botanical Name: Salvia colorata. Common Name: Red Sage or purple topped sage. Medicinal Properties: Emmenagogue, diuretic, nervine, stimulant, tonic, diaphoretic, stomachic, mild astringent, aromatic, detergent, aphrodisiac.

Red Sage is a wonderful remedy for many diseases. It could almost be called a "cure-all." It might be said that you never go amiss when you take red sage.

Is very good for any lung trouble, asthma, coughs, colds, bronchitis, inflammation of the lungs, fevers of all kinds, la grippe, sore throat, tonsillitis. Gargle with a strong tea and swallow some; for diphtheria, gargle with a strong tea or swab the throat until the false membrane loosens.

Fine remedy for female troubles, will increase menstruation when too scanty and check it when profuse.

Is a splendid stomach remedy, prevents gas, fermentation, and biliousness. Is slightly laxative. Excellent liver cleanser. Is fine for nervousness, and nervous headache. Good for poultices, for inflammation of all kinds; very useful for typhoid and scarlet fevers, measles, and smallpox.

For any serious throat trouble add red root half and half, or wood betony. Ordinary dose is one heaping teaspoonful to a cup of hot water, steep thirty minutes, strain and take three or four cups a day one hour before meals and upon retiring, more or less as the case requires. Children according to age.

SANICLE
(Root and leaves)

Botanical Name: Sanicula marilandica. Common Names: Sanicle, black sanicle, black snake root, wood sanicle, sanicle root. Medicinal Properties: Vulnerary, astringent, alterative, expectorant, discutient, depurative.

Wood sanicle has powerful medicinal properties and many uses. This is one of the herbs that could well be called a "cure-all," because it possesses powerful cleansing and healing virtue, both internally and externally. Both the leaves and roots are used.

It is a powerful herb to heal both internal and external wounds and tumors. Use a heaping teaspoonful of the granulated herb to a cup of water. Let it steep for twenty or thirty minutes. Drink five or six cups a day. If the powder is used, put a good half teaspoonful to a cup of hot or cold water.

It will help to check women's courses if too free. It is also good to check hemorrhages from the lungs or bowels, and ulcerations of the kidneys. It will stop pain in the bowels. It is excellent in gonorrhea and syphilis, as it is powerful to cleanse the body from mucous and poisonous waste matter. It is very healing for sores in the mouth, for sore throat, quinsy, to cleanse throat of mucus when used as a gargle with a strong tea. It is very healing to ulcers in the stomach, and is an effective remedy to cure ulcers of the lungs and for the dreadful disease, consumption. The following combination is very effective:

> 2 oz. Sanicle
> 1 oz. Marshmallow Root

1 oz. Mullein Herb
1 oz. Golden Seal
½ oz. Myrrh

Of this mixture, take a heaping teaspoonful to a cup of boiling water. Let steep twenty or thirty minutes, and drink one cupful one hour before each meal and one before going to bed.

If powdered herbs are used, make a mixture using the same proportions, and take small half teaspoonful to a cup of hot or cold water. For external use, make a strong tea and bathe the affected parts four or five times a day.

In scurvy, erysipelas, scald head, tetters, and rashes it is effective to use externally.

SARSAPARILLA
(Root)

Botanical Name: Smilax officinalis. Common Names: Jamaica sarsaparilla, guay-quill sarsaparilla, red sarsaparilla. Medicinal Properties: Alterative, diuretic, demulcent, anti-syphilitic, stimulant, antiscorbutic.

Very useful in rheumatism, gout, skin eruptions, tetters, ringworm, scrofula. An excellent antidote after taking a deadly poison. Drink copiously after thoroughly cleaning out the stomach with an emetic. Excellent for internal inflammations, colds, catarrhs, and fever. Will increase the flow of urine. Good eyewash. Will promote profuse perspiration when taken hot. Powerful to expel gas from the stomach and bowels. One of the best herbs to use for infants infected with venereal disease. They can be cured with this without the use of mercurials. Wash the local pustules or sores with a tea made of the root, and administer inwardly by mixing the powdered root with their food.

SASSAFRAS
(Bark of the root)

Botanical Name: Sassafras officinale. Common Names: Ague tree, saxifrax, cinnamon wood, saloip. Medicinal Properties: Aromatic, stimulant, alterative, diaphoretic, diuretic.

Often called a spring medicine to purify the blood and cleanse the entire system. Good to flavor other herbs which have a disagreeable taste, and much used in combination with other blood-purifying herbs. Useful as a tonic to stomach and bowels. Will relieve gas. Taken warm, is an excellent remedy for spasms. Valuable in colic, and all skin diseases and eruptions. Good wash for inflamed eyes. Good for kidneys, bladder, chest, and throat troubles. Oil of sassafras is excellent for toothache. Good in varicose ulcers. Wash externally and take internally.

SAW PALMETTO BERRIES
(Fresh or dried berries)

Botanical Name: Serenoa serrulata. Common Names: Pan palm, dwarf palmetto. Medicinal Properties: Antiseptic, sedative, cardiac.

A very useful article in asthma and all kinds of throat troubles, especially when there is excessive mucous discharge from the head and nose, colds, bronchitis, la grippe, whooping cough, and where the throat is irritated and painful. Valuable in all diseases of the reproductive organs, ovaries, prostate, testes, etc. Very useful in Bright's disease and diabetes.

SEAWRACK
(Whole plant)

Botanical Name: Fucus versiculosus. Common Names: Bladder fucus, seaweed, bladder wrack, sea oak, kelpware, black tany. Medicinal Properties: Alterative, diuretic.

The best remedy for obesity. Good in all glandular affections, goiter, and scrofula. Has an excellent effect on the kidneys. Steep a heaping teaspoonful to a cup of boiling water for thirty minutes. Drink three or four cups a day an hour before meals, and one hot upon retiring.

SELF-HEAL
(Whole plant)

Botanical Name: Prunella vulgaris. Common Names: Wound wort, all heal, heal all, Hercules wound wort, brownwort, sickle wort, blue curls, panay, hook heal, hood weed. Medicinal Properties: Pungent, tonic, antispasmodic, vermifuge, diuretic, astringent, styptic, vulnerary.

Excellent for fits, convulsions, falling sickness, and obstructed liver. Will expel worms. Especially useful for internal and external wounds. For internal wounds, take the tea. Use as a poultice. Used as a wash in all external wounds and sores. Will stop bleeding. Also very cleansing. Will cleanse and heal ulcers of the mouth. Good for ulcerated private parts. An old Italian proverb says: "He that hath Self-Heal and Sanicle needs no other physician."

SENNA
(Leaves)

Botanical Name: Cassia marilandica. Common Names: American senna, locust plant, wild senna. Medicinal Properties: Laxative, vermifuge, diuretic.

Senna is a valuable, mild, and effective laxative, sometimes causing griping, therefore should be combined with an aromatic herb. Excellent for worms, biliousness, halitosis (bad breath), and bad taste in the mouth. Most effective for worms when combined with other herbs indicated for worms. Steep a teaspoonful in a cup of boiling water.

for thirty minutes, strain, and drink a cupful a day, more or less, according to needs.

SCULLCAP
(Whole plant)

Botanical Name: Scutellaria lateriflora. Common Names: Blue scullcap, blue pimpernel, hoodwart, hooded willow herb, side-flowering scullcap, mad dogweed, mad weed, helmet flower, American scullcap. Medicinal Properties: Antispasmodic, nervine, tonic, diuretic.

Is one of the best nerve tonics, often combined with others. Very quieting and soothing to the nerves of people who are easily excited. In delirium tremens will produce sleep. Good in neuralgia, aches and pains. Useful in St. Vitus's dance, shaking palsy, convulsions, fits, rheumatism, hydrophobia, epilepsy, and bites of poisonous insects and snakes. Splendid to suppress undue sexual desire. The following combination is a positive remedy for wakefulness: equal parts scullcap, nerve root, hops, catnip, and black cohosh. Take a tablespoonful of each, mix together, and use a heaping teaspoonful to a cup of boiling water. This combination is very useful in aiding a morphine addict to sleep. Scullcap as a substitute for quinine is more effective and is not harmful as quinine is.

SHEPHERD'S PURSE
(Whole plant)

Botanical Name: Capsella bursa pastoris. Common Names: Cocowort, shepherd's heart, pickpocket, toywort, pick purse, poor man's pharmacetty, St. James' weed, St. James' wort, St. Anthony's fire, pepper grass. Medicinal Properties: Astringent, detergent, vulnerary, diuretic.

Most excellent in cases of hemorrhage after child birth, and all other internal hemorrhages. Has been successful in such cases when all other remedies have failed. Good for bleeding of the lungs. One of the best remedies to check profuse menstruation. Excellent in intermittent fever, bleeding piles, and hemorrhoids. Steep a heaping teaspoonful to a cup of boiling water for thirty minutes, and drink cold two or more cupfuls a day as needed, a large mouthful at a time. Is also an excellent remedy for diarrhea.

Nearly every wheat field is full of this herb. It grows over the entire United States. When you chew the green grass, it has a very pleasant peppery taste.

SKUNK CABBAGE
(Roots and seed)

Botanical Name: Ictodes foetidus. Common Names: Meadow cabbage, skunk weed, collard, stinking poke, fedit hellebore, pole cat weed, swamp cabbage. Medicinal Properties: Sudorific, expectorant, pectoral, antispasmodic, stimulant, diaphoretic.

One of the old-fashioned, well-known remedies. Very reliable in tuberculosis, chronic catarrh, all bronchial affections, lung affections, whooping cough, spasmodic asthma, hay fever, pulmonary consumption, pleurisy. Excellent remedy in chronic rheumatism, nervous troubles, dysentery, spasms, convulsion, dropsy, hysteria, epilepsy, and for use during pregnancy. Good made into an ointment for external tumors and for all sores; greatly eases the pain.

SOLOMON'S SEAL
(Root)

Botanical Name: Convallaria polygonatum. Common Name: Solomon's seal. Medicinal Properties: Tonic, expectorant, astringent, mucilaginous.

A fine remedy for all kinds of female troubles. Excellent as a wash for poison ivy, erysipelas, and other sores on the body. Will allay pain and heal piles. Inject four or five tablespoonfuls of the tea several times a day into the rectum. Take internally as other tea for neuralgia. Solomon's seal makes an excellent poultice for external inflammations and wounds.

SORREL
(Leaves and root)

Botanical Name: Rumex acetosa. Common Names: Common field sorrel, red top sorrel, garden sorrel, meadow sorrel, sourgrass. Medicinal Properties: Diuretic, antiscorbutic, refrigerant, vermifuge.

The leaves are used like greens, as spinach, and are very high in life-giving properties.

It kills putrefaction in the blood, expels worms, and is warming to the heart. The root boiled is good for profuse menstruation or stomach hemorrhage. Also expels gravel from the kidneys, and is good in jaundice. A tea from the flowers is good in internal ulcers and black jaundice; also scurvy, scrofula, and all skin diseases. A poultice is excellent for cancer, boils, and tumors.

The leaves eaten as a salad in the spring are an excellent preventive for scurvy.

SPEARMINT
(Whole plant)

Botanical Name: Mentha viridis. Common Name: Mint. Medicinal Properties: Antispasmodic, aromatic, diuretic, diaphoretic, carminative.

A highly esteemed remedy for colic, gas in the stomach and bowels, dyspepsia, spasms, dropsy, and is very useful in nausea and vomiting, also for gravel in the bladder. Will relieve suppressed, painful, or scalding urine. Excellent local application for piles. Inject in small amounts into the rectum for painful piles. Good in inflammation of the kidneys and bladder. Excellent to stop vomiting in pregnancy. Very good to quiet and soothe the stomach after an emetic. Very soothing and quieting to the nerves. NEVER BOIL SPEARMINT. No home should be without this excellent home remedy.

SPIKENARD
(Root)

Botanical Name: Aralia racemosa. Common Names: American spikenard, pretty morel, life of man, spignet, Indian aralia bark. Medicinal Properties: Pectoral, diaphoretic, stimulant, alterative, balsamic.

One of the old-fashioned remedies. It makes childbirth easy and shortens the ordeal. Take the tea for some time before labor. Is an excellent blood purifier. For use in venereal diseases combine with the following: equal parts of spikenard, dandelion, burdock, yellow dock. Flavor with one of the following by using equal part: catnip, peppermint, wintergreen or sassafras. Good in all skin diseases, pimples, eruptions, etc. Very useful in coughs, colds, and all chest affections.

SQUAW VINE
(Whole plant)

Botanical Name: Mitchella repens. Common Names: Partridge berry, checkerberry, deerberry, winter clover, oneberry, hive vine, partridge berry, one-berry leaves. Medicinal Properties: Diuretic, astringent, tonic, alterative, parturient.

This herb was very highly esteemed by the Indian women. It is an excellent medicine to take during pregnancy, and will make childbirth wonderfully easy. It is better than red raspberry leaves, but it is good to combine the two. An excellent wash for sore eyes in infants. For this purpose combine with equal parts of raspberry leaves and witch hazel leaves. If the witch hazel leaves cannot be secured, use wild strawberry leaves. This is also an excellent injection for mild leucorrhea, dysentery, and gonorrhea. This herb is good for gravel, urinary troubles, uterine troubles, female complaints, and increases the menstrual flow. A strong tea made from the berries is good to bathe sore nipples. Add a little olive oil or cream. Stir thoroughly and apply.

ST.-JOHN'S-WORT
(Tops and flowers)

Botanical Name: Hypericum perforatum. Common Names: Johnswort. Medicinal Properties: Aromatic, nervine, astringent, resolvent, sedative, diuretic, vulnerary.

Powerful as a blood purifier. Very good in cases of tumors and boils. Very good in chronic uterine troubles, after pain in childbirth, suppressed urine, diarrhea, dysentery and jaundice. Will correct irregular menstruation. Good in hysteria, and nervous affections. Excellent for pus in the urine. Good used externally in the form of fomentation and ointment for caked breast, all wounds, ulcers, and old sores. Will correct bed-wetting in children when proper diet is given. The seeds steeped in boiling water will expel congealed blood from the stomach caused by bruises, falls, or bursting veins. For this purpose use a heaping teaspoonful of the seeds to a cup of boiling water.

STRAWBERRY
(Leaves)

Botanical Name: Fragaria vesca. Common Names: Mountain strawberry, pine apple strawberry, wood strawberry, common strawberry, wild strawberry. Medicinal Properties: Astringent, tonic, diuretic. Fruit: Diuretic, refrigerant.

This is the common, well-known strawberry leaf that is in every garden. All should become thoroughly acquainted with the medicinal properties and value of strawberry leaves. If a tea made of the leaves were used in place of tea and coffee, it would prove a blessing. It tones up the appetite and system generally. It is good for various bowel troubles, and cleanses the stomach. Is an excellent remedy for children. Good for eczema used internally and as a wash externally. Will prevent night sweats. Very useful in diarrhea and dysentery, and weakness of the intestines. Should be taken internally and also used as an enema.

SUMACH BERRIES

Botanical Name: Rhus glabrum. Common Names: Scarlet sumach, smooth sumach, dwarf sumach, upland sumach, Pennsylvania sumach, sleek sumach, mountain sumach. Medicinal Properties: Bark and leaves: Tonic, astringent, alterative, antiseptic: Berries: Diuretic, refrigerant, emmenagogue, diaphoretic, cephalic.

A remedy valuable in the cure of gonorrhea and syphilis when others have failed is the following: Equal parts sumach berries and bark, white pine bark, and slippery elm. This tea is very cleansing to the system, and is very useful in leucorrhea, scrofula, and for inward sores and wounds. A tea of sumach berries alone is excellent for bowel complaints, diabetes, all kinds of fevers, and for sores and canker in the mouth there is no superior. Use also as a gargle and wash for the mouth.

SUMMER SAVORY
(Whole plant)
Botanical Name: Satureja hortensis. Medicinal Proper-

ties: Aromatic, stimulant, carminative, condiment, emmenagogue, aphrodisiac.

A specific remedy for wind colic. Taken warm is excellent for suppressed menstruation, and is very useful in colds. The oil dropped into a tooth will relieve toothache.

As a culinary herb, the leaves are used for flavoring, usually combined with sage.

SWEET BALM
(Whole herb and flowers)

Botanical Name: Melissa officinalis. Common Names: Lemon balm, bee balm, blue balm, balm mint, sweet balm, citronelle, cure all, dropsy plant. Medicinal Properties: Aromatic, emmenagogue, diaphoretic, cephalic.

Very effective taken hot for la grippe, colds, and fevers. Excellent in all cases of nausea and vomiting, and will quiet and settle the stomach. Very useful in kidney and bladder troubles, headache, and suppressed urine. Useful in painful menstruation and female complaints.

TANSY
(Whole herb)

Botanical Name: Tanacetum vulgare. Common Names: Hindheel, common tansy. Medicinal Properties: Aromatic, tonic, emmenagogue, diaphoretic, vulnerary. Seed: Vermifuge.

An old well-known family remedy used to tone up the system and soothe the bowels. Excellent taken hot in colds, fevers, la grippe, and agues.

Good for dyspepsia. One of the best remedies to promote menstruation. Tansy seed will expel worms. Useful in hysterics, jaundice, dropsy, worms, and kidney troubles. Strengthens the weak veins. Hot fomentations wrung out of tansy tea is excellent for swellings, tumors, inflammations, bruises, freckles, sunburn, leucorrhea, sciatica, tooth-ache, and inflamed eyes. Good in heart trouble. Will check palpitation of the heart in a very short time.

THYME
(Whole plant)

Botanical Name: Thymus vulgaris. Common Names: Common garden thyme, mother of thyme. Medicinal Properties: Tonic, carminative, emmenagogue, resolvent, antispasmodic, antiseptic.

One of the old-time, household remedies. One can use it freely with benefit. Excellent taken hot for obstructed or suppressed menstruation. Good in fevers. Will produce profuse perspiration when taken hot. A reliable nervine, and excellent for nightmare. Valuable in whooping cough, asthma, and lung troubles. For small children, give small and frequent doses. Good remedy for weak stomach, dyspepsia, gas, griping, cramps in the stomach, and diarrhea. Better taken cold for these purposes. Will relieve headache.

TURKEY CORN
(Root)

Botanical Name: Corydalis formosa. Common Names: Wild turkey pea, staggerweed, dieyltra, turkey pea, squirrel corn, choise dieyltra. Medicinal Properties: Tonic, alterative, diuretic, antisyphilitic.

An excellent remedy in syphilis, scrofula, and all skin diseases. For boils, it is most effective when used in combination with hot baths and salt glows. An excellent tonic in all enfeebled conditions. One of the most valuable alteratives in the herbal kingdom. Take as a tea like other herbs.

TWIN LEAF
(Root)

Botanical Name: Jeffersonia diphylla. Common Names: Ground squirrel pea, rheumatism root, helmet pod, yellow root, twin leaf root. Medicinal Properties: Diuretic, alterative, antisyphilitic, antirheumatic, antispasmodic, tonic.

Very useful in chronic rheumatism, nervous, and spasmodic affections. Very successful in neuralgia, cramps, and syphilis. Splendid gargle for throat troubles. Fine in scarlet fever, scarletina, and indolent ulcers. Applied as a poultice or a hot fomentation wrung out of the strong tea, will relieve pain anywhere in the body. In severe pains, take hot internally. Steep a teaspoonful in a cup of boiling water thirty minutes, simmer ten minutes, strain, drink one cupful, and follow with small frequent doses.

UVA URSI
(Leaves)

Botanical Name: Arctostaphylos uva ursi. Common Names: Bearberry, upland cranberry, universe vine, mountain cranberry, mountain box, wild cranberry, bear's grape, kinpikinn ick, mealberry, sagckhomi. Medicinal Properties: Diuretic, astringent, nephreticum, tonic.

Very useful in diabetes, Bright's disease, and all kidney troubles. Excellent remedy for dysentery, piles, hemorrhoids, excessive menstruation, for the spleen, liver, pancreas, and when there are mucous discharges from the bladder with pus and blood. Excellent in gonorrhea, ulceration of the neck of the womb, and other female troubles. Take internally, and use also as a douche. Steep a heaping teaspoonful in a pint of boiling water thirty minutes, and drink one-half cupful every four hours.

VALERIAN
(Root)

Botanical Name: Valeriana officinalis. Common Names: English valerian, German valerian, great wild valerian, vermon valerian, vandal root, all heal, set wall, American English valerian (grown in U.S.). Medicinal Properties: Aromatic, stimulant, tonic, anodyne, antispasmodic, nervine.

Excellent nerve tonic—very quieting and soothing. Useful in hysterics. Will promote menstruation when taken hot. Excellent for children in measles, scarlet fever, and restlessness. Give two tablespoonfuls two or three times daily. Good for convulsions in infants. Useful in colic, low fevers, to break up colds, and also gravel in the bladder. Healing to ulcerated stomach, and very powerful to prevent fermentation and gas. The tea is very healing applied to sores and pimples externally, and must also be taken internally at the same time. Relieves palpitation of the heart. DO NOT BOIL THE ROOT.

VERVAIN
(Whole plant)

Botanical Name: Verbena hastata. Common Names: American vervain, wild hyssop, blue vervain, false vervain, simpler's joy, traveler's joy. Medicinal Properties: Tonic, sudorific, expectorant, vulnerary, emetic, nervine, emmenagogue, vermifuge.

Vervain is one of the most wonderful gifts of God in the healing of diseases. This herb should be in every home ready for use immediately when needed. Very powerful to produce profuse perspiration. Excellent in fevers. Will often cure colds overnight. Take a warm cup of the tea often. An excellent remedy in whooping cough, pneumonia, consumption, asthma, ague, will expel phlegm from the throat and chest. In fevers take a cup of the hot tea every hour, also for epilepsy and fits. Good in all female troubles. Will increase menstrual flow. Also good in scrofula and skin diseases. Will often expel worms when everything else fails. Take freely until the worms pass. Very useful in nervousness, delirium, insanity, sleeplessness, and nervous headache. Will tone up the system in convalescence from heart diseases. Will remove obstructions in the bowels, colon, and bladder. Good in stomach troubles, when the breath is short and there is wheezing. Used in combination of equal parts, smart weed, and peppermint leaves. Is excellent for appendicitis. In fevers use in combination with boneset, willow bark, or smart weed. The tea is very healing applied to external sores. Much better than quinine for the purposes for which quinine is used.

VIOLET
(See BLUE VIOLET)
(Virgin's Bower)

Botanical Name: Clematis virginica. Common Names: Common virgin's bower, traveler's joy. Medicinal Properties: Leaves and flowers: Stimulant, diuretic, sudorific, vesicant.

Will give relief to severe headaches. Combine with other herbs in poultices for cancer, ulcers, and bed sores. Combine with other herbs in ointments for cancer, itch, and ulcers. Internally steep a heaping teaspoonful in a cup of boiling water thirty minutes, strain, take a tablespoonful four to six times a day.

WAHOO
(Bark of the root)

Botanical Name: Euonymus atropurpureus. Common Names: Whahow, wauhoo, wahoo, Indian root, Indian arrow, Indian arrow wood, burning bush, bitter ash, arrow wood, spindle tree, strawberry tree, pegwood. Medicinal Properties: Tonic, laxative, expectorant, diuretic, alterative.

A splendid laxative. Excellent in chest and lung affections. Useful in fevers, dyspepsia, torpid liver, also pancreas and spleen. Good remedy for dropsy. Steep a small teaspoonful in a cup of boiling water thirty minutes. Take two or three cups a day, an hour before meals. Better than quinine.

WATER PEPPER
(Whole plant)

Botanical Name: Polygonum punctatum. Common Names: American water pepper, smart weed. Medicinal Properties: Astringent, diaphoretic, tonic, stimulant, emmenagogue, antiseptic.

Useful remedy for scanty menstruation, all womb troubles, gravel in the bladder, colds, coughs, bowel complaints, and kidney troubles. Can be used internally and externally. A poultice made of charcoal, moistened with water pepper tea is an excellent remedy for pain in the bowels, also ulcers. Is one of the best known remedies for this purpose. Take internally. Apply in a charcoal poultice. Give high enemas, fruit juice, a liquid diet for a few days; is a most wonderful remedy in appendicitis.

A fomentation wrung out of the hot tea and applied over the abdomen is very useful in cholera, also given in enema. Use the tea as a wash in erysipelas, and as a mouth wash for sore mouth in nursing mothers.

WHITE CLOVER
(Blossoms)

Botanical Name: Trifolium repens. Common Names:

White shamrock, shamrock. Medicinal Properties: Depurative, detergent.

Common white clover blossoms are an old-fashioned remedy to cleanse the system. A very fine blood purifier, especially in boils, ulcers and other skin diseases. The tea made strong is very healing to sores applied externally. Equal parts white clover, and yellow dock makes an excellent salve.

WHITE OAK BARK
(Whole plant)

(Leaves and bark—inner white bark is best)

Botanical Name: Querous alba. Common Name: Tanner's bark. Medicinal Properties: Tonic, astringent, antiseptic.

A very strong astringent. A strong tea made from white oak bark is excellent in leucorrhea and womb troubles. Will expel pin worms. Simmer a tablespoonful in a pint of water ten minutes. Drink three cups a day. One of the best remedies for piles and hemorrhoids, hemorrhages, or any trouble in the rectum. Use internally, and take in enema. For enemas and douches, steep a heaping tablespoonful in a quart of boiling water thirty minutes, and strain through a cloth. Use as hot as possible. Stops hemorrhages in the lungs, stomach, and bowels, spitting of blood, and bleeding at the mouth. Very helpful to prevent nocturnal emissions or night losses due to excessive sexual desire or a weakened condition. Increases the flow of the urine, and removes gallstones and kidney stones. Checks excessive menstrual flow. The tea is good for use in bathing scabs and sores. In fevers it brings the temperature down. It is helpful for ulcerated bladder or bloody urine.

Very useful in goiter and hardened neck. Excellent for varicose veins. Take the tea internally, and bathe the veins externally with a strong tea. In goiter, fold a small towel, or fold some cheesecloth several times to make a compress, and moisten in the tea as made for enemas. Tie around the neck, leaving all night, and covering well with a woolen or flannel cloth. The tea taken internally normalizes the liver, kidneys, and spleen, also is good for inward tumors and swellings. Bathe varicose veins three or four times a day, reducing the tea a little if there are any open sores. It is also good to moisten a cloth with the tea, wrap around the legs, and cover well with flannel. This will also reduce the swelling in hard tumors.

WHITE POND LILY
(Root)

Botanical Name: Nymphaea odorata. Common Names: White water lily, sweet-scented pond lily, sweet-scented water lily, toad lily, pond lily, water lily, cow cabbage, sweet water lily, water cabbage. Medicinal Properties: Deobstruent, astringent, vulnerary, discutient, demulcent, antiseptic.

This is one of the old-fashioned, home remedies. Very astringent. Use as a douche in leucorrhea. Take internally for leucorrhea, diarrhea, bowel complaints, scrofula. Excellent remedy in mucous troubles, and inflamed tissues in various parts of the body, and bronchial troubles. Very effective in dropsy, and kidney troubles, catarrh of the bladder, irritation of the prostate. Excellent for infant bowel troubles. Very healing to inflamed gums. In making poultices for painful swellings, boils, ulcers, etc., mix the ingredients with a strong tea of this herb. Valuable as a gargle for canker and sore throat. The leaves are very healing to wounds and cuts. Apply by poultice.

WHITE WILLOW

Botanical Name: Salix alba. Common Names: Willow salacin willow, willow bark, withe, withy. Medicinal Properties: Febrifuge, antiperiodic.

Useful in all stomach troubles, sour stomach, and heartburn. Excellent in intermittent fevers, all kinds of fevers, chills, ague, and acute rheumatism. The tea made from the leaves or buds is good in gangrene, cancer, and eczema. Use internally and externally. Good for bleeding wounds, nosebleed, or spitting of blood, as an anti-emetic, eye wash, and to increase flow of urine. Excellent to use in place of quinine, and far more effective.

WILD ALUM ROOT
(Root)

Botanical Name: Geranium maculatum. Common Names: Cranesbill, geranium, tormentil, spotted geranium, wild dovefoot, American tormentil, storksbill, wild cransbill, alum root, crowfoot, American kino root. Medicinal Properties: Astringent, styptic, antiseptic.

A powerful astringent. Very useful in cholera, diarrhea, and dysentery. Should be used both internally and externally. Rinse the mouth often with a strong tea for sores in the mouth and bleeding gums. Useful in piles. Inject a little of the strong tea several times a day. When there is bleeding from extracted teeth, rub some of the powder on. Excellent in hemorrhage, bleeding wounds, nosebleed, and profuse menstruation. The dry powder sprinkled on a wound or cut will stop bleeding immediately. Useful in old chronic ulcers. In womb troubles, give as a douche. A strong solution of the tea rubbed over the breast will dry up milk, or just over the nipples will harden them. For internal piles, inject two or three tablespoonfuls several times a day, and after each stool. Excellent for mucus and pus in the bladder and intestines, and for leucorrhea, or mucous discharges in any part of the body. Very useful in diabetes and Bright's disease. In mucous discharges it is excellent to use with an equal part of golden seal. Use a teaspoonful each to a pint of boiling water. Let steep thirty minutes. Use this liquid as an injection for piles or any trouble in the rectum, as a douche, or take internally, a tablespoonful four to six times a day. For general use, steep a heaping teaspoonful in a cup of boiling water thirty minutes. Drink one or more cupfuls a day, a large mouthful at a time. Children less according to age.

WILD CELANDINE (See CELANDINE)
WILD CHERRY
(Inner bark)

Botanical Name: Prunus virginiana. Common Names: Wild black cherry, black cherry, black choke, rub cherry, cabinet cherry. Medicinal Properties: Tonic, pectoral, sedative, stimulant.

Tones up the system. Loosens phlegm in the throat and chest. Good for colds, la grippe, tuberculosis, stomach troubles, dyspepsia, fevers, and daily recurring fevers, also high blood pressure. Will cure asthma.

WILD OREGON GRAPE
(Root)

Botanical Name: Berberis aquifolium. Common Names: Holly-leaved barberry, mahonia, California barberry. Medicinal Properties: Root: Tonic, alterative.

Useful in liver, kidney troubles, rheumatism, leucorrhea, or whites. Is good blood purifier, and useful in scrofulus and chronic skin diseases such as psoriasis, eczema, chronic uterine diseases, and constipation.

WILD YAM
(Root)

Botanical Name: Dioscorea villosa. Common Names: Colic root, China root, yuma, devil's bones. Medicinal Properties: Antispasmodic, antibilious, diaphoretic, hepatic.

Very relaxing and soothing to the nerves. Useful in all cases of nervous excitement. Will expel gas from the stomach and bowels. Good in cholera. Useful in neuralgia of any part. Excellent for pains in the urinary tract. One of the best herbs for general pain during pregnancy. Take during the whole period of pregnancy. Will allay nausea in small frequent doses. Excellent for cramps during the latter part of pregnancy. Combined with ginger will greatly help to prevent miscarriage. Use a teaspoonful of wild yam, one-fourth teaspoon ginger. Also good to combine with squaw vine for use during pregnancy. Valuable in affections of the liver, spasms, and rheumatic pains. Steep a heaping teaspoonful in a cup of boiling water thirty minutes. Drink cold one to three cupfuls a day, a large swallow at a time. Children less according to age.

WINTERGREEN
(Leaves)

Botanical Name: Gaultheria procumbens. Common Names: Spring wintergreen, candad tea, partridge berry, checkerberry, boxberry, wax cluster, spice berry, mountain tea, beerberry, spicy wintergreen, aromatic wintergreen, chink, ground berry, grouse berry, red pollom, redberry tea, hillberry, ivory plum. Medicinal Properties: Stimulant, antiseptic, astringent, diuretic, emmenagogue.

This is an old-fashioned remedy. Taken in small frequent doses will stimulate stomach, heart, and respiration. Useful in chronic inflammatory rheumatism, also rheumatic fever, sciatica, diabetes, catarrh of the bladder, and all bladder troubles, scrofula, and skin diseases. Valuable in colic and gas in the bowels. Helpful in dropsy, gonorrhea, stomach trouble, and obstructions in the bowels.

The oil of the wintergreen is used internally and externally. It is very useful in liniments.

As a poultice, it is good in boils, swellings, ulcers, felons, and inflammation. A douche of the tea is excellent in whites and leucorrhea. The tea is also very beneficial as a gargle in sore throat and mouth. Good wash for sore eyes.

WITCH HAZEL
(Bark and leaves)

Botanical Name: Hamamelis virginica. Common Names: Winter bloom, striped elder, spotted elder, hazelnut, snapping hazel, pistachio, tobacco wood. Medicinal Properties: Astringent, tonic, antiphlogistic, sedative.

This is an old-fashioned remedy. The writer has used witch hazel for over thirty years with most remarkable results. It is unsurpassed for stopping excessive menstruation, hemorrhages from the lungs, stomach, uterus, bowels, etc. Very useful in diarrhea, taken internally and as an enema. In nosebleed, snuff the tea up the nose. For piles, inject a teaspoonful several times a day and after each stool. Excellent local application in gonorrhea. Will restore perfect circulation. As a poultice or wash is excellent for painful tumors, all external inflammation, piles, bed sores, and sore and inflamed eyes. Excellent gargle in throat troubles. In piles and dysentery, or diarrhea, give enemas. In gonorrhea, leucorrhea, and whites, give as a douche. Internally, steep a heaping teaspoonful in a cup of boiling water thirty minutes. Take one or more cupfuls during the day as needed, a large mouthful at a time. Children less according to age.

WOOD BETONY
(Leaves)

Botanical Name: Betonica officinalis. Common Names: Lousewort, betony. Medicinal Properties: Aperient, stomachic, nervine, tonic, antiscorbutic.

Excellent for the stomach. Mildly stimulating to the heart. Unsurpassed for headache, insanity, neuralgia, all pains in the head or face, heartburn, indigestion, cramps in the stomach, jaundice, palsy, convulsions, gout, colic pains, all bilious and nervous complaints, dropsy, colds, la grippe, consumption, worms, delirium, poisonous serpents, insect bites. Open obstructions of liver and spleen. More effective than quinine.

Formula:—Two parts wood betony, one part scullcap, one part calamus root.

WOOD SAGE
(Whole plant)

Botanical Name: Teucrium scorodonia. Common Name: Garlic sage. Medicinal Properties: Tonic, vermifuge, alterative, diuretic, slightly diaphoretic.

Will promote appetite. Good external wash to cleanse old sores, combined with chickweed. Makes an excellent poultice for old sores, indolent ulcers, swellings, and boils. As a poultice for cancer and tumors combine with comfrey and ragwort. This will often cure. Very useful in palsy, quinsy, sore throat, colds, fevers, kidney and bladder troubles. Increases urine flow and menstrual flow.

(331)

WOOD SANICLE—(See SANICLE)
WORMWOOD
(Whole plant)

Botanical Name: Artemisia absinthium. Common Name: Absinthium. Medicinal Properties: Aromatic, tonic, antiseptic, febrifuge.

An old and good remedy for bilious and liver troubles, jaundice, and intermittent fevers. Excellent appetizer. Will expel worms. Good in chronic diarrhea and leucorrhea. Good in poor digestion. The oil of wormwood is an excellent ingredient for liniments, for use in sprains, bruises, lumbago, etc.

Fomentations wrung out of the hot tea are excellent for use in rheumatism, swellings, and sprains.

Internally, steep a heaping teaspoonful in a cup of boiling water, for thirty minutes. Drink one or two cups a day, a large swallow at a time. Children less according to age.

YARROW
(Plant)

Botanical Name: Achillea millefolium. Common Names: Milifoil, noble yarrow, nosebleed, millefolium, ladies' mantle, thousand leaf. Medicinal Properties: Astringent, tonic, alterative, diuretic, vulnerary.

The writer has used yarrow very extensively as it grows very abundantly in the northern part of Wisconsin where he was born and reared. It also grows in many other parts of the United States.

Excellent for hemorrhages and bleeding from the lungs. If taken freely at the beginning of a cold with other simple remedies, it will break it up in twenty-four hours. A fine remedy in all kinds of fevers, taken hot. Most effective remedy for suppressed urine, scanty urine, and where there are mucous discharges from the bladder. An ointment of yarrow will cure old wounds, ulcers, and fistulas. Excellent douche for leucorrhea. Very useful in measles, smallpox, and chicken pox. Good for dyspepsia and hemorrhages of the lungs and bowels.

For piles and hemorrhages, use an enema of the tea after the bowels have been cleansed with a cleansing enema. Also inject two tablespoonfuls several times a day, and after each stool. When there is a bad condition of piles and hemorrhoids, take a cleansing and yarrow enema each day. When there is much pain have the water 112° to 115° F. Yarrow has a very healing and soothing effect on the mucous membranes. It is a very successful remedy in typhoid fever. For diarrhea and dysentery it is effective. Is excellent for diarrhea in infants. For very small infants inject a cupful, and more according to age. Successful in female troubles, in womb troubles. Inject right into the womb. Good to expel gas from the stomach. Very useful in diabetes and Bright's disease. Yarrow is more effective than quinine. In fevers drink hot. Steep a heaping teaspoonful in a cup of boiling water for thirty minutes. Drink three or four cups a day an hour before meals, and one upon retiring. Children less according to age.

YELLOW DOCK
(Root)

Botanical Name: Rumex crispus. Common Names: Sour dock, curled dock, narrow dock, garden patience. Medicinal Properties: Alterative, tonic, depurative, astringent, antiscorbutic, detergent.

Excellent and effective remedy in the following diseases: Impure blood, tones up the entire system, good in eruptive diseases, scrofula, glandular tumors, swellings, leprosy, cancer, ulcerated eyelids, syphilis, running ears, and for itch. Makes a valuable ointment for itch and sores. For glandular tumors and swellings, apply fomentations wrung from the hot tea. Most wonderful blood purifier.

YERBA SANTA

Botanical Name: Eriodyction glutinosum. Common Names: Consumptive weed, gum plant, bear's weed, mountain balm, tar weed. Medicinal Properties: Tonic, expectorant.

This is a well-tried and much-used remedy in chronic laryngitis, bronchitis, and various lung troubles. Effective when there is excessive discharge from the nose. Good in rheumatism.

CHAPTER XXX

DEFINITIONS OF MEDICINAL PROPERTIES OF HERBS

Alterative: Producing a healthful change without perceptible evacuation

Anodyne: Relieves pain

Anthelmintic: An agent which expels worms

Aperient: Gently laxative, without purging

Aromatic: Stimulant, spicy

Astringent: Causes contraction and arrests discharges

Antibilious: Acts on the bile, relieving biliousness

Antiemetic: Stops vomiting

Antiepileptic: Relieves fits

Antiperiodic: Arrests morbid periodical movements

Anthilitic: Prevents the formation of calculi in the urinary organs

Antirheumatic: Relieves or cures rheumatism

Antiscorbutic: Cures or prevents scurvy

Antiseptic: Opposed to putrefaction

Antispasmodic: Relieves or prevents spasms

Antisyphilitic: Having effect on or curing venereal diseases

Carminative: Expels wind from the bowels

Cathartic: Evacuating to the bowels

Cephalic: Used in diseases of the head

Cholagogue: Increases the flow of bile

Condiment: Improves flavor of food

Demulcent: Soothing, relieves inflammation

Deobstruent: Removes obstructions

Depurative: Purifies the blood

Detergent: Cleansing to boils, ulcers, and wounds

Diaphoretic: Produces perspiration

Discutient: Dissolves and removes tumors

Diuretic: Increases the secretion and flow of urine

Emetic: Produces vomiting

Emmenagogue: Promotes menstruation

Emollient: Softening and soothing to inflamed parts

Esculent: Eatable as food

Exanthematous: Remedy for skin eruptions and diseases

Expectorant: Facilitates expectoration

Febrifuge: Abates and reduces fevers

Hepatic: Remedy for diseases of the liver

Herpatic: Remedy for skin eruptions, ringworm, etc.

Laxative: Promotes bowel action

Lithontryptic: Dissolves calculi in the urinary organs

Maturating: Ripens or brings boils, tumors, and ulcers to a head

Mucilaginous: Soothing to inflamed parts

Nauseant: Produces vomiting

Nervine: Acts specifically on the nervous system, allaying nervous excitement

Opthalmicum: A remedy for disease of the eye

Parturient: Induces and promotes labor at childbirth

Pectoral: Remedy to relieve chest affections

Refrigerant: Cooling

Resolvent: Dissolves and removes tumors

Rubifacient: Increases circulation, produces red skin
Sedative: Tonic effect on nerves, also quieting
Sialagogue: Increases the secretion of saliva
Stomachic: Strengthens and gives tone to the stomach
Styptic: Arrests hemorrhage and bleeding
Sudorific: Produces profuse perspiration
Tonic: Remedy which is invigorating and strengthening
Vermifuge: Expels worms

CHAPTER XXXI

HERBS INDICATED FOR SPECIFIC DISEASES

The following pages give a number of diseases and a list of nonpoisonous herbs which are especially good for these diseases. Study the description of each one of these herbs as given in this book, also directions for use of nonpoisonous herbs.

APPETITE
(Herbs to improve appetite)

Agrimony, beech, calamus, camomile, colombo, gentian root, ginseng, golden seal, origanum, strawberry, wood sage, wormwood, balomy, marjoram.

ACHES

Scullcap, motherwort, valerian, catnip, peppermint, angelica.

ADENOIDS

Bayberry bark, bloodroot, golden seal, myrrh, echinacea, red root.

AGUE

Gentian root, sorrel, tansy, vervain, willow, broom, camomile.

APPENDICITIS

Buckthorn bark, vervain, water pepper, lady's-slipper, body cleanser and laxative (as given in this book).

ASTRINGENTS

Bistort root (strongest astringent known), fire weed, white oak bark, wild alum root, bayberry bark.

(338)

ABCESSES

Carrot (poultice), lobelia, mugwort, slippery elm, charcoal, potato (poultice).

ANEMIA

Comfrey, dandelion, fenugreek, barberry bark, agrimony, century, raspberry leaves, quassia chips.

APOPLEXY

Masterwort, black cohosh, hyssop, vervain, blue cohosh, catnip, antispasmodic tincture, scullcap.

ASTHMA

Black cohosh, comfrey, coltsfoot, horehound, hyssop, Indian hemp, lobelia, masterwort, milkweed, mullein, myrrh, pleurisy root, prickly ash, saw palmetto berries, skunk cabbage, thyme, vervain, wild cherry, flaxseed, masterwort, balm of Gilead, red root, red sage, boneset, cubeb berries, elecampane.

BLADDER

Celandine, aloes, juniper berries, comfrey, apple tree bark, balm, beech, broom, carrot, camomile, cleavers, corn silk, cubeb berries, fleabane, golden seal, hydrangea, hyssop, nettle, peach leaves, birch, buchu, pimpernel, queen of meadow, sassafras, slippery elm, spearmint, sweet balm, uva ursi, valerian, vervain, water pepper, white pond lily, wild alum root (pus in bladder), wintergreen, wood sage, yarrow, hemlock, bethroot.

BREASTS (SORE, SWOLLEN, CAKED)

Comfrey, parsley, St. John's-wort (caked), poke root (caked).

BOWEL TROUBLES

Water pepper, white pond lily, wintergreen, dandelion, wood sanicle, bethroot, chickweed, myrrh, witch hazel, echinacea, bayberry bark, birch, bitterroot, blue violet, caraway seed (expels wind), catnip (for acids), chickweed, comfrey, coriander, cubeb berries, fenugreek, golden seal, gum arabic, hyssop, magnolia, masterwort, milkweed, mugwort, mullein, origanum, pileworth, rhubarb, rue, sage, sanicle, sassafras, slippery elm, spearmint, strawberry, sumach berries, tansy, vervain, marshmallow.

BILIOUSNESS

Apple tree bark, senna, poke root, camomile, red sage (excellent), wood betony, queen of the meadow, hyssop, agrimony.

BED SORES

Plantain, balm of Gilead, bayberry bark, bloodroot, witch hazel, golden seal.

BRIGHT'S DISEASE

Golden seal (combined with peach leaves, queen of the meadow, clover, and corn silk), Indian hemp, queen of the meadow, saw palmetto berries, uva ursi, wild alum root, yarrow, peach leaves, blossoms or twigs, peppermint.

BLOOD PURIFIER

Bittersweet, blue cohosh, burdock, chickweed, dandelion, elder, fire weed, gentian root, hyssop, nettle, prickly ash, red clover, sanicle, sassafras, sorrel, spikenard, St.-Johns'-wort, turkey corn, white clover, yellow dock, borage, cleavers, echinacea, blue flag, wild Oregon grape, fringe tree, poke root (greens), holy thistle, dandelion, elecampane, sarsaparilla.

BED-WETTING

Plantain, St.-John's-wort, buchu, corn silk, cubeb berries, fennel seed, milkweed, wood betony.

BILE

Bitterroot (increases secretion); hops (increases secretion), cascara sagrada, fringe tree, celandine (will remove bile from gall bladder.)

BACKACHE

Nettle, pennyroyal, tansy, uva ursi, buchu, wood betony.

BLEEDING

Self-heal, mullein (stops bleeding from lungs), shepherd's purse (for lungs, stomach, kidneys and bowels), wild alum root.

BRUISES AND CUTS

Buglewood (for internal bruises), comfrey, hyssop, lobelia, mugwort, giant Solomon seal, St.-John's-wort, bittersweet (combined with camomile as ointment), pennyroyal, tansy, balm of Gilead, burnet.

BLOOD POISONING

Chickweed, plantain, echinacea, golden seal, myrrh, burdock, bloodroot, smart weed and charcoal poultice.

BURNS

Bittersweet, burdock, calamus, chickweed, elder, poplar, onions (bruised), comfrey, liniment (See Table of Contents).

Immerse burned part in real cold water and keep the water cold by changing or adding more ice or cold water. Keep covered with water until fire is all drawn out and there will not be any blister.

BRONCHITIS

Chickweed, coltsfoot, cubeb berries, golden seal, lungwort, mullein, myrrh, white pine, pleurisy, sanicle, saw palmetto berries, skunk cabbage, slippery elm, white pond lily, yerba santa, bloodroot, ginger, blue violet, bethroot, red root, red sage, elecampane.

BEVERAGES
(Herbs used as beverages)

Red clover blossoms, sage, mint, sassafras, strawberry leaves, peppermint, spearmint, fennel, red raspberry leaves, hyssop, chickweed, catnip, wintergreen, sarsaparilla, wild cherry bark or small twigs, birch bark or small twigs, chicory, dandelion, yellow dock, camomile, hops, calamus root (sweet flag), meadow sweet, juniper berries, alfalfa, green celery leaves, horsemint, rue.

BOILS AND CARBUNCLES

Balm poultice, powdered bayberry bark, poultice, burdock, chickweed, comfrey, coral, flaxseed, hops, lobelia, origanum, slippery elm, sorrel, St.-John's-wort, turkey corn, white clover, white water lily, wintergreen, wood sage, echinacea, birch bark or small twigs, plantain, wild cherry bark or small twigs.

CARBUNCLES

Carrot (poultice), lobelia (poultice), mugwort, echinacea, burdock, origanum.

CANKER IN MOUTH

Bayberry bark, bistort (combined with equal parts of red raspberry leaves), golden seal, gold thread, myrrh, pilewort, red raspberry, rock rose, self-heal, sumach berries, white water lily, wild alum root, birch, burdock, pennyroyal, rosemary, prickly ash, hemlock, wood sanicle, red root.

CANCER

Blue violet (with rock rose and red clover blossoms), chickweed, cleavers, coral, red clover (combined with blue violet, burdock, yellow dock, dandelion root, rock rose, and golden seal), rock rose, slippery elm, sorrel, virgin's bower, willow, wood sage, yellow dock, poplar, golden seal, poke root(poultice, also tea), comfrey, blue flag.

CRAMPS

Blue cohosh, cayenne (stomach cramps), coral, fennel, motherwort, rue, thyme, twin leaf, wood betony, masterwort, pennyroyal.

CROUPS

Mullein, white pine, antispasmodic tincture (as found in Table of Contents).

CORNS AND CALLOUSES

Bittersweet and camomile combined into an ointment, liniment (See Table of Contents).

COUGHS

Blue violet, comfrey, coltsfoot, ginseng, horehound, hyssop, lungwort, myrrh, origanum, white pine, water pepper, (smart weed), black cohosh, bloodroot, borage, flaxseed, marjoram, rosemary, spikenard, balm of Gilead, bethroot, red sage.

CHEST TROUBLE

Ginseng, hops, hyssop, myrrh, pimpernel, white pine, sassafras, giant Solomon seal, vervain, wahoo, wild cherry, spikenard, comfrey, shepherd's purse, yarrow, elecampane, horehound.

CONVULSIONS

Black cohosh, catnip, fit root, rue, scullcap, self-heal, skunk cabbage, valerian, gentian, pennyroyal, mistletoe, antispasmodic tincture (to stop convulsions), wild yam, lady's-slipper, peppermint, fennel seed, sweet balm, sweet weed, hyssop.

CATARRH

Bayberry bark, coltsfoot, golden seal, Indian hemp, lungwort, marshmallow, mullein, white pine, sanicle, skunk cabbage, sarsaparilla, bloodroot, comfrey, fringe tree, buchu.

CIRCULATION (INCREASE)

Cayenne, gentian, golden seal, hyssop, witch hazel, holy thistle. Combination: Golden seal, scullcap, cayenne, bayberry bark.

CHOLERA INFANTUM

Birch, poplar, yarrow, wild cherry bark, red raspberry leaves and lady's-slipper as enema, bayberry bark (as enema, and also to take internally), wild alum root.

COLDS

Bayberry bark with yarrow, catnip, sage, peppermint, wood betony, angelica, blue violet, butternut bark, ginseng, Indian hemp, lungwort, nettle, white pine, pleurisy root, prickly ash, rosemary, saffron, summer savory, sweet balm, tansy, valerian, vervain, water pepper, wood sage, yarrow, blood root, elder, ginger, gentian, golden seal, hyssop, masterwort, pennyroyal, sarsaparilla, saw palmetto berries, spikenard, wild cherry.

COLIC

Blue cohosh, caraway seed, carrot seed, catnip, dill, fennel, masterwort, origanum, pennyroyal, peppermint, prickly ash, rosemary, rue, sassafras, spearmint, summer savory, wintergreen, wood betony, flaxseed, valerian, fringe tree, angelica, motherwort.

COLON TROUBLE

Colombo, fire weed, fleabane, peppermint, vervain, aloes, slippery elm bark, bayberry bark, white oak bark, golden seal, myrrh.

CONSUMPTION (TUBERCULOSIS)

Coltsfoot, plantain, sanicle, skunk cabbage, slippery elm, vervain, colombo, comfrey, marjoram, pennyroyal, rosemary, wood betony, bethroot, red root, sanicle, wild cherry, myrrh, golden seal, horehound, elecampane root.

CHILLS

Cayenne pepper, bayberry bark tea with pinch of cayenne, myrica, peppermint, willow, peach, sage, catnip, anti-spasmodic tincture (to stop chill).

CHOLERA

Bistort root, cayenne, colombo, elder, fire weed, fleabane, peppermint, prickly ash, wild alum root, wild yam, ginger, water pepper (smart weed, red clover, geranium).

CHOLERA MORBUS

Peach leaves, bistort, queen of the meadow, raspberry leaves, peppermint, rhubarb, charcoal (Pulverize, and take two heaping teaspoonfuls in cup of water every two hours.)

CHILDBIRTH (TO MAKE EASY)

Black cohosh, blue cohosh (brings on labor pains when time), shepherd's purse, spikenard (taken some time before, shortens the ordeal), squaw vine (taken some time before, shortens the ordeal), red raspberry leaves—a teacupful with juice of one orange squeezed in three cups daily through last month will make childbirth easy. Combine with squaw vine. Angelica to expel afterbirth.

CONSTIPATION

Balomy, buckthorn bark, cascara sagrada, chickweed, ginger, mandrake, origanum, psylla, white ash, elder, blue flag, wild Oregon grape, rhubarb root, butternut bark.

DIABETES

Beech, blue cohosh, golden seal, Indian hemp, white pine, poplar, queen of meadow, saw palmetto berries, sumach berries, uva ursi, wild alum root, wintergreen, yarrow, buchu (first stages of diabetes), dandelion root (especially good), bittersweet, white pine with: uva ursi, marshmallow, poplar bark. Red root, blueberries and blueberry leaves (especially good), raspberry leaves (very good), pleurisy root.

DYSENTERY

Balm, mullein, bethroot, bayberry bark, birch, bistort, comfrey, colombo, fire weed, fleabane, magnolia, marshmallow, masterwort, nettle, peppermint, pilewort, plantain, pleurisy root, red raspberry, rhubarb, skunk cabbage, slippery elm, squaw vine, St.-John's-wort, strawberry, uva ursi, witch hazel, purse, ginger (preferably African ginger), hemlock, geranium.

DIZZINESS

Peppermint, catnip, rue, wood betony.

DANDRUFF

Burdock, nettle (bull), sage.

DEAFNESS

Chickweed, origanum, marjoram, angelica, wintergreen (oil of), rosemary, oil of sassafras, oil of hemlock, tincture of myrrh, tincture of lobelia.

DROPSY

Wood betony, hemlock, buchu, blue flag, celandine, juniper berries, holy thistle, lobelia, iris (excellent), bitterroot, black cohosh, blue cohosh, broom, buckthorn bark, carrot, celery, cleavers, dandelion, elder, hydrangea, Indian hemp, milkweed, mullein, nettle, origanum, parsley, queen of meadow, skunk cabbage, spearmint, tansy, twin leaf, wahoo, white ash, white pond lily, wintergreen, camomile, hyssop, marjoram, masterwort, pennyroyal, plantain, lily of the valley, dwarf elder (excellent.)

DIARRHEA (See BOWEL TROUBLE)

Bayberry bark, birch, bistort root, comfrey, colombo, elder, marshmallow, mullein, nettle, peppermint, pilewort, poplar, red raspberry, rhubarb, St.-John's-wort, slippery elm, strawberry, thyme, white pond lily, witch hazel, wild alum root, yarrow, wormwood, ginger, rock rose, hemlock, bethroot, cinnamon, shepherd's purse, plantain, blackberry root, cranesbill, charcoal pulverized. One heaping teaspoonful every two hours.

DIPHTHERIA

Golden seal, Indian hemp, myrrh, echinacea, lemon juice, red sage, jaborandi, eucalyptus, capsicum (red pepper), make a gargle of it (very effective), lobelia.

DYSPEPSIA

Beech, buckbean, calamus, cayenne, colombo, gentian root, golden seal, gold thread, horehound, magnolia, origanum, peach leaves, quassia, sage, spearmint, tansy, thyme, wahoo, wild cherry, yarrow, balomy, blood root, camomile, Peruvian bark, ginger.

DELIRIUM AND DELIRIUM TREMENS

Motherwort, vervain, wood betony, mistletoe, hops, lobelia, scullcap, lady's-slipper, hyssop, quassia chips, black cohosh, valerian, antispasmodic tincture (for quick relief).

ENEMA

Catnip, chickweed, bayberry bark, white oak bark, shepherd's purse, wild alum root, echinacea, strawberry leaves, raspberry leaves.

EARS (RUNNING)

Yellow dock, lemon juice diluted one-half, oil of origanum, peroxide of hydrogen (Put in ear warm).

EMETICS AND ANTIEMETICS

Bayberry bark, buckbean, lobelia (large doses), small doses will stop spasmodic vomiting, mint (antiemetic), mustard, myrica, peach leaves (antiemetic), peppermint, (antiemetic), giant Solomon seal (antiemetic), spearmint, (antiemetic), white willow, colombo (antiemetic), ragwort (emetic).

EARACHE

Hops, origanum, pimpernel, lemon juice (pure), burnet.

EYES

Rosemary, borage (inflamed or sore eyes), camomile cataract, chickweed, elder, fennel, golden seal, hyssop, marshmallow, rock rose, sarsaparilla, sassafras, slippery elm, squaw vine, witch hazel, wintergreen, yellow dock, plantain, golden seal and burnt alum, tansy, white willow, chickweed, angelica.

ECZEMA

Balomy, beech, cleavers, dandelion, golden seal, nettle, strawberry, willow, bloodroot, wild Oregon grape, poke root, white poplar bark, plantain, yellow dock.

ERYSIPELAS

Chickweed, coral, elder, golden seal, lobelia, magnolia, plantain, Solomon's seal, giant Solomon's seal, water pepper (smart weed), wood sanicle, echinacea, slippery elm powder (sprinkled on), cayenne pepper.

EPILEPSY

Black cohosh, elder, mistletoe, Peruvian bark, vervain, valerian, scullcap, lady's-slipper, antispasmodic tincture.

FEVER

Catnip, sage, shepherd's purse, sumach berries, sweet balm, tansy, thyme, valerian, vervain, wahoo, wild cherry, willow, wintergreen, wood sage, wormwood, yarrow, borage, dandelion, Peruvian bark, apple tree bark (intermittent fever), bitterroot (intermittent fever), buckbean (intermittent fever), camomile, cinchona bark, cleavers, colombo, butternut bark (all fevers), calamus, intermittent fevers, coral, elder, fenugreek, fire weed, fit root, gentian root, hyssop, masterwort, Indian hemp, lobelia (excellent), magnolia, mandrake, nettle, parsley, pennyroyal, peppermint, pleurisy root, poplar, quassia, mugwort, cayenne, fringe tree, echinacea, angelica, yarrow (break up fever in 24 hours), sarsaparilla, red sage, boneset, lily of the valley, cedron (intermittent fever).

FLOODING

Bayberry bark tea, ginger and cinnamon tea (checks), yarrow, shepherd's purse, wood betony, burnet, cayenne pepper, red sage, celandine (checks flooding), bistort.

FAINTING

Lavender (prevents), cayenne, peppermint, antispasmodic tincture, motherwort.

FELONS

Bittersweet (poultice made of the berries), lobelia, origanum, wintergreen.

FEMALE TROUBLE

Black cohosh, milkweed, motherwort, mugwort, parsley, prickly ash, queen of meadow, ragwort, rosemary, slippery elm, Solomon's seal, giant Solomon's seal, squaw vine, sweet balm, vervain, yarrow, comfrey, Peruvian bark, dandelion root, gentian root, bethroot, red sage.

FERMENTATION AND GAS (SEE HEARTBURN)

Anise, calamus, caraway seed, catnip, dill, fennel, mint, origanum, peppermint, sage, sarsaparilla, sassafras, spearmint, thyme, wild yam, wintergreen, yarrow, ginger, nutmeg, valerian, angelica, wood betony.

GALLSTONES

Bitterroot, cascara sagrada, milkweed, camomile, parsley, fringe tree, mandrake, goose grass and sweet weed, cherry bark, rhubarb, wood betony.

GOITRE

Bayberry bark, white oak bark, internally and externally, kidneys, echinacea, Irish moss, polk root, seawrack.

GANGRENE

Camomile, comfrey, myrrh, willow, poplar, hemlock, echinacea (golden seal, smartweed, pleurisy root, good combined in hot fomentations).

GARGLE

Bayberry bark, bistort root, hyssop, myrrh, pilewort, rock rose, sage, golden seal, Kloss's liniment (diluted or full strength).

GRAVEL

Broom, carrot, hyssop, marshmallow, apple tree bark, hydrangea, nettle, queen of meadow, ragwort, sorrel, spearmint, valerian, water pepper, hops, masterwort, mugwort, parsley, squaw vine, hemlock, buchu.

GOUT

Blue violet, birch, burdock, gentian root, mugwort, rue, sarsaparilla, broom, buckthorn bark, ginger, mugwort, pennyroyal, plantain, wood betony, balm of Gilead.

GONORRHEA

Bittersweet, black willow, burdock, cleavers, cubeb berries, golden seal, hops, parsley, rock rose, sanicle, squaw vine, sumach berries, uva ursi, witch hazel, wintergreen, poplar, bistort root (combined with plantain), sanicle, red root, juniper berries.

GLEET

Cubeb berries, juniper berries, wild alum root, yarrow, bloodroot, elder, plantain, yellow dock, saw palmetto, Oregon grape, red clover, echinacea, prickly ash, golden seal, rock rose.

GLANDULAR ORGANS

Bittersweet, mullein, parsley, seawrack, yellow dock, myrica, poke root (echinacea, slippery elm, both internally and as a poultice), queen of the meadow.

GALL BLADDER

Golden seal combined with equal parts: red clover, yellow dock, dandelion, parsley. Milkweed excellent to correct bile.

GRIPING IN BOWELS

Anise, caraway seed, catnip, coriander, ginger, pennyroyal, thyme, nutmeg, balm, bay leaves.

PROSTATE GLAND

Corn silk, golden seal, saw palmetto berries, white pond lily, buchu, garlic.

GENITALS
(Burning, Itching)

Raspberry leaves, marshmallow, slippery elm, pleurisy root (Take these internally for itching.), peach leaves (for dropsy), chickweed (internally and as a wash for burning, itching).

HYDROPHOBIA

Lobelia, scullcap, balm, gentian, white ash, antispasmodic tincture (See Table of Contents).

HICCOUGHS

Blue cohosh, dill, Indian hemp, orange juice.

HAIR

Indian hemp (stimulates growth), nettle, rosemary (prevents hair from falling out), sage peach, burdock.

HAY FEVER

Mullein, poplar, skunk cabbage, coltsfoot, black cohosh.

HEARTBURN (See FERMENTATION AND GAS)

Willow, wood betony, angelica, burnet (excellent), origanum (excellent to strengthen the stomach and for gas).

HEART

Angelica, blue cohosh (for palpitation of the heart), borage (strengthens heart), cayenne (stimulant), coriander, golden seal, peppermint, sorrel, valerian, vervain, wintergreen, wood betony, bloodroot, motherwort, sorrel, mistletoe, holy thistle, tansy. Combination: Golden seal, scullcap, cayenne.

HEMORRHOIDS

Burdock, golden seal, myrrh, nettle, psylla, shepherd's purse, uva ursi, white oak bark, yarrow, pilewort, aloes, bloodroot, bittersweet.

HEADACHE

Blue violet, catnip, coltsfoot, peppermint, rhubarb, rosemary (pain in the head), rue, sweet balm, thyme, vervain, virgin's bower, wood betony (pain in head), elder, marjoram, calamint (pain in head and water on brain), pennyroyal, fringe tree, red root, holy thistle, mountain balm, yerba santa, camomile, tansy.

(352)

HOARSENESS

Marshmallow, golden seal, lobelia, wild cherry, hyssop, horehound, mullein, coltsfoot, skunk cabbage.

HEMORRHAGES

Bayberry bark, comfrey, fleabane (bowels and uterus), golden seal (hemorrhages of rectum), nettle, pilewort, shepherd's purse, sorrel, St.-John's-wort, white oak bark, wild alum root, witch hazel, yarrow. Lemon juice diluted taken cold as possible. Capsicum (red pepper), taken internally, take one double 00 capsule of it and immediately drink a glass or two of as hot water as can be drunk freely.

HEAD TROUBLE—HYDROCEPHALUS
(Water on brain)

Sage, rue, rosemary, calamint, calamus, broom, catnip, red sage, rosemary, marjoram, wood betony, pennyroyal, scullcap. Can combine any of these.

HYSTERIA

Skunk cabbage, saffron, scullcap, valerian, mistletoe, peppermint, vervain, catnip, black cohosh, blue cohosh, antispasmodic tincture (quick relief), motherwort, pennyroyal, tansy, rue.

HALITOSIS (Offensive breath)

Rosemary, myrrh, golden seal, echinacea, body cleanser and laxative (See Table of Contents).

HIGH BLOOD PRESSURE

Broom, black cohosh, blue cohosh, hyssop, wild cherry bark, valerian, vervain, sanicle, body cleanser and laxative, (See Table of Contents), boneset, scullcap, golden seal, myrrh.

INDIGESTION—GAS AND FERMENTATION

Balomy, bay leaves, beech, bitterroot, buckbean, cayenne, gentian root, ginseng, golden seal, gold thread, poplar,

(353)

peruvian bark (coltsfoot, gas and fermentation), lobelia, (gas and fermentation), wild cherry bark (gas and fermentation), bayberry bark, (gas and fermentation), scullcap, (gas and fermentation), nutmeg (gas and fermentation), balm, bloodroot, marjoram, rosemary, wood betony, wormwood, red root.

INFLUENZA

Indian hemp, peppermint, white pine, poplar.

INFLAMMATIONS

Fenugreek, golden seal, hops, lobelia, marshmallow, mugwort, sarsaparilla, slippery elm, Solomon's seal, sorrel, tansy, white water lily, witch hazel, smartweed, and charcoal poultice, flaxseed oil, hyssop, chickweed, gum arabic, cayenne pepper.

INSANITY

Catnip, peppermint, rosemary, rue, vervain, wood betony, holy thistle, scullcap.

INSECT BITES OR STINGS

Black cohosh, lobelia, parsley, plantain, scullcap, balm, bistort root, borage, fennel, gentian, hyssop, marjoram, pennyroyal, wood betony, echinacea, basil sweet.

INTESTINES

Fenugreek, golden seal, mint, nettle, pennyroyal, psylla, slippery elm, giant Solomon's seal, strawberry, wild alum root, cascara sagrada.

ITCH

Buckthorn bark (ointment), origanum, virgin's bower, yellow dock (excellent), borage, marjoram, pennyroal, plantain, poke root (fine), chickweed.

IVY POISON

Lobelia, golden seal, myrrh, echinacea, bloodroot, Solomon's seal. Equal parts strong tea of white oak bark and lime water is very good for poison ivy or poison oak. Apply a bandage wet with this solution and change as often as it becomes dry. Apply antiphlogistine cold and renew every twelve hours for poison ivy or poison oak. Spread on one-half inch thick and cover the surrounding healthy skin which will prevent it from spreading.

JAUNDICE (Yellow)

Bayberry bark, balomy, bittersweet, buckbean, cleavers, dandelion, gentian root, horehound, Indian hemp, mandrake, peach leaves, poplar, sorrel, St.-John's-wort, tansy, wormwood, origanum, bistort root, bloodroot, borage, broom, sorrel, camomile, hyssop, lungwort, marjoram, parsley, pennyroyal, plantain, wood betony, henna leaves, fringe tree, celandine, chicory, fennel.

KIDNEYS

Cayenne, chicory, water pepper, white oak bark, white pond lily, wood sage, birch, black cohosh, bloodroot, buckbean, masterwort, parsley, hemlock, cayenne, wood sanicle, bethroot, wild Oregon grape, fringe tree, poke root, juniper berries, balm, beech, bitterroot, bittersweet, broom, carrot, camomile, comfrey, cleavers, corn silk, dandelion, elder, golden seal, hydrangea, hyssop, marshmallow, celandine, holy thistle, milkweed, mustard (plaster), nettle, white pine, pleurisy root, poplar, queen of meadow, sage, sanicle, sassafras, seawrack, sorrel, spearmint, sweet balm, tansy, uva ursi, aloes.

LAXATIVE

Golden seal, horehound, hyssop, mandrake, mullein, peach leaves, psylla, rhubarb, sage, senna, wahoo, elder, blue flag, wild Oregon grape, fringe, aloes, body cleanser and laxative (See Table of Contents.)

LA GRIPPE

Butternut bark, lungwort, nettle, peppermint, pleurisy root, poplar, saffron, sweet balm, tansy, ginger, golden seal, saw palmetto berries, wild cherry, wood betony, sage, angelica, hyssop.

LUNGS

Bayberry bark, chickweed, comfrey, coltsfoot, ginseng, lobelia, lungwort, marshmallow, mullein, mustard, myrrh, nettle, pimpernel, white pine, sanicle, shepherd's purse, skunk cabbage, slippery elm, thyme, wahoo, witch hazel, yarrow, yerba santa, pennyroal, wood sanicle, bethroot, holy thistle, angelica, red sage, black cohosh.

LUNG FEVER

Pleurisy root, blood root, coltsfoot, red sage.

LAME BACK—LUMBAGO

Queen of meadow, shepherd's purse (excellent), uva ursi, vervain, black cohosh, liniment, (See liniment in Table of Contents).

LOCK JAW

Silver weed, red pepper, lobelia, antispasmodic tincture, scullcap, fit root, cayenne pepper.

LEPROSY

Bittersweet, burdock, red clover, yellow dock, pennyroyal, henna leaves, queen's delight.

LIVER

Bitterroot, black cohosh, bloodroot, buckbean, fennel, parsley, plantain, wood betony, fringe tree, celandine, aloes, chicory, holy thistle, angelica, beech, bittersweet, butternut bark, carrot, cascara sagrada, celery, cleavers, dandelion, elder, golden seal, lobelia, magnolia, mandrake, milkweed, motherwort, poplar, prickly ash, rhubarb, sage, self-heal, wahoo, white oak bark, wild yam, wormwood, balm, blue flag, wild Oregon grape, red root, poke root, gentian root, red sage, hops, uva ursi.

LEUCORRHEA OR WHITES

Bayberry bark (douche), bistort root, comfrey, cubeb berries, golden seal and myrrh (for douche and also take internally), magnolia, pilewort, plantain, ragwort, slippery elm, squaw vine, sumach berries (white oak bark, douche), white pond lily, wild alum root, wintergreen, wormwood, yarrow, (increases menstrual flow), blue cohosh, tansy, ragwort (combined with lily), hemlock, buchu, bethroot and cranes' bill (douche), wild Oregon grape, juniper berries.

LIQUOR HABIT

Lady's-slipper, lobelia, equal parts; scullcap, one ounce valerian or lady's-slipper, one-half ounce given every half hour in hot water until results are obtained, then continue taking until taste for liquor is gone. Quassia chips, magnolia bark, ivy (five-leaf).

LOSS OF SPEECH

Rosemary, prickly ash, red pepper, golden seal, myrrh, wild cherry, sumach.

MEASLES

Cleavers, pleurisy root, saffron, valerian, yarrow, bistort root, red sage, raspberry leaves.

MENSTRUATION (To decrease flow)

Bayberry bark, pilewort, shepherd's purse, sorrel, uva ursi, wild alum root, bistort root, plantain, red raspberry, witch hazel, sanicle, bethroot, burnet, wood betony, red sage, yarrow, lungwort.

MENSTRUATION (To increase flow)

Squaw vine, aloes, angelica, fennel, balm, bittersweet, black cohosh, camomile, catnip, coral, gentian root, ginger, horehound, marjoram, masterwort, mugwort, nettle, origanum, pennyroyal, pleurisy root, ragwort, rue, saffron, St.-John's-wort, summer savory, sweet balm, tansy, thyme, valerian, vervain, water pepper (smart weed), yarrow, carrot, coral with blue cohosh, squaw mint, red sage, motherwort.

MUCOUS MEMBRANES (Diseases of)

Bitterroot, coltsfoot, golden seal, gum arabic, hyssop, myrica, red raspberry, white pond lily, wild alum root, yarrow, fire weed.

NAUSEA

Ginger, lavender, mint, origanum, peach leaves, pennyroyal (but should not be taken during pregnancy), peppermint, red respberry, spearmint, sweet balm, wild yam, anise, giant Solomon's seal, golden seal (will allay nausea during pregnancy.)

NASAL TROUBLE

Black willow (combined with palmetto berries or scullcap, witch hazel (bleeding nose), wild alum root (bleeding nose), white willow, bloodroot.

NOSEBLEED

Witch hazel, wild alum root, buckthorn, bayberry bark.

NOCTURNAL EMISSIONS

Black willow (combined with palmetto berries or scullcap), sage, saw palmetto berries.

NIGHTMARE

Bugleweed, thyme, lily of the valley, catnip, peppermint.

NIGHT SWEATS

Coral, sage, strawberry leaves.

NEURALGIA

Bitterroot, blue cohosh, celery, hops, nettle, origanum, peppermint, poplar, queen of meadow, scullcap, Solomon's seal, giant Solomon's seal, twin leaf, wild yam, wood betony, Peruvian bark.

NERVOUSNESS

Camomile, celery, cinchona bark, dill, fit root (scullcap with golden seal and hops), lobelia, motherwort, origanum, peach leaves, pennyroyal, queen of meadow, red clover, rosemary, rue, sage, scullcap, skunk cabbage, spearmint, squaw vine, St.-John's-wort, thyme, twin leaf, valerian, vervain, wild cherry, wood betony, blue violet, sanicle, buchu, mistletoe, red sage, catnip, peppermint, marshmallow root, mugwort, (antispasmodic tincture for quick results).

OVARIES

Saw palmetto berries, pennyroyal, black cohosh, blue cohosh, bayberry bark (pleurisy root, for inflammation of ovaries), burdock, peach leaves.

OBESITY (SEE REDUCE FLESH)

Seawrack, white ash, fennel, Irish moss, chickweed, burdock, sassafras.

PNEUMONIA

Marshmallow, vervain, bloodroot, Peruvian bark, sage, red sage, black cohosh, willow, coltsfoot, skunk cabbage, comfrey, elecampane, wild cherry, spikenard, horehound combined.

PREVENTION OF DISEASES

Juniper berries (prevent contagious diseases), holy thistle, angelica, (gentian, wonderful), garlic, dandelion and dandelion greens, blueberries and leaves, lemon juice. (Take the juice of four lemons daily, diluted one-half with water.)

PIMPLES

Spikenard, valerian, gentian, plantain, bistort root.

PLEURISY

Coral, Indian hemp, lobelia, pleurisy root, skunk cabbage, flaxseed, cayenne, chickweed, elder, yarrow, boneset.

POULTICES

Balm, flaxseed, gum arabic, hyssop, marshmallow, mustard, slippery elm, virgin's bower, wintergreen, chickweed, poke root, cayenne pepper, flaxseed meal, smart weed and charcoal, red sage, burdock, lobelia, comfrey.

PILES

Bittersweet, chickweed, fire weed, golden seal, mullein, myrrh, nettle, plantain, shepherd's purse, Solomon's seal, spearmint, uva ursi, white oak bark, witch hazel, wild alum root, yarrow, bloodroot, pilewort, pimpernel, aloes.

PHLEGM

Hyssop, nettle, white pine, vervain, wild cherry, borage, pennyroyal, coltsfoot.

PARALYSIS

Hydrangea, black cohosh, valerian, vervain, scullcap, ginger (prickly ash, excellent), lady's-slipper, cayenne.

PANCREAS

Bittersweet, dandelion, golden seal, uva ursi, wahoo, cayenne, blueberry leaves, huckleberry leaves.

PAIN

Catnip, fit root, mint, mullein, nettle, scullcap, skunk cabbage, Solomon's seal, giant Solomon's seal, twin leaf, wood betony, camomile, dill.

PERSPIRATION INDUCERS

Bayberry bark, elderberry leaves, coral, sage, holy thistle, horehound, hyssop, Indian hemp, marjoram, pennyroyal, saffron, thyme, vervain.

PARALYSIS OF THE TONGUE

Ginger, prickly ash (especially good), red pepper, black cohosh, valerian, vervain, scullcap, rosemary.

PALSY

Masterwort, scullcap, elder, wood betony, wood sage.

QUININE SUBSTITUTES (Better than quinine)

Fit root, golden seal, magnolia, white poplar (bark), yarrow (willow excellent), Peruvian bark, scullcap, gentian root, peach, sage, vervain, wahoo, wood betony, willow bark and red pepper (act quickly: they are tonic and stimulating without any reaction), boneset, capsicum (red pepper), turnips, grated, skin and all, given in tablespoonful doses whenever a dose of quinine is indicated is better than quinine. Dogwood blossoms.

QUINSY

Hyssop, sage, sanicle, ragwort, sumach berries, agrimony, red sage, raspberry leaves, slippery elm bark, hyssop, cudweed. These are all to be taken internally and as a gargle.

RUPTURES

Comfrey, giant Solomon's seal, bistort root.

RELAXANTS

Lobelia, boneset, queen of the meadow, pleurisy root, antispasmodic tincture (See Table of Contents.)

RINGWORM (Skin disease in circular patches)

Golden seal, lobelia, blood root, borage, plantain, sarsaparilla.

RHEUMATISM

Buchu, balm of Gilead, blue flag, wild Oregon grape, cayenne, birch, bitter root, bittersweet, black cohosh, blue cohosh, buckbean, buckthorn bark, burdock, celery, elder, hydrangea, Indian hemp, lobelia, mugwort, nettle, colombo, origanum, peppermint, white pine, pleurisy root, poplar, prickly ash, quassia, queen of meadow, sarsaparilla, scullcap, skunk cabbage, twin leaf, wild yam, willow, wintergreen, wormwood, yellow dock, wild Oregon grape.

SINUS TROUBLE

Plantain, saw palmetto berries, golden seal, bayberry bark.

STINGS

Plantain, barage, echinacea, marjoram, Kloss's liniment, cedron.

SKIN DISEASES (SEE RINGWORM)

Beech, bittersweet, blue violet, buckthorn bark, burdock, chickweed, cleavers, coral, dandelion, elder, golden seal, magnolia, rock rose, saffron, sarsaparilla, sassafras, sorrel, turkey corn, vervain, white clover, wintergreen, blood root, pennyroyal, plantain, blue flag, wild Oregon grape, poke root, prince's pine, hyssop, red root, red clover, spikenard.

SCALD HEAD

Sanicle (apply raspberry leaves, lobelia, make tea of 2 oz. leaves, 1 qt. water, steep thirty minutes, add ½ oz.

lobelia powder, both morning and evening), with hazel extract to allay itching. (Take a good blood purifier.)

ST. VITUS'S DANCE
Black cohosh, scullcap, mistletoe (excellent).

SUMMER COMPLAINT (SEE DIARRHEA)
Fire weed, fleabane, shepherd's purse, bayberry bark, white oak bark, colombo.

SPERMATORRHEA
Sage, buchu, juniper berries, cubeb berries, uva ursi, black willow.

SWELLINGS
Burdock, comfrey, elder, fenugreek, hops, Indian hemp, mugwort, origanum, parsley, tansy, white oak bark, white lily, wintergreen, wood sage, wormwood, yellow dock, camomile, dill.

STOMACH, INDIGESTION AND GAS
Angelica, strawberry, thyme, valerian, vervain, witch hazel, wild cherry, willow, wintergreen, wood betony, camomile, marjoram, echinacea, bethroot, chickweed, aloes, chicory, bayberry bark, balomy, blue violet, buckbean, calamus, caraway seed, catnip, cayenne, cinchona bark, comfrey, colombo, cubeb, fennel, ginseng, golden seal, golden thread, cayenne, sage, sassafras, slippery elm, giant Solomon's seal, spearmint, St.-John's-wort, gum arabic, hyssop, milkweed, mint, mugwort, nettle, origanum, (especially sour stomach), peach leaves, pimpernel, plantain, rue, anise, bay leaves, cedron.

SCALDING URINE
White poplar bark, burdock seed, spearmint, cubeb meadow, peach leaves, clives. For cystitis or any inflammatory condition of the urinary organs. If there is bleeding, use shepherd's purse.

SYPHILIS

Bitterroot, bittersweet, bloodroot, buglewood (for syphilitic sores), burdock, elder, golden seal, plantain, prickly ash, rock rose, sumach, (berries or leaves) turkey corn (and bark) twinleaf, yellow dock, poplar, bayberry bark, barberry, blue violet, sanicle, echinacea, blue flag, red root, poke root, white pine bark, palmetto, Oregon grape, red clover, yellow parilla, milkweed, parsley.

SPRAINS

Comfrey, lobelia, origanum, wormwood, bittersweet combined with camomile as ointment.

SORE THROAT

Bayberry bark, bistort root, bloodroot, blue violet, cayenne, fenugreek, ginger, horehound, hops, hyssop, mullein, origanum, white pine, rock rose, sage, sassafras, saw palmetto berries, twinleaf, vervain, white water lily, wild alum root, wintergreen, wood sage, borage, wood sanicle, echinacea, red root, golden seal, red sage.

SLEEP INDUCER

Hops, motherwort, mullein, vervain, scullcap (Combination: Equal parts scullcap, nerve root, hops, catnip, black cohosh), peppermint.

SORES

Peach, pimpernel, poplar, blue violet, hemlock, echinacea, poke root, aloes, cayenne, bayberry bark, bittersweet, calamus, carrot (poultice), camomile, chickweed, comfrey, elder, flaxseed, golden seal, mullein, myrrh, plantain, sage, sanicle (prickly ash, apply powder), self-heal, skunk cabbage, Solomon's seal, St.-John's-wort, sumach berries, valerian, vervain, virgin's bower, white clover, witch hazel, wood sage, yellow dock, bistort root, borage, masterwort, bloodroot.

SPASMS

Blue cohosh, catnip, cayenne, fit root, masterwort, red clover, rue, sassafras, skunk cabbage, spearmint, twinleaf, wild yam, red root, antispasmodic tincture, fennel, cedron.

SPINAL MENINGITIS

Black cohosh, golden seal, lobelia.

SPLEEN

Bittersweet, dandelion, golden seal, uva ursi, wahoo, white oak bark, balm, broom, fennel, gentian root, hyssop, marjoram, parsley, wood betony, cayenne, red root, aloes, chicory, angelica.

SNAKEBITES

Black cohosh, borage, scullcap, bistort root, fennel, gentian root, hyssop, marjoram, pennyroyal, wood betony, echinacea, plantain, basil sweet, cedron.

SORE GUMS

Buglewood, myrrh, golden seal, bistort root, and herbal liniment, as given in this book.

SEXUAL DESIRE (EXCESSIVE, TO CORRECT)

Black willow, hops, sage, scullcap, lily root, star root, rocky mountain grape root.

SCARLETINA

Rock rose, twinleaf, bloodroot.

SCALDS AND BURNS

Bittersweet, chickweed, elder, onions (bruised), kerosene, herbal liniment, linseed oil. Submerge a burn in real cold water, keeping the water cold, and hold it in until it stops burning. If this is done, it will not form a blister.

STIMULANTS

Cayenne, elder, prickly ash, peppermint, ginger, cloves, red sage, raspberry, nettle, pennyroyal, rue shepherd's purse, valerian.

SCROFULA

Bayberry bark, buckbean, burdock, calamus, comfrey, cleavers, coltsfoot, coral, dandelion, elder, gentian root, hyssop, milkweed, nettle, plantain, king's evil, prickly ash, rhubarb, rock rose, sarsaparilla, seawrack, sorrel, sumach berries, turkey corn, vervain, white pond lily, wintergreen, yellow dock, blue violet, wild Oregon grape, poke root, juniper berries, figwort, echinacea.

SCURVY

Buckbean, chickweed, cleavers, coral, dandelion, hydrangea, nettle (scorbutic), origanum, white pine, sanicle, sorrel, marjoram, wood sanicle, lemon juice.

SCIATICA

Rue, wintergreen, broom, burdock, tansy.

SMALLPOX

Yarrow, bistort root, red sage, raspberry leaves (golden seal mixed with vaseline and applied will prevent pitting.) Lemon juice allays itching. Apply full strength.

SCARLET FEVER

Cayenne, cleavers, golden seal, pleurisy root, saffron, twinleaf, valerian, red sage.

THYROID GLAND

Poke root (Use green root when possible.), bayberry bark, white oak bark, scullcap, black cohosh.

TESTES (THE TESTICLES)

Chickweed, mullein, saw palmetto berries, to be taken when swollen and painful. The following herbs to be used as a mixture for poultice, or taken internally, in the usual manner: Burdock, 2 oz.; clivers, 1 oz.; sanicle, 1 oz.; bittersweet root, 1 oz.

TETTER

Borage, plantain, sarsaparilla, sanicle, raspberry leaves, gentian. Healing lotion, as given in this book, applied externally. Golden seal, mixed with borax and vaseline, to be used in the first stages.

TYPHOID FEVER

Bitterroot, camomile, golden seal, yarrow, bloodroot, red sage, myrrh.

TONSILLITIS

Mullein, white pine, echinacea, red root, sage, golden seal, tansy. (Use the strong tea, gargle every few minutes, and swallow a mouthful.)

TOOTHACHE

Hops, origanum (essence), sassafras (oil of), cloves (oil of), summer savory, balm, broom, marjoram, mullein, pennyroyal, plaintain, pimpernel, tansy, liniment.

TUMORS

Blue violet, chickweed, coltsfoot (for scrofulous tumors), coral, elder, hops, mugwort, mullein, rock rose, sanicle, skunk cabbage, sorrel, St.-John's-wort, tansy, white oak bark, witch hazel, wood sage, yellow dock, flaxseed, sanicle, celandine. Red root taken internally will destroy tumors.

TUBERCULOSIS

Comfrey, myrrh, skunk cabbage, wild cherry bark, sanicle, golden seal, bayberry bark, burdock root, coltsfoot, yellow dock, elecampane.

TOBACCO HABIT

Calamus, magnolia, myrtle leaves and seeds, scullcap, vervain, peppermint, catnip, valerian, motherwort, quassia chips, angelica, black cohosh, blue cohosh, sweet flag, and use burdock for cleansing the blood stream.

TO DRY UP MILK IN NURSING MOTHERS

Sage, wild alum root (the strong tea rubbed over breast), camphor applied to breast.

TYPHUS

Coral, pleurisy root, culver's root, boneset, borage, camomile.

TONIC HERBS

Camomile, celery, coriander, colombo, elder, fire weed, gentian root, hyssop, lavender, magnolia, marjoram, prickly ash, sassafras, turkey corn, wild cherry bark, yellow dock, fringe tree, poke root, angelica, barberry, Oregon grape root, apple tree bark, heal-all, red clover blossoms, boneset, sweet flag, scullcap, wood betony, vervain.

UTERUS (PROLAPSED)

Witch hazel, black cohosh, white oak bark (used in douche), bayberry bark (douche), slippery elm (douche). Tampons saturated in a strong tea made of bayberry bark or white oak bark tea, combined with slippery elm, make a very fine medicinal support for prolapsed uterus. Witch hazel bark may also be used.

URINARY (SEE ALSO SCALDING URINE)

Mugwort, squaw vine, white willow, hemlock, buchu, chicory, juniper berries, angelica, mandrake, blue cohosh, broom, carrot, celery, comfrey, cleavers (or clivers), corn silk, cubeb berries, dandelion, elder, gentian root, ginseng, fleabane, marshmallow, milkweed, mint, nettle, origanum, parsley, peach leaves, poplar bark, queen of the meadow, ragwort, sarsaparilla, spearmint, St.-John's-wort, sweet balm, white ash, wild yam, yarrow, burdock, hops, marjoram, masterwort, tansy, fennel.

ULCERS

Bistort root, borage, lungwort, pennyroyal, poplar, blue violet, hemlock, wood sanicle, chickweed, celandine, angelica, cayenne, beech, buglewood, calamus, carrot (poultice), chickweed, comfrey, fenugreek, golden seal, gold thread, hops, mullein, myrrh, pilewort, prickly ash, pyslla, rock rose, sage, sanicle, sorrel, St.-John's-wort, twinleaf, valerian, virgin's bower, water pepper, white clover, white water lily, wild alum root, wintergreen, wood sage, yarrow, and use chickweed tea to heal ulcers and sores; externally use as a wash, and take internally.

VARICOSE VEINS

White oak bark, witch hazel, bayberry bark, wild alum root, burnet.

VAGINAL DOUCHE

Fit root and fennel, gum arabic, marshmallow, slippery elm, uva ursi, white oak bark, white pond lily, wild alum root, fenugreek, bayberry bark.

VOMITING (PREVENTIVE)

Basil sweet, colombo, peach leaves, white poplar bark, clover, spearmint. Use equal parts white poplar bark and clover, to stop vomiting in pregnancy, lobelia is also good, given in small doses. Peppermint and peach leaves, given in small doses.

WOMB TROUBLES

Slippery elm, bayberry bark (douche), black cohosh, blue cohosh, fit root and fennel, gum arabic (in inflammation of uterus), mandrake, peach leaves, rue, squaw vine, St.-John's-wort, witch hazel, fenugreek, bethroot, wild Oregon grape, shepherd's purse (to stop excessive flow), yarrow (increases menstruation), smartweed, uva ursi. For douches, use wild alum root, or white oak bark.

WHOOPING COUGH

Black cohosh, blue violet, coltsfoot, lobelia, peach leaves, red clover, saw palmetto berries, skunk cabbage, thyme, vervain, red root, red clover, blue cohosh, bloodroot, slippery elm, elecampane. Drink the tea generously; is excellent. Antispasmodic tincture, taken according to directions (See Table of Contents.).

WARTS

Buckthorn bark, mullein, celandine.

WOUNDS

Burdock, carrot (poultice), camomile, chickweed, comfrey, fenugreek, plantain, prickly ash, sage, self-heal, Solomon's seal, St.-John's-wort, white water lily, wild alum root, yarrow, bistort root, pilewort, pimpernel, poplar, wood sanicle, echinacea, balm of Gilead, aloes, beech.

WORMS

Birch, bitterroot, buckbean, buckthorn bark, butternut bark, carrot, camomile, horehound, hops, nettle, quassia, rue, sage, self-heal, senna, sorrel, tansy, vervain (take three days), white oak bark, wormwood, bistort root, catnip, hyssop, motherwort, peach, poplar, wood betony, aloes.

CHAPTER XXXII

DIRECTIONS FOR USE OF NON-POISONOUS HERBS

Granulated or finely cut herbs.—Steep a heaping tea-spoonful of the herbs in a cup of boiling water for twenty minutes, strain, and take one cup one hour before each meal and one cup on retiring. You may take more or less as the case requires. If too strong, use less herbs per cup.

Roots and barks.—Roots must be simmered one-half hour or more in order to extract their medicinal value. Do not boil hard.

When you gather the roots and bark yourself, cut or crush them fine. If you raise or gather herbs and barks, use good judgment in making teas; if you get it too strong, add more water.

Flowers and leaves.—Flowers and leaves should never be boiled. Steep them in boiling water in a covered dish for twenty minutes, just as you would make common tea. Boiling evaporates the aromatic properties.

Powdered herbs.—The powdered herbs may be mixed in hot or cold water. Use one-half teaspoonful to one-fourth glass of water. Follow by drinking one glass water, either hot or cold. The herbs take effect quicker if taken in hot water.

Golden seal may be taken in three ways, as follows:

1. One-fourth to one-half teaspoonful dissolved in one-fourth glass water. Follow by drinking one glass of water. Take one to four doses a day.

2. Steep a heaping teaspoonful in a pint of boiling water twenty minutes, stir thoroughly, let settle, and pour off the clear liquid. Take eight tablespoonfuls a day, taking two tablespoonfuls fifteen minutes before each meal and the remainder upon retiring. You may double the above amount and take even more with benefit.

3. Take in gelatin capsules and drink one glass of water after taking the capsules. Gelatin capsules may be purchased at most retail or wholesale drug stores. I make most use of No. 1, No. 0, No. 00 sizes, but there are smaller sizes. As a rule, take two of the No. 00 size for a dose, more or less according to needs.

In warm weather the tea must be made fresh every day to prevent souring.

Good judgment must be exercised in the amount of herbs taken, usually four cups a day—one cup, one hour before each meal, and one cup upon retiring. Each person has a different constitution; therefore, if good results are not obtained by taking as directed, increase or decrease as may be best. For instance, if the herbs are not laxative enough, increase the dose; if too laxative, decrease the dose. The bowels should move three times a day, if three meals are eaten.

Persons who have very sensitive stomachs, ulcerated stomach, etc., at times may become nauseated and sick after taking some of the best old-fashioned herbs. If this is experienced, do not become alarmed. It is not the herbs that are at fault but the sensitive condition of the stomach.

In some cases where the stomach is very sensitive, start by taking teaspoonful doses of tea, often—say, every fifteen minutes—and increase the amount until able to take the required amount.

Powdered herbs may be mixed with food stuffs, such as mashed potatoes, or mashed vegetables of any kind, sweet fruits, as figs or dates, ground.

To the herb tea you can add a little honey or malt sugar, especially for children, to make it more palatable. DO NOT USE CANE SUGAR.

NEVER TAKE DRUGS WHEN TAKING NON-POISONOUS HERBS. THE TWO DO NOT WORK TOGETHER.

DO NOT PREPARE HERBS OR FOOD IN ALUMINUM COOKING UTENSILS.

To Make Syrups

A simple syrup.—Dissolve three pounds of brown sugar in a pint of boiling water, boil until thick. To this you may add any medicinal substance.

Malt honey, bee's honey, or karo syrup may be used in making syrups. To make an herb syrup, simply add the cut herbs (or if using granulated, sift them so there will not be any dust or sediment), boil to the syrupy consistency, and strain through a double cheesecloth, and bottle.

Syrup of lemons.—Boil one pint of lemon juice ten minutes, strain, add three pounds of brown sugar, and boil a few minutes longer.

Wild cherry syrup.—2 oz. wild cherry bark
　　　　　　　　　2 oz. cubeb berries
　　　　　　　　　2 oz. mullein
　　　　　　　　　2 oz. skunk cabbage
　　　　　　　　　2 oz. lobelia herb

Add four quarts boiling water, simmer ten minutes, and let stand until nearly cold, then strain through a double cheesecloth. Put in a porcelain cooking dish, add four pounds of brown sugar. Boil this down to a medium thick syrup—it must be thick enough so it will not sour. Add the juice of four lemons and let boil two or three minutes longer. Strain again. If a tar flavor is desired, you may add two tablespoonfuls purified oil of tar, when adding the brown sugar. When cool, it is ready for use, or bottling.

To Make Herb Salves

Use fresh leaves, flowers, roots, barks, or the dried granulated, or powdered herbs. If you gather the herbs yourself, and use them fresh, be sure to cut up finely.

Use one pound of herbs, to one and a half pounds cocoa fat, or any pure vegetable oil, and four ounces beeswax. It is necessary to use a little more beeswax in the warmer climates, as this is the ingredient that keeps the salve firm.

Mix the above together, cover, and place in the hot sun or oven, with the fire turned low, for three or four hours. Strain through a fine sieve or cloth. When it is cold, it will be firm and ready for use. It can be used, however, before it is cold.

Poultices

Do not warm over a poultice once used. Do not allow a poultice to become cold. Have a second poultice ready immediately upon removing the first one.

To make the following poultices it is best to have the herbs in a ground or granulated form. When using the herbs in powdered form, mix with just enough water to make a thick paste. When using them granulated, mix with water, cornmeal, or flaxseed meal to make a thick paste. If fresh green leaves are used, beat them up, steep, and apply to the affected parts.

Poultices are most excellent for enlarged glands of any kind, such as neck, breast, groin, prostate, etc. Also for eruptions, boils, carbuncles, and abcesses. An excellent thing to do in any case where poultices are to be used is to bathe the affected part thoroughly with mugwort tea first. If you do not have this, cleanse it with hydrogen of peroxide before applying the poultice. It must be remembered that many herbs are used for poultices, so, study the herbs and use those best suited to the condition, or those recommended for that condition.

Slippery elm poultice.—This poultice has no superior in the line of poultices, either used alone or combined as follows:

Lobelia and slippery elm poultice.—Take one-third part lobelia, two-thirds part slippery elm. Very excellent for blood poisoning, also for boils, and abcesses. Use for rheumatism.

Charcoal and hops poultice.—Will remove gallstone pain quickly.

Charcoal and smartweed poultices.—Is excellent for inflammation of the bowels or inflammation in other parts of the body. When using for old and inflamed ulcers and sores, add powdered echinacea, golden seal, or myrrh, or a small amount of the three. They are all powerful to heal and are disinfectant.

Polk root and cornmeal poultice.—It is very excellent for caked and inflamed breast. Also good for white swelling and blood poison.

Burdock leaf poultice.—Burdock leaf poultice is very cooling and drying. It is good to use on old ulcers and sores. A poultice made of the root, adding a teaspoonful of salt, eases the pain of a wound caused by the bite of a mad dog.

Plantain poultice.—Excellent in mad dog bites and to prevent blood poisoning.

A poultice made of any of the following herbs, is very good in dissolving tumors: Origanum, nettle, wintergreen, fenugreek, and mullein.

Garden carrots, grated raw, and applied as a poultice, will cleanse old sores and ulcers. Follow with an application of healing lotion, or a wash of golden seal and myrrh solution.

To bring a boil to a head quickly, apply poultices at a temperature of 100° F. and repeat as often as necessary to keep the temperature above body heat. When a soothing effect is desired, as in painful wounds, bee stings, etc., apply agreeably warm, and renew sufficiently often to prevent souring or becoming dry.

In applying poultices the aim is to have the warmth and moisture retained as long as possible.

In making a yeast poultice, dilute ordinary yeast with enough liquid to make a stiff batter. It can be diluted with strong infusions of the desired herb tea, and cornmeal to make a stiff batter. In sluggish conditions, such as gangrene, old sores, etc., mix either myrrh, charcoal, ginger, or golden seal with the batter before applying.

To check discharges from ulcers, add witch hazel or wild cherry bark tea. When there is much inflammation and tenseness, sprinkle lobelia over the poultice, either the herb or crushed seeds.

Potato poultice.—Scrape or grate a raw Irish potato and apply to any feverish part, such as a carbuncle or boil. It has a very soothing and cooling effect and will draw it to a head.

Bayberry poultice.—Use in the treatment of foul ulcers, old sores, and cancerous sores.

White pond lily poultice.—This poultice, either used alone or combined with slippery elm or linseed, is one of the best for old sores, inflamed tumors, etc.

Sage poultice.—Excellent for sore breast, or any inflamed gathering.

Charcoal and slippery elm poultice.—Use equal parts to make the poultice, use for gangrenous sores.

Slippery elm and yeast.—Make a regular slippery elm poultice. Mix the yeast cake with warm water and add to the slippery elm. The poultice will bring boils and abcesses to a head and keep gangrene from setting in.

Hyssop poultice.—A small handful of this herb (use fresh), boiled in water for a few minutes, then drained and applied, will remove discoloration from bruises, and will remove the discoloration from a black eye. If you use the dried herbs, steep in boiling water.

Comfrey, ragwort, and woodsage poultice.—Use equal parts of these three herbs; steep in boiling water. Apply poultice to external cancers and tumors. They are most beneficial and will give excellent results.

Bread and milk poultice.—A poultice of bread and milk, with a little lobelia added, is very soothing and will bring boils to a head.

Bran poultice.—Use enough hot water to make a paste of the bran; apply as hot as can be borne. Use for inflammations of any kind, sprains, or bruises. When there is great pain, use equal parts lady's-slipper and lobelia with the bran. Cover the poultice with several thicknesses of

(377)

flannel or oiled silk to retain the heat. This is an unusually excellent poultice.

Slippery elm poultice.—Stir ground slippery elm bark in water or any strong herb tea suitable, to the consistency of thick paste. Excellent for irritable sores.

Carrot poultice.—Boil carrots until soft, or they can be used raw, mash to a pulp, add some vegetable oil to keep from hardening, spread on a cloth, and apply. Excellent for offensive sores.

Onion poultice.—Make in the same way as carrot poultice. Very stimulating to indolent sores, and for slow boils.

Lobelia poultice.—1 oz. powdered lobelia, 1 oz. powdered slippery elm. Excellent for wounds, fistula, boils, felons, erysipelas, insect bites and stings.

Elderberry poultice.—The elderberry leaves bruised or steamed just enough to wilt them, add a little pure olive oil. This makes an excellent poultice for inflammations, such as, piles and hemorrhoids, etc., apply as warm as can be borne, for the space of an hour or more when suffering.

Charcoal

For medicinal purposes, fresh charcoal made from the finest woods should be used. The best charcoal is obtained from boxwood, shells of cocoanuts, willow, pine, and other soft woods.

Charcoal is an absorbent; it will absorb and condense many times its own volume of various gases. It is very useful as an antiseptic, due to its absorbent and oxidizing qualities. It is excellent taken internally in acid dyspepsia, also for gas, fermentation, and heart-burn.

Dose.—One heaping teaspoonful after each meal. Put the charcoal in a cup, add water enough to make a paste, dilute, and drink at once. More can be taken with benefit.

Charcoal is a valuable remedy in cases of colic due to decomposition of foods in the stomach and bowels, and can be used as a preventive or curative. Give a tablespoonful in half a glass of hot water. As a preventive, take a teaspoonful after each meal in a little hot water.

For inflammation of the bowels or dysentery, give a tablespoonful in half a glass of hot water, and repeat as often as necessary. Give charcoal poultices over the bowels and stomach.

Charcoal mixed in a strong smartweed tea, makes an excellent poultice for bruises, also for internal or external inflammations.

A charcoal poultice is good to relieve inflammation of the eyes. It is also a most excellent poultice for gangrene, old ulcers, and sores.

I have used charcoal mixed with olive oil to the consistency of paste, or so that it is easy to take. It is very good for some kinds of indigestion. Charcoal mixes easily with soybean milk, and may be taken in this way for indigestion.

Old charcoal is made more effective if heated before using.

Charcoal can be purchased at drugstores; it is best to buy it in bulk, then you know it is pure charcoal.

(See Table of Contents for Charcoal Poultices.)

Herbal Liniment

Uses.—For all pains, painful swellings, bruises, boils, skin eruptions of any kind, pimples, etc., apply the liniment every few minutes for an hour or two. It will stop a stye from developing on the eye in a short time if used freely. Be careful not to get it in the eye.

It is also very useful in headaches. Apply to the temples, back of the neck, and to the forehead. It is very effective for rheumatism. For toothache, apply in the cavity and all around on the gums, and outside the jaw if necessary; it will take the swelling and soreness out. It is excellent for pyorrhea and sores in the mouth. Saturate a piece of cotton and thoroughly wash the mouth, or take a mouthful and rinse the mouth with it; spit out. It is very effective for pain or cramps in any part of the body. Is good for athletic foot trouble. Apply frequently, saturating the affected parts thoroughly.

How to Make Herbal Liniment

Combine two ounces powdered myrrh, one ounce powdered golden seal, one-half ounce cayenne pepper, one quart rubbing alcohol (70 per cent). Mix together and let stand seven days; shake well every day, decant off, and bottle in corked bottles. If you do not have golden seal, make it without.

Herbal Laxative

To make herbal laxative, combine equal parts buckthorn bark, rhubarb root, cascara sagrada bark, calamus root, fennel seed. Mix thoroughly. These herbs are non-poisonous and are soothing to the stomach and will help to prevent gas and fermentation.

Dose.—One small fourth teaspoonful in a fourth glass of water. Follow with a glass of hot water. Take after each meal if the digestion is slow, or you can take a half teaspoonful in the same manner upon retiring. Increase or decrease the amount taken to suit your personal need, but take enough so that you have three good eliminations every day. Children proportionately less according to age.

This laxative should be made of the powdered herbs, then it can also be used in the gelatin capsules. Two No. 00

are the usual dose for an adult. If making a tea of granulated herbs, you would steep a teaspoonful to a cup of boiling water for thirty minutes, and drink.

If you do not have on hand or cannot obtain all the herbs used in the above laxative, any one of the following three will bring good results used singly in the same dose as given above: buckthorn bark, rhubarb root and cascara bark.

A Nervine and Tonic

Combine equal parts gentian root, scullcap herb, burnet root, wood bethony, and spearmint herb.

This will prove a blessing to everyone who takes it. It is soothing and relaxing, quieting to the nerves, has many good qualities, and is perfectly harmless.

Dose.—One-half teaspoonful mixed in one-half glass of cold water, followed by a glass of hot water, one hour before each meal and upon retiring. This can be put in gelatin capsules Two No. 00 capsules would contain the required amount for one dose. More can be taken with benefit.

Composition Powder

Composition powder is a fine remedy for colds, flu, hoarseness, colic, cramps, sluggish circulation, beginning of fevers, etc. It should be kept in every home, and used when the need arises. It is safe and effective.

In fevers and colds, give a cup of composition tea every hour until the patient perspires freely. This will clear the body of colds, and bring the fever down.

How to make composition powder:
     4 oz. Bayberry
     2 oz. Ginger
     1 oz. White pine

1 dr. Cloves
1 dr. Cayenne

Use all powdered herbs. Mix and put through a fine sieve twice. Steep one teaspoonful in a cup of boiling water fifteen minutes, covered. Drink the clear liquid poured off from the sediment.

Antispasmodic Tincture

Antispasmodic tincture may be used either internally or externally. It is very effective for cramps in the bowels, taken internally. Take eight to fifteen drops in a half glass of hot water in cases of snake bites and mad dog bites, or any dangerous illness. Increase the dose to one teaspoonful every two or three hours. Children less according to age. It is a stimulant, without any reaction, as it is non-poisonous. It is very effective for pyorrhea and sores in the mouth, and is an excellent remedy for tonsillitis, diphtheria, or any other throat trouble. Use as a gargle using one-half teaspoonful to a glass of water. Gargle with this solution until the throat is perfectly clear. Repeat as often as necessary. It will cut all the mucus, and kill the poisons. It is also a very good voice tonic.

Apply externally to any kind of swelling, cramps; is very beneficial in rheumatism, lumbago, etc. It is an excellent remedy for lockjaw. Put it into the mouth, getting it between the teeth, so that it will get on the tongue. It will invariably unlock the jaw in a few minutes. For small children, when it is hard to get it between the teeth, bathe the neck and jaws frequently with it until relief is obtained.

How to Make Antispasmodic Tincture

1 oz. Lobelia seed, granulated
1 oz. Scullcap, granulated
1 oz. Skunk cabbage, granulated

1 oz. Gum myrrh, granulated
1 oz. Black Cohosh, granulated
½ oz. Cayenne, powdered

Take one pint boiling water, and one pint apple vinegar (cider vinegar). Steep the herbs in the pint of boiling water one-half hour, strain, add the apple vinegar, and bottle for use.

Emetics

Emetics have been used from time immemorial. Hippocrates called them "upward purges." When Rome was the chief city of the earth, the fashionable had their palaces built with a room especially to take "upward purges" in.

Sick rooms were called "vomitories." In these vomitories there was a marble rail, where, after they had eaten a feast, they would go and lean over, and have a slave tickle their throats, after drinking some warm water or decoction. Then they would go back and finish their feast.

An emetic is given when it is necessary to empty the stomach or cleanse it. In nausea, when there is a lot of undigested food, it must be cleaned out. When a person has been bitten by a mad dog, or poisonous snake, or poisons of any kind have been taken internally, an emetic is one of the remedies. It is also good to take a high enema, and rid the body of as much poison as possible in that way. Worn-out materials in the body, excess of starch, dead blood corpuscles, are much more easily thrown out by emetics than any other means. Anyone who is weak, or subject to hemorrhages of the stomach, should not take emetics. The stomach, in those cases, should be cleaned out by fasting, mild herb laxatives, and enemas used to cleanse the rest of the system.

How to take an emetic.—Drink five or six cups of lukewarm water. It vomiting does not occur freely, touch the back of the throat far down. This will bring up the contents of the stomach. In some cases it may be necessary to drink more. This should be repeated until the stomach is entirely cleansed and the water comes back clear. The addition of a teaspoonful of salt is very helpful.

Herb emetics are very beneficial. Use a tea made of boneset, pennyroyal, Canada snake root, or lobelia.

A cup of peppermint, spearmint, or catnip tea, taken after an emetic, has a soothing and settling effect on the stomach. Golden seal taken afterwards is very healing, and destroys mucus and foul matter in the stomach.

After the emetic, and an herb tea has been taken to settle and soothe the stomach, take a tonic herb, such as wild cherry bark, scullcap, valerian, or calamus root. Make tea according to directions given for use of non-poisonous herbs. Take one-half cupful every two hours.

Chapter XXXIII

TREATMENT OF DISEASES

Diagnosis

Following are a number of diseases, their causes, symptoms, and treatment by natural methods which I have used for many years in connection with competent physicians.

No one should try to do the work of a physician. When you are sick, call your family physician, or some other competent physician, and have a correct diagnosis made of your symptoms.

Acidosis

Causes.—Meats, fish, fowl, tea, coffee, tobacco, alcohol, pepper, mustard, spices, vinegar, excessive use of salt, baking powder, soda, jellies, sweet desserts, candy, preserves, pancakes, hot breads, pastries, fried foods, irregular eating, eating late at night, excess starch, improperly cooked foods, starchy or poorly baked bread, foods too hot or too cold, and foods cooked in aluminum utensils.

Symptoms.—Loss of appetite, headaches, sleeplessness, acid urine, acid or strong perspiration, acid mouth, sour stomach, lassitude, vomiting.

How to correct.—Soybean products are excellent to remedy acid condition. A diet of soybean milk or buttermilk for a few days or a week, or orange juice, would be excellent. Avoid constipation. Use zwieback or soybean bread. The drier the food is eaten, the sooner acid condition can be overcome. Chew! Chew! CHEW! so that your food is liquified before swallowing. Be sure that your food is thoroughly saturated with saliva, as it is highly alkaline, and rich in vitamins. Do not drink with meals. Do not eat between meals!

After taking the diet, have one good vegetable meal every day, preferably at noon. Be careful of combinations. Do not eat fruits and vegetables at the same meal. Do not use any of the foods listed under acidosis, as, when these are used, acidosis will again occur.

All these conditions are the result of years of wrong living. You must not expect them to disappear immediately. It will require persistence, and persistence alone will win, but you will be well rewarded.

Sodium and magnesium foods should be eaten in abundance, such as:

oranges	apples
beets	cherries
carrots	strawberries
celery	cocoanuts
cucumbers	figs
okra	string beans
radishes	spinach

Burnet, sanicle, golden seal, wood betony, calamus, peppermint, and other herbs are very beneficial. Golden seal, taken one-fourth teaspoon in a glass of hot or cold water an hour before meals, is very beneficial.

Appendicitis

Causes.—Constipation is one of the causes of appendicitis to an extent, and of course, wrong diet, which diet would include the use of devitaminized foods, such as white flour products, cane sugar, and cane-sugar products, greasy and fried foods, tea, coffee, chocolate, and wrong combination of foods. These must be strictly avoided in appendicitis, as must alcoholic drinks, tobacco, and all stimulating food and drink.

Symptoms.—Nausea, pain and distress around the navel, constipation, quick pulse, and perhaps a rise in temperature to 100° or 102° F. There may be tenderness to the right of the navel and below, which is increased by pressure or movement. The patient frequently flexes the right knee to ease the pain.

Treatment.—Cleanse the colon thoroughly with an enema, preferably herb, take as much water as possible, as hot as possible. This treatment is of great value and will often relieve the pain immediately. If using an herb enema, use either spearmint, catnip, white oak bark, bayberry bark, or wild alum root. When herbs are not available, use plain water. After the colon has been somewhat cleansed by enemas, if pain continues, a very warm enema of catnip alone will greatly relieve. Then apply hot and cold fomentations to the region of the appendix and the full length of the spine. This will aid in the cleansing process, and relieve pain. At night, apply a poultice. Prepare as follows, using granulated or crushed mullein leaves. Take a large handful, add a tablespoonful of granulated or powdered lobelia, and sprinkle with ginger. Mix the herbs together with boiling water, making it thick enough to spread as a paste by adding powdered slippery elm or cornmeal. Apply the poultice as warm as the patient can stand, leave on until cool, then repeat.

When suffering an attack of appendicitis, go on a liquid diet, drinking alkaline broths, fruit juices, and drink several glasses of slippery elm every day. When over the attack, use the nourishing diet as given in this book.

Asthma

(A disease which affects the bronchial tubes)

Causes.—It is caused by the system being filled with waste matter, and mucus. To find that there is some difficulty in the stomach, intestine, kidneys, or bowels is not infrequent in asthma sufferers. Eating foods that are hard to digest sometimes brings on an attack.

Symptoms.—Difficult breathing, and wheezing, the patient sometimes fearing he may choke to death. The severest attacks frequently occur in the night, when the person will feel he must fight for air, and will get up and go to an open window, or some place where there is a great deal of fresh air. In severe cases the patient may become almost black in the face, or the complexion will be livid.

Treatment.—An emetic is always beneficial, particularly when the attack follows shortly after a meal. I have found the following emetic to be very effective. Pour one pint of boiling water over one teaspoonful of lobelia herb, allow to steep a few minutes, and drink several cups lukewarm. If vomiting does not occur freely, place your finger far back in the throat until vomiting occurs. If lobelia is not on hand, drink lukewarm water with a little salt in it, one cup after another until vomiting occurs. The addition of a little mustard will be found beneficial in cleansing the stomach and lungs, a tablespoonful to a glass of water. When the stomach has been cleansed in one of these ways, there is relief at once. Then drink a cup of hot spearmint or peppermint tea or hot lemonade (sour) to settle the stomach. Give hot fomentations over the stomach, liver, and spleen. You may also give them over the lungs. Then place the patient in a tub of hot water, just above body temperature, and have him remain in the tub forty-five minutes to an hour or longer. Do not let the water cool off but keep adding hot water. Finish the bath by sponging with cool water, or a cool shower. Cold morning baths are very valuable in the treatment of asthma, particularly applying cold water to the neck and shoulders in the mornings.

Herbs.—It will be well to use some tonic herbs. A mixture that I have found excellent is the following: Equal parts of lobelia, wild cherry bark, scullcap, gentian, valerian, calamus, and cubeb berries. Mix thoroughly and use a heaping teaspoonful to the cup of boiling water. Drink a cupful of this three or four times a day an hour before meals, and a cupful hot upon retiring. If you do not have all these herbs, use the two, three, or more that you have. If constipated, use herbal laxative as given in this book, taking at night.

Any of the following herbs may be used for a tea the same as those given above, and are indicated for asthma: hyssop, vervain, skunk cabbage, coltsfoot, mullein, horehound, poplar, black cohosh, yerba santa, milkweed, jaborandi, boneset, chickweed, lungwort, masterwort, pleurisy root, thyme, blue cohosh, calamus, and cubeb berries. Select any one, two, or more and mix in equal parts. Take as given above. For children the amount should be less according to age, or make the tea weaker and give frequently. I have had good results when only using one herb indicated in asthma, so read their descriptions and take the one or ones best suited to your case.

Antispasmodic tincture, recipe for which is given in this book, is valuable, as is also the herbal cough preparation given in this book.

Diet.—Diet is a very important factor in helping asthma cases. A simple, nourishing, non-stimulating diet is always helpful. It is better to have the heavier meal in

(389)

the middle of the day and a small or light meal in the evening. A fruit diet for a few days is highly recommended, after which partake only sparingly of nourishing foods, and few mixtures at a meal. Zwiebach, and soybean milk are excellent. French toast, as given in this book, or whole wheat flakes with soybean milk. Vegetables may be eaten, the leafy ones being especially good. Potatoes, steamed with the jackets on, or baked and mashed as given in this book, may be eaten. Natural brown rice, cooked in very little water, three-minute oatmeal, eaten with a little honey or soybean butter.

Remember, the bowels must be kept open (at least three movements a day). Take baths as much as possible, get plenty of outdoor exercise, and practice deep breathing. Have good ventilation in the sleeping room. The water treatments and high enemas should be kept up for some time. Follow the above treatment faithfully, and you will obtain splendid results.

Catarrh

Causes.—Foods robbed of life-giving properties; poor circulation; lowered vitality; lack of sunshine, fresh air and exercise; eating wrong combinations of foods; too much soft foods and drinking with meals; along with poor elimination.

Symptoms.—The mucus membrane thickens, making nose breathing difficult. Secretions are thick and abundant, and sneezing is common. There is dryness of the throat, mouth breathing, snoring at night, frontal headaches, and impairment of hearing. The turbinated bones of the nasal cavity enlarge at times to such an extent as to completely obstruct one side. This may cause nosebleed, neuralgic pains, and a dull, aching pain between the eyes.

Treatment.—The mucus membrane of the nose must be kept clean, for when mucus gathers around the turbinated bones and is not cleaned out, it becomes putrid and causes trouble. The first thing to do is to wash the nose out thoroughly, and here is a safe and effective way of doing it. Take a pint of soft lukewarm water and put one teaspoonful of salt in it. Bend over a wash bowl, pour your hand full of this water, and snuff it up the nose. Keep repeating this until the water comes out of the mouth. Then blow the nose, holding one passage shut and then the other. Repeat this process until the passage is entirely clean and no more mucus comes out. To hold one passage shut while blowing the other has a tendency to suck the mucus out of the cavity of the cheek and also out of the cavity of the forehead. After the nose passages are clean, gargle well with the same solution to clean the throat. Make a solution of one teaspoonful of powdered golden seal to a pint of boiling water. Let it steep for a few minutes and then pour the liquid carefully off. Add one-half teaspoonful boric acid and snuff this up the nose the same as the salt water. Then gargle with this solution. This is not only cleansing, but soothing and healing. It is a very effective remedy when done thoroughly, along with other things, such as proper eating, outdoor exercise, proper elimination, and deep breathing. Should the nose be stopped up so that the water cannot be drawn through, practice for a few minutes what is called the jumping-jack exercise. I have seen a nose that would not open up otherwise, do so when this was done.

Attention must be given to the diet, and it should be simple but nourishing. A fruit diet for a few days will do much to cleanse the system of mucus. Pineapple juice in particular is beneficial, but all fruit juices are good for this condition. Such foods as milk, proteins, etc., cause mucus. When eating other foods, eat them dry and chew them thoroughly. The bowels must be kept open and active. Take at least one high herb enema a day for awhile. They cannot hurt you, and they will do much to cleanse the intestines and colon of mucus. Bayberry bark would be suitable. Take tonic cleansing herbs, such as black cohosh, calamus, and valerian, according to directions for using non-poisonous herbs. Golden seal should be taken, a teaspoonful to a pint of boiling water. Let it steep, and take two or three swallows several times during the day.

Any one of the following herbs is good for this condition: Lungwort, coltsfoot, jaborandi, skunk cabbage, buckthorn, wild cherry bark. Look them up in the Table of Contents and take those best suited.

The faithful taking of exercises, plenty of fresh air, etc., will often prevent catarrh from going into hay fever, asthma, or tuberculosis. Using the wash for the nose and gargling will prevent the cold from going down.

Cholera

The danger of cholera is greater in hot climates than elsewhere.

Symptoms.—Cholera usually begins with a watery diarrhea, but can be checked at once by the use of a high enema, as hot as can be borne. Use an enema made of the following: Use two tablespoonfuls each, bayberry bark, white oak bark, sumach or wild cherry. Use the granulated herbs, and steep this mixture in four quarts of boiling water for thirty minutes, strain, and use. Give hot fomentations over the bowels and also the full length of the spine. Often there is vomiting of mucus, accompanied by great pain. If this is the case, give weak peppermint tea, or spearmint tea, lukewarm, and drink a pint to a quart, as much as you can possibly take. Then place the finger far down in the throat until you vomit. After you have thoroughly cleansed the stomach out in this manner, drink a cupful of hot peppermint tea, made strong. This will settle the stomach and relieve the distressed feeling. If the vomiting of mucus returns, or pains, repeat.

A weak person, or invalid, might not be able to do this, in which case, give a cup or two of very hot peppermint, catnip, or camomile tea. This will relieve the stomach.

Two hours after the peppermint tea has been taken, it would be well to take a cup of golden seal, gentian, or bayberry. This would greatly strengthen the stomach and kill the poisons in it.

In cholera, as well as in diarrhea, the patient should be kept quiet in bed. Frequent doses of antispasmodic tincture, recipe for which is given in this book, may be taken often with benefit. Take eight to fifteen drops in one-half glass of water, followed by more water, if desired.

The stools and all discharges should be disinfected or burned, as this disease is contagious. No one should touch articles used by patient without disinfecting.

Diet.—The best diet to use in cholera is oatmeal water, slippery elm water, which is highly nourishing, and soybean milk. (See Diets in Table of Contents.)

Colic in Infants

Causes.—Faulty feeding, teething, hot weather, and unhygienic surroundings.

Symptoms.—Incessant vomiting; frequent stools that are thin, watery, and have a musty odor; sunken eyes; hollow cheeks; pinched features. Symptoms develop rapidly and become dangerous in from six to twelve hours. There may be prostration and great weakness. Children may be restless, and may go into a stupor or have convulsions.

Treatment.—Give catnip or bayberry enema immediately, of about 102° to 105° F. If you do not have the catnip on hand, give a water enema, but catnip will relieve and soothe the pain. A high enema should be given once a day. Keep the patient absolutely quiet and give plenty of fresh air. Give hot fomentations to both abdomen and back. Give a warm bath at 100° F. The temperature may be made warmer, if desirable. Give a tea of white oak bark, bayberry bark, or red raspberry, using one teaspoonful of the herb to a cup of boiling water. Steep and give a tablespoonful five or six times a day. A little honey may be added if a child objects to taking it. Antispasmodic tincture may be given three or four drops to a fourth glass of water for an infant. Increase the dose for older children. Liniment, recipe for which is given in this book, applied to abdomen and back, will relieve the pain. Rice water will check the diarrhea.

The diet should consist of liquids for at least a day. Slippery elm tea should be given freely. When taken half a cup with orange juice or some fruit juice, it is more palatable for children. Soybean milk, cooked a little with oatmeal, is nourishing and alkaline. If dairy milk is used at all, it should be diluted by adding oatmeal water or barley water or one tablespoonful lime water to every glass of milk.

Colic in Children

Causes.—Indigestion, improper food, constipation.

Symptoms.—Crying out, pulling knees up to stomach, red face, distended stomach.

Treatment.—Warm catnip tea given in bottle, and also a catnip tea enema will be beneficial. Spells of crying come on at regular intervals, and if a very warm bath is given an hour before the expected attack, the attack can sometimes be prevented. Have catnip tea on hand to use in an emergency.

A hot foot bath or hot fomentation over the abdomen will give relief. If the baby is fed from a bottle, dissolve wheat flakes by pouring boiling water over them, put through a sieve, and add soybean milk to make the desired consistency. Potassium broth and oatmeal gruel, as given in the Table of Contents, are also very good for nourishment.

Circulation—Increase

Relieve the bowels by a high enema. Take deep breathing exercises each morning and evening and during the day. In the morning, cold towel rubs, followed by a thorough rubbing with a dry, coarse towel, are beneficial. Take plenty of outdoor exercise, breathing deeply while taking the exercise. For constipation, which is one great cause of poor circulation, take an eliminating diet and herbal laxative as given in this book.

The following herbs are good to increase the circulation: Gentian root, scullcap, colombo, rue, valerian, vervain, peppermint, catnip, spearmint. (See directions for use of non-poisonous herbs in Table of Contents.) Take African red pepper in No. 1 size gelatin capsules, one capsule one hour before each meal, drinking a full glass of water with each capsule. This can be taken any time during the day or with other herbs. It is fine to increase the circulation.

Constipation

Nearly the entire race is afflicted with constipation. Waste matter is left entirely too long in the body.

Causes.—Wrong diet is the main cause. Eating foods that do not contain enough roughage or bulk and also foods which are devitalized; lack of muscular tone in the bowels; improper mastication of food; meat diet; too many varieties of food at one meal; eating food that is too concentrated; using coffee, tea, and liquor of all kinds; irregular habits of attending to the calls of nature; sedentary life; and lack of exercise are other contributing factors to this almost universal ailment.

The life-giving properties which would aid digestion are removed from the foods we eat, or are spoiled by improper cooking and wrong combinations. Excessive use of drugs and patent medicines is a frequent cause of constipation, tumors, etc.

Symptoms.—Coated tongue, foul breath, backache, headache, mental dullness, depression, insomnia, loss of appetite, and various pains. Infants are irritable and cross if bowels are irregular.

Treatment.—Regulate the diet. Take high enemas of red raspberry leaves, wild cherry bark or leaves, or bayberry bark, using one heaping teaspoonful to a quart of water. This is a very good disinfectant and stimulant to bring back the peristaltic action of the colon. Take an enema every evening. (For directions look in Table of Contents under High Enemas.)

Eat your food as dry as possible. If food is eaten dry and thoroughly saturated with saliva, it is a wonderful help to lubricate the bowels, it will make the system alkaline, and will greatly increase the rapidity of digestion.

Do your drinking one hour before or two or three hours after eating. Drinking with meals is very harmful. No liquid of any kind should be taken with the meals. Eat freely of fresh and stewed fruits, apples, figs, peaches, oranges, bananas, blueberries, selecting the fruits that agree best with you. Fruits and vegetables should not be eaten at the same meal.

Take plenty of outdoor exercise, brisk walking, horse-back riding, rowing, bicycling, swimming, and deep breathing. Practice deep breathing while walking; and in the morning before getting up, lie on your back, knees flexed, and pant, breathing in short, rapid gasps. Roll on your right side, face, and left side, and continue panting. This exercise massages the bowels.

The bowels should move three or four times a day. Visit the toilet regularly after each meal to train the bowels. Food should digest readily and the waste matter be eliminated from the body promptly. If it stays too long in the colon, it kills the peristaltic action. Look in Table of Contents for "Bran Water" and "Oatmeal Water." These two articles, which may be used in many food stuffs and in baking, are an effective means of making the bowels active.

Plenty of baths and massages to the bowels are also excellent to overcome constipation. A happy mental attitude is very helpful.

The following is an excellent formula for a laxative: Mix thoroughly one tablespoonful each of mandrake, buckthorn bark, rhubarb root, fennel seed, and calamus root, and one teaspoonful of aloes. This is a real body cleanser. Mandrake is one of the finest herbs to cleanse the liver. If powdered, take one-fourth teaspoonful in a half glass of cold water, followed by a glass of hot water. This can be taken after meals or upon retiring. Take more or less than the one-fourth teaspoonful, according to your individual needs.

Moderate exercise after meals is very helpful. Never lie down or go to sleep immediately after meals. Practice deep breathing just before and right after eating. The oxygen thus gained is one of the greatest factors in helping digest your food and in making red blood. It is impossible to get the full benefit of your food without exercise.

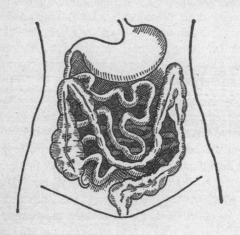

PROLAPSED COLON

Another laxative herb formula which is very good is this: Mix thoroughly one ounce mandrake root, one ounce cascara sagrada bark, one ounce buckthorn bark, one ounce fennel seed, one ounce calamus root, and one-fourth ounce aloes. To put this mixture through a fine sieve is a good way to mix it thoroughly. The above herbs are in powdered form. Take one-fourth teaspoonful, or one No. 00 capsules with a glass full of hot water upon retiring. Increase or decrease the amount taken so as to have three good bowel movements every day.

Colitis

Causes.—Faulty diet; constipation; too many mixtures which irritate the stomach and bowels; too much cane sugar, grease, white-flour and cane sugar products; eating too hastily; too much liquid and very soft foods; taking of cathartics; and food cooked in aluminum vessels.

Symptoms.—Running off of the bowels, or constipation. Mucous passes in feces and discharges are stringy. There is a feeling of weakness through the abdomen, at times headache, often great pain and dizziness, emaciation, weakness, and pains in various parts of the body.

Treatment.—The following treatment is very beneficial. Take a high enema made of one tablespoonful of bayberry bark to every quart of water. Yellow dock root or burdock root are good also and are very healing. Cover and let simmer for a few minutes. Steep for fifteen or twenty minutes. After the herbs settle, pour off the tea and take as hot as you can stand (from 100° to 108°F.—in some cases hotter). Wild alum root, golden seal, or myrrh, are also excellent herbs to use as an enema. Use a heaping teaspoonful of golden seal and a heaping teaspoonful of myrrh to four quarts of boiling water. Steep and let the mixture settle.

A liquid diet for a short time is advisable. When eating solid food, thoroughly chew and liquify it with saliva, using no liquids with meals. All roughage and foods containing skins and seeds should be avoided until the condition is better. Puree the vegetables until the condition clears up. Soybean milk and wheat flakes is an excellent diet used with zwieback.

(399)

Herbs to be taken internally.—Use a teaspoonful of golden seal and one-fourth teaspoonful of myrrh to a pint of boiling water. Let it steep and take a tablespoonful of this mixture six or eight times a day. If the case is severe, take a tablespoonful every hour; or take from one-fourth to one teaspoonful, as per directions for taking herbs, one hour before each meal and upon retiring.

In many cases where sumach grows, a tea may be made from either the bark, leaves, or berries. For an enema take a handful of either of these in four quarts of water and steep for an hour. This also makes an excellent douche. (See list of herbs given in this book for Colitis).

Convulsions or Spasms

Causes.—Children are the most frequent sufferers; and worms, indigestion, teething, rickets, fever, whooping cough, and congestion of the brain may be the cause. Some articles of food, such as candy; ice cream; cake; pies; meat and gravy; and heavy, indigestible foods, are causes. Undernourished, nervous children are apt to be troubled with convulsions. Children of this type should be given plenty of fresh air and light, nourishing food.

Symptoms.—The child straightens out and becomes stiff; breathing seems to be stopped; eyes are fixed and staring or turned upwards; and head is drawn back. Several attacks in succession are dangerous, and the child may never awaken. However, it is reassuring to know that death seldom results from the convulsions unless the child is very weak. If a child is much disturbed at night, grits his teeth, and rubs his nose, it is a sign of worms. Give the treatment for worms.

If these signs are not very prominent and yet the child is not well, it would not be amiss to give the worm treatment, as that is very beneficial to the system and does no harm.

The convulsion comes on suddenly and many times without warning. Frequently there is froth at the mouth. Often the extremities are cold, and the child usually becomes unconscious.

Treatment.—The first thing to do is to loosen the clothing and give plenty of fresh air. Put the child in a full bath at 100°F. and increase the heat by adding hot water. Wring a towel out of cold water and put around the neck and on the head. Produce vomiting by placing the finger down the throat. If gums are hot and swollen, give cold water and rub gums with a cloth that has been held on ice. Keep the child in the bath from ten to twenty minutes, as may seem best. Dry thoroughly, wrap in a warm blanket, put into bed, keep quiet, and give plenty of fresh air. If the child goes to sleep, let it sleep as long as it will.

If the child is constipated, give immediately a warm injection of catnip tea, made by putting a heaping teaspoonful of catnip in a quart of boiling water. Let it steep for fifteen minutes, strain, cool to tepid, and use. Keep the bowels rather loose, seeing that there are at least three good movements every day. If catnip is not at hand, give warm water enema with a little Ivory soap in it, giving as much as the child can hold.

Always have antispasmodic tincture on hand. The dose for children is eight drops in a tablespoonful of water. Follow by drinking more water. Look under herbs for convulsions in Table of Contents, and use according to instructions for use of non-poisonous herbs. The herbs may be sweetened with a little malt honey, honey, or malt sugar to make them more palatable.

For nourishment give potassium broth, as given in this book, fruit juices of all kinds, and oatmeal gruel, to which some soybean milk has been added. After giving a liquid diet for two or three days, give vegetable puree, mashed potatoes as given in this book, and baked potatoes. A light, nourishing diet is best for some time, as often the diet is to blame for the convulsions.

If there is no sign of convulsions after the child has had the first one; if all solid food is withheld for a few days and the child is given plenty of catnip tea and warm catnip injections; if the bowels are kept regular and the worm treatment is given, it is not likely that there will be a recurrence.

This same treatment applies to adults. Often in very severe convulsions the antispasmodic tincture will stop it at once. A dose for adults is fifteen drops to one teaspoonful in a glass of warm water. It may be repeated as often as necsssary.

Croup

Causes.—Usually overeating. When the system is overloaded with food, it is very easy to catch cold. The fermentation in the stomach causes phlegm, which in turn causes coughing and choking spells. It is often caused by worms. This is not real croup, but the symptoms are similar. In true croup there is generally inflammation of the bronchial tubes.

Symptoms.—In case of fake croup, which is generally caused by stomach disorders and worms, there is less liability of fever, but in true croup there is often high fever. The child's face is flushed and the eyes are bloodshot, sometimes bordering on diphtheria. No time should be lost in doing all that is possible for the patient. The attacks seem to be much worse at night. The child seems unable to get his breath, being awakened suddenly by a spasmodic cough. At times it seems like the child is strangling. When the child takes a breath, there is a whistling sound.

Treatment.—During the day if the child is peevish, an attack can be modified or prevented by a warm bath or hot foot bath. Vick's Vaporub, rubbed on the chest, throat, and back, is helpful, and can be obtained almost everywhere. The child must be watched at night and be kept warm and well covered. Give a catnip tea enema, and then keep the bowels open with laxative herbs, given in proportion to the age. Take a teaspoon of senna pods, or granulated senna, coltsfoot, horehound, white cherry bark, cubeb berries, or black cohosh, and mix these well together. Take one teaspoon to a cup of boiling water, let steep one-half hour, and then give the child a tablespoonful every hour until the bowels move naturally. If you do not have all these herbs, use senna with cubeb berries. This mixture will cut the phlegm and relieve spasms of the throat.

Give a prolonged hot bath, but be sure that the child does not go out and take more cold afterwards. Giving a thorough rubbing with oil of some kind, such as olive oil or cocoafat, is a good preventive against catching more cold. When the child is very ill, he must be kept in bed in a well-ventilated room. Keep water in a dish on the stove or radiator to keep the air moist.

Make a tea of cubeb berries, horehound and lobelia, equal parts, and put the tea in a kettle, letting it steam in the room, so that the child will inhale the fumes. This will sometimes give immediate relief. If this is done before the child goes to sleep, and is continued during sleep, it will sometimes prevent him from having an attack in the night. Hot and cold applications to the chest often bring speedy relief. Antispasmodic Tincture, as given in this book, applied to the throat as a liniment, will give relief. This can be taken internally, three or four drops to a teaspoonful of water for infants, increasing the dose for older children. Give every fifteen minutes, if necessary.

Diet.—The child's diet should be regulated. Give a fruit diet for a few days, as, for example, baked apples, pine-apple juice, grape juice, orange juice, etc. There is nothing that is more nourishing or better than soybean milk, either with toast or whole wheat flakes. This is very easily digested. If cow's milk is used at all, boil a little oatmeal in it and strain. When using cow's milk, put a tablespoonful of lime water to the glass. For young infants about five or six months old, dissolve four tablespoonfuls of whole wheat flakes in a little hot water and add either soybean milk or cow's milk. This will keep the child from losing weight and strength. Potassium broth is excellent, as it is nourishing and is a medicine to cleanse the system and tastes good.

Diabetes

Causes.—Diabetes is essentially a disease of physical degeneration, due to some part of the digestive tract failing to function properly. When the digestive tract fails to function normally you have diabetes. Ascertain the cause. Call on your family physician for an examination and diagnosis. In Diabetes Mellitus, starchy foods turn into sugar in the body, and nature is trying to rid the body of excess sugar.

It is generally understood that diabetes has something to do with the function of a large gland, called the pancreas, which lies just under the stomach near the outlet. From study and searching out of the cause of diabetes, it is found to be a fact that the pancreatic duct is not the only organ responsible for this condition. One of the causes of diabetes is an unbalanced diet, largely consisting of sugars, fats and starches, prepared so as to delight the eye and palate, and which are to a great extent denatured. The greater part of the food as eaten by the majority of people from day to day is denatured in one way or another.

Resulting from a large consumption of meat, sugar, white flour products, etc., diabetes has become a common disease in the United States. Diabetes will continue to increase as long as people partake of artificial sweets, white flour products, tea, coffee, tobacco, liquor, coca-cola, soft drinks, and all denatured food and harmful drinks.

Many of the food preparations that are used daily are prepared with baking powder and soda. Soda decreases the activity of the pancreatic juices, which juices are used in the body to digest protein, fats, and carbohydrates. The pancreas is one of the most important organs of digestion. Foods cooked in aluminum cooking dishes are also a cause of diabetes.

Symptoms.—Constant hunger, frequent urination, great thirst, progressive weakness, loss of flesh, inordinate appetite, mental depression, dyspepsia and a dry, red tongue. The patient is irritable, restless, and morose. Not all these symptoms are present in every case.

Treatment.—There is not a known remedy that will cure diabetes wtihout a reformation along the lines that cause it. Generally, there is some colon trouble; therefore, using either powdered burdock root, yellow dock root, or bayberry bark, a high enema, should be taken every day as it will help to cleanse and heal the colon. Pour four quarts of boiling water over one tablespoonful of the powdered herb, stir thoroughly and use. Daily hot baths, followed by cold towel rubs, are very beneficial. For best results, take the enema before the bath. Lying in a tub of hot water for one-half hour to two hours (as long as the patient can stand) will greatly help to eliminate the sugar and waste matter from the system. Excellent results are obtained in diabetes, by having the water as hot as the patient can comfortably stand, and have patient drink a hot tea made either from red raspberry leaves, blueberry leaves, dandelion root, or pleurisy root, while in the tub. Raise the patient up when he feels too warm, or if there is slight palpitation of the heart, and sponge off with cool water. If you have a shower bath, have the patient stand, and shower off with cool water getting right back into the hot water. Repeat a number of times, then finish with a cool shower, and vigorous towel rub.

A salt glow is very beneficial. I recommend this highly as it will increase the circulation and remove the old dead skin from the body so that the pores are open and the skin more active. Much of the poison in the system will escape through the skin. A general massage after the bath is very restful and beneficial as it also helps the circulation. When massaging always rub towards the heart.

Fomentations, followed by short cold, should be applied to the spine, also over the stomach, liver, spleen and pancreas daily. Do not fail to take cold morning baths, thoroughly rubbing the body with a cold wet towel, then vigorously with a dry towel. Take upon arising.

The bowels must be kept loose, with at least three good eliminations every day. This is imperative to cure diabetes. Do not take harsh cathartics. Use herbal laxative compound, as given in this book, or other laxative herbs.

Diet.—The general health must be improved if the patient expects to recover. Correct the diet, which is one cause of diabetes. The food question is an important item to be considered in the treatment of this disease. There are many herbs which have medicinal properties that can be used, and will greatly aid the vegetables and fruits in supplying the needed alkaline elements for the body. All foods that can be enjoyed in their natural state are best adapted for normal nutrition. Meat of all kinds must be excluded from the diet; milk, and eggs should be reduced to a minimum. Stimulating foods (which are given under this heading in Table of Contents) are strictly forbidden, as well as such foods as oysters, chickens, clams, crabs, etc. Avoid all starches, sugars, except natural sweets, such as, juice of ripe fruit.

Bran, oatmeal, and slippery elm water are very beneficial in diabetes. A very wholesome dish, high in life-giving properties and an alkaline food is the soybean. Prepare by using soybeans which have been sprouted a half inch or more. Boil until tender, then place in a baking dish, and bake a little. Flavor with vegetable extract, onions, garlic, or tomatoes to suit the taste.

The following list of foods is very good in diabetes: greens of all kinds, Chinese cabbage, red cabbage, cauliflower, watercress, cucumbers, okra, Brussels sprouts, asparagus, onions (baked or boiled), sprouted lentils, peas (tender young), ripe olives, lettuce, beets and tops (tender young), string beans, carrots, and carrot juice is excellent, celery, spinach, eggplant, radishes, endive, parsnips, sprouted lima beans, green corn (very tender), soybean milk, soybean cottage cheese, whole wheat zwieback, buttermilk, cream, baked Irish potatoes, cocoanut milk (see directions in Table of Contents for making), peanuts, almonds, walnuts, pecans, and Brazel nuts. Do not eat peanuts roasted, or peanut butter made from roasted peanuts. Raw peanuts, and butter made from them is good. Avocados are excellent in diabetes; when thoroughly ripe they are almost a specific.

Use all kinds of fresh fruits that are ripened on the tree, in the sun, as: strawberries, oranges, apricots, currants, blueberries, peaches, pears, pineapples, apples, lemons, red raspberries, huckleberries, grapefruit, cherries, and limes.

Fruits should never be sweetened with sugar. Cane sugar, raw, or natural brown sugar, and all sugar syrups are harmful. Natural sugars as contained in grapes and other fruits are beneficial. A small amount of *malt* sugar may be used.

Never eat fruits and vegetables at the same meal. Eat as many raw fruits and vegetables as possible. Those requiring cooking should not be cooked more than just enough to make them palatable. It is best to steam or bake vegetables, but when boiled, boil in as little water as possible, so there will not be any to throw away.

Your tender beet tops and young tender beets are very desirable. The full grown beets or old beets contain an excessive amount of sugar and should not be eaten by diabetics.

Deep breathing and as vigorous outdoor exercise as the condition of the patient will permit, must be taken.

Blueberry leaves, red root, and dandelion root tea are especially beneficial in diabetes.

The following list of herbs are helpful and beneficial in diabetes. Study them separately and use one or a combination of several that best suit your needs. (See Table of Contents how to use non-poisonous herbs.) Beech, blue cohosh, golden seal, Indian hemp, white pine, poplar, queen of the meadow, saw palmetto berries, sumach berries, uva ursi, wild alum root, wintergreen, yarrow, buchu (in first stages of diabetes), dandelion root (especially good), bittersweet, white pine combined with: uva ursi, marshmallow, and poplar bark, equal parts. Raspberry leaves (very good), and pleurisy root.

Diabetes Insipidus requires very much the same treatment as Diabetes Mellitus. If the kidneys and nerves are in bad condition or affected, use one of the following herbs: cornsilk, cubeb berries, fennel, scullcap, wild cherry bark, and nerve root.

Dysentery or Summer Complaint

Causes.—Inflammation of the rectum and large intestines; insufficient food, and improper diet, drinking with meals, overeating, wrong combinations, stimulating foods, and all liquors, the use of tea, coffee, tobacco, and drinking of impure water. Unhygienic surroundings, and eating of foods which have begun to decompose, either fruits or vegetables, and foods that have been standing in pantries that are not well ventilated. Habitual constipation.

Symptoms.—(mild) Frequent, small and painful passages from the bowels with slimy mucous, streaked with blood. A constant desire to evacuate the bowels. Great straining. More or less fever, loss of appetite, sleeplessness, and restlessness at night. Sometimes the abdomen is swollen.

Severe Symptoms.—Fever continues, great thirst, tongue becomes red, abdomen collapses in some cases, straining ceases and the bowels become relaxed and protrude. The urine is hot and scanty. Slow pulse, rapid breathing, generally the patient is pale and looks emaciated. Do not let this condition become chronic. Give the following treatment in either mild or severe cases, and good results will be obtained.

Treatment.—First, give a high enema, using either white oak bark, bayberry bark, or wild alum root tea, either one is astringent. Give the enemas as hot as can be borne, 102°F. to 108°F. It may be hard to retain the tea at this temperature, but it will give great relief. It may be given hotter in very severe cases.

(409)

Give hot fomentations to the abdomen and spine, continuing for a half hour, and if the case is severe give three or fours times a day. These are indispensable.

The liniment, as given in this book, thoroughly applied to the abdomen and spine after the fomentations, is excellent.

The diet must be light. Use potassium broth, soybean milk, oatmeal water, and drink at least a pint a day of slippery elm water, and barley water. Whole wheat flakes can be completely dissolved in soybean milk—a diet of this would be most nourishing and highly alkaline. It contains all the elements the system requires. For solid foods, see cleansing diet, in Table of Contents. Chew your food thoroughly, until it is a cream, before swallowing.

Take equal amounts of slippery elm, lady's-slipper, gentian, wild yam, bayberry bark and scullcap. Mix thoroughly. Use a heaping teaspoonful to a cup of boiling water, steep one-half hour, drink a half cupful every half hour until relieved, and then take three or four cups a day. The addition of calamus root will prevent griping, fermentation and gas.

Another excellent combination of herbs are—equal parts red raspberry leaves, and witch-hazel leaves. If the kidneys are affected, add peach leaves. Mix thoroughly together, use a heaping teaspoonful to a quart of boiling water, and drink four or five cups a day, as hot as possible.

Delirium Tremens
(From intoxication)

Cause.—Habitual intoxication.

Symptoms.—Loss of appetite; nausea; vomiting; pulse feeble and rapid; wild expression on face; delusions; fright because of horrible fancies, such as snakes. It is sometimes hard to control the patient who is full of such fears. When the patient is very bad, it takes two strong persons to take care of him. In such a case, the patient must be shut in where he cannot do himself or anyone else harm. Sometimes patients have convulsions, talk incessantly, and are not able to sleep. Nearly all cases have a bad stomach and poor elimination.

Treatment.—The first thing to do is to give a high enema. If the colon is bad, give herbal enema. (See list of herbs for enemas in Table of Contents). Use herbal laxative, as given in this book, for constipated condition. Take enough of it so as to have three good bowel movements every day. Take a teaspoonful of golden seal, steeped in a pint of boiling water, strain, and give two or three swallows four or five times during the day. This will be very beneficial to the stomach. To destroy the taste for liquor, give quassia chips, scullcap, and cayenne. Take a teaspoonful of hops to a cup of boiling water with a little lobelia added, steep, strain, and give this hot. It will prove very quieting and produce sleep. Give more than one cup if necessary.

Place the patient in a neutral bath and keep him there as long as possible—two or three hours or more. While he is still in the bath, give him drinks of hot, soothing, quieting herbs, such as the following: Valerian, gentian, catnip, peppermint, spearmint, calamus root, sweet balm, scullcap. Do not make the tea too strong. Use a small teaspoonful of herbs to a cup of water. Keep the head cool with towels wrung out of cold water. Put these around the neck and on the head. Give either shower or sponge bath, short and cold, several times during the warm bath. Just before finishing, give a good brisk salt glow. Put the patient in the warm water afterwards, letting him become thoroughly warmed through; then give the final cold shower or rub.

(411)

Dry thoroughly, rubbing vigorously with a rough, Turkish towel. Put him to bed.

Give a light, nourishing diet. The stomach is usually in such a condition that it cannot retain much food at a time and digest it. It is best to give a liquid diet for a while, such as oatmeal water, potassium broth (See Table of Contents), soybean milk, fruit juices, etc.

Take the patient out in the open air for exercise and have him practice deep breathing. For violent cases of this kind, when they are treated at home, tie the hands and feet with wide bandages made of towels or sheets. There is also what is called a "straight jacket" that may be used. Kind, gentle treatment and kind soothing words will help a great deal to hasten a speedy cure. You will absolutely have success if this treatment is strictly followed.

Select one or more of the following herbs and take as directed: (See Table of Contents for use of herbs). Antispasmodic Tincture (for quick relief), valerian, black cohosh, quassia chips, hyssop, lady's-slipper, scullcap, lobelia, mistletoe, wood betony, vervain, motherwort, hops.

Diphtheria

Most common in children, diphtheria is a poisonous, contagious disease affecting the throat and upper air passages. The first thing to do is to call a competent physician.

Causes.—Impure blood, unhygienic measures, contaminated milk and foods, excessive starchy diet. Starch clogs the body unless there are enough acids to dilute it, and there seldom are. Sore throat, when not properly treated, sometimes runs into diphtheria. Many cases of acute sore throat and acute tonsillitis are mistaken for diphtheria and vice versa.

Symptoms.—Slight chills, sometimes vomiting and diarrhea; always fetid breath; more or less difficulty in swallowing; hoarseness. Children usually complain first of being tired and sleepy, and the tonsils appear inflamed and dark red, unevenly swollen, and white patches that look like parchment, appear on them. The glands of the neck swell in most cases. This tenacious membrane in the throat and on the tonsils spreads very rapidly unless checked. The membrane may appear yellowish or greenish. It is not always the same. In severe cases it is gangrenous. In a very short time, if something is not done, this false membrane will cover the back of the throat and the entire cavity of the mouth. When this membrane spreads down into the air passages, it shortens the breath and the patient has a frightened look. If there are no white patches or exudation, the disease is not diphtheria.

Treatment.—If you have a sore throat of any kind, whether there is any danger or not of its being diphtheria, the treatment given below may be used with benefit. Do not wait until the actual symptoms have developed.

Steep one teaspoonful of powdered golden seal and one teaspoonful of powdered myrrh, with a pinch of cayenne, in a pint of boiling water for one-half hour. Gargle and swab the throat thoroughly with this solution. It will kill the poisons that are there. Do this until you have the throat clean. A hot fomentation to the throat, followed by a cold compress, will give great relief.

If there is any danger of paralysis, give hot and cold applications to the spine, stomach, and liver. Thoroughly saturate that throat and spine with the liniment as given in this book. Take ten or twelve drops of Antispasmodic Tincture in a glass of water five or six times a day, or every ten or fifteen minutes if the case is bad. This will ward off paralysis. A hot tub bath or sitz bath is a very valuable measure.

(413)

The patient must be kept in a well ventilated room, but must be kept warm until the most serious stage of the disease is over.

Give two high enemas each day. Herb enemas are preferable because herbs will kill poisons. Use either bayberry bark or red raspberry leaves tea. (See High Herb Enemas). Use laxative herbs and keep the bowels open. There should be at least three or four movements a day.

I have used bayberry bark and lobelia with splendid results as an emetic. Bayberry bark and lobelia clean off the mucous membranes. After you have vomited once, it must be repeated until the stomach and throat are entirely clean. Treat children the same way, using only about half the amount of the tea that you would use for adults. Bayberry not only cleans the membrane, but destroys the odor, and is stimulating, so that poisonous exudation can be thrown off. It is also healing and antiseptic. It is also good to add a little capsicum or ginger to the bayberry, as these are both excellent stimulants. (See Emetics).

Sleepiness is not a good symptom. Always give the emetic and stimulating herbs with the enema before you allow either a child or adult to sleep, if you wish to save them. After the throat and colon have been thoroughly cleansed and the patient has been given at least three cups of prickly ash bark tea, if, after a sleep, there is wheezing or choking, wake the patient up and give a dose of red raspberry leaf tea and bayberry until the nose and throat are clean. Give fresh or unsweetened pineapple juice.

Red clover, yellow dock, sweet flag, prickly ash berries, golden seal, myrrh, and jaborandi are also excellent to take internally. Use only liquid foods, fuit juices, etc., until the patient is well cleaned out, the exudation has stopped, and the throat is clean.

When the patient begins to recuperate, the following diet may be used: Baked apples, potassium broth, soy-bean milk, fresh fruits, and vegetables (properly cooked).

Diphtheria is a very poisonous disease and no time must be lost in giving this treatment night and day until it is conquered. If this treatment were thoroughly given, especially the emetic, most cases would recover.

Dyspepsia

Causes.—Non-nourishing and devitaminized food, such as white-flour and cane-sugar products and polished rice; eating too much soft foods; drinking with meals; hasty eating; late suppers; irregular meals; food seasoned too highly; poor mastication; iced tea; coffee; all iced drinks; overeating. People who lead a sedentary life should take plenty of outdoor exercise and rest, and should breathe deeply.

Symptoms.—Heartburn, headache, heaviness in the stomach, irregularity of bowels, cold feet, weak pulse, and general prostration in chronic cases. In cases of long standing there will be a hacking cough, intermittent fever at times, and palpitation of the heart. Irritability is another symptom.

Treatment.—When overeating is the cause, a mild emetic to empty the stomach will often bring immediate relief. This can be done by drinking as much warm water with a little salt in it as the stomach can hold. Put the finger down the throat after drinking the water, and you will be surprised at the matter that comes up. This will not strain if plenty of water is taken. (See Herb Emetics.) The taking of soda and magnesia are very injurious. Antispasmodic Tincture, as given in this book, given eight to ten drops in a glass of water, will give relief. Golden seal, taken one-quarter of a teaspoonful to a glass of water an hour before meals, will help the digestion greatly; or a teaspoonful of it can be steeped in a pint of boiling water. Drink one-half cupful an hour before meals. A cup of scullcap of gentian tea, taken every three hours, will prove most beneficial, as many cases of dyspepsia are primarily caused by nervous troubles.

The herbs listed below will prove soothing and add tone to the system. Any one, two, or three of them may be used together, and will be of great advantage in treating this ailment.

tansy	gentian root	thyme
wild cherry	boneset	summer savory
origanium	buckbean	yarrow
magnolia	horehound	golden seal
sweet flag	quassia	white oak
masterwort	spearmint	peach leaves
golden thread	wahoo	myrrh

Diet.—The old idea of starving dyspepsia is a wrong one. Ordinarily dyspeptics should eat more than the usual amount of food, but it should be light, nourishing, and easy to digest, so as to give plenty of nourishment and not burden the stomach. Quick elimination is essential. The following foods are recommended: Whole wheat zwieback, mashed potatoes as given in this book, soybean cottage cheese, asparagus, tender corn, cauliflower, eggplant, a good grade of string beans, tender canned peas (if the fresh cannot be obtained), spinach, lettuce (the curly head or leaf lettuce is better than the iceburg. Vegetables are best baked. Season a little with soybean butter. Crisp whole-wheat or bran crackers are good. If raw vegetables, such as spinach, lettuce, and celery, do not agree with you, do not eat them; for in this kind of a diet you obtain all the vitamines that are needed. Bran muffins and soybean muffins, as given in this book, and potassium broth are excellent for a weak stomach. Masticate thoroughly. Never eat in a hurry, be regular in eating, and eat no late meals. If hungry when going to bed, drink fruit juice, hot soybean milk, or soybean coffee. Be happy, relax at mealtime, and avoid nervous tension.

Dropsy

Causes.—Dropsy is an accumulation of watery fluid in the cellular tissues or in any of the cavities of the body, as the chest or abdomen, and may be due to disease of the heart, lungs, liver, kidneys, or peritoneum. Anything that will cause the blood to become poisoned or the red corpuscles to die may result in dropsy. In most cases it is caused by a crippled heart or kidneys. Sometimes the liver and gall bladder are so diseased and inflamed that they will not function normally, and a dropsical condition will arise, causing the abdominal cavity to fill up with fluid. It may be that the kidneys are the cause. In the case of Bright's disease, when the kidneys are not able to function properly, dropsy will result.

Treatment.—Generally a complete change should be made in the diet, leaving off all alcoholic drinks, cocoa, chocolate, tea, coffee, coca-cola, and all other such drinks. No flesh foods, pies, cakes, or rich pastries should be indulged in. All foods should be eaten as dry as possible, thereby causing the patient to chew his food thoroughly. No fluid should be taken with the meals, but water can be taken one hour after meals. Do not use any salt. Fruits or tomatoes should compose a large part of the diet. One vegetable meal a day (preferably at noon) should compose the diet of all patients. Never eat fruit and vegetable at the same meal. Sprouted lentils and sprouted soybeans are very good as well as all the soybean preparations mentioned in this book. Eat freely of vegetables, as eggplant, young beets, parsley, celery, okra, kale, asparagus, collards, mustard, lettuce, spinach, parsnips, onions, cucumbers, watercress, pumpkin, potatoes, peas, yellow corn, Swiss chard, cauliflower, endive, fresh beans, and peas.

Fresh grapes should be eaten freely in season, and if they cannot be had, the dried ones should be used. Thoroughly ripe bananas may be eaten often. Nuts or nut preparations should take the place of meat. Cocoanut is also good. If a patient cannot take the whole cocoanut, the cocoanut milk as given in this book is excellent. (See Table of Contents for Cocoanut Milk.) Whole wheat zwieback should be eaten instead of fresh bread. Never eat bread made with soda or baking powder.

Drink plenty of water and fruit juices to flush the kidneys and bladder. A hot bath daily (preferably at night) to produce perspiration will help rid the body of impurities. Cold morning baths and the washing of the limbs and abdomen two or three times a day with cold water are also very beneficial.

Drinking plenty of herb tea of red raspberry or pleurisy root will produce perspiration. If this is in powdered form, take a half teaspoonful to one cup of boiling water. Let it steep thirty minutes, and drink; or the powder may be taken in capsules four to six times a day. An excellent herb combination for this purpose is one-half teaspoonful each of wild yam and black cohosh, with a pinch of cayenne pepper added, to a cup of water. Keep the bowels active, so that they move at least three times a day, by using the herbal laxatives as given in this book. (See Table of Contents.) A tea made of the following may be taken freely, as much as four to six cups a day with benefit: Wild carrot (blossoms or seeds ground), dandelion root, yarrow, burdock root, queen of the meadow, dwarf elder, and broom.

This may be mixed equal parts, using one teaspoonful to a cup of boiling water, and steeping twenty or thirty minutes.

Burdock and broom make a good combination. They are also prepared in the same way. Dwarf elder is especially good, since it cleanses the kidneys.

The following remedy has been known to cure dropsy many times: Take grapevine root and burn to ashes. Use one dessert spoonful of this in a glass of water three or four times a day, always drinking plenty of water with it. The inner bark of the vine is good too, prepared in the same way.

Frequent bathing in the ocean is very helpful for dropsy. If one cannot do this, take one pound Epsom Salts and one pound table salt and add to your bath.

Wild carrot, which grows so abundantly in many of the states of the United States, has been known to cure dropsy, together with the proper diet after leaving off the harmful drinks, foods, and habits.

Epileptic Fits
(Or Falling Sickness)

Causes.—Main cause is wrong diet, which in turn has caused stoppage of the bowels and affected the sympathetic nerves, which in turn affects the cerebro-spinal nerves. This condition calls all the blood away from the head, which at times almost stops the heart and causes the face to become very pale, or purple, and the body limp. It is often caused from trouble in the bowels and intestines, or can be caused by falls, blows, fractures and other injuries. Many epilepsy cases have worms.

Symptoms.—The patient usually becomes unconscious, gnashing the teeth. The eyes roll us and become fixed. Foaming at the mouth. The patient ursually falls forward.

Before an attack, there is a peculiar sensation over the body, dizziness, twitching of the muscles, sudden perspiration. If you feel any of these unnatural sensations, do not wait until you fall, lie down immediately.

Treatment.—Have some antispasmodic tincture on hand, and give from eight to fifteen drops in one-half glass of water. If the patient cannot drink, put a few drops on the tongue. This will check the fit at once. Give a high enema of catnip tea immediately to relieve and cleanse the bowels thoroughly.

When the attack first comes on, or during the duration of the fit, have the patient lie down, have plenty of fresh air in the room. In bad cases where there is danger of biting the tongue, place a hard piece of wood or rubber between the teeth. When possible give the antispasmodic tincture before the attack.

To make an excellent tea for use in epilepsy, mix equal parts of the following herbs: black cohosh, valerian, lady's-slipper, and scullcap. Steep a heaping teaspoonful of this mixture in a cup of boiling water for thirty minutes. Have the patient drink two or three cups of this just as warm as possible when they feel the attack coming on. This tea should be continued after the attack also.

If the patient complains of pain in the bowels, apply Liniment, as given in this book, rub it in freely and thoroughly.

Many times I have had bad cases—gave them the foregoing herbs or some of the following list, combined with a simple, nourishing diet, high enemas, and plenty of fresh air, and many times there has not been a recurrence of the attacks.

When using the herb teas, enemas and baths, you must stop eating the things which have caused epilepsy. If you do not, those same things that brought on the attacks in the first place, will bring them on again. Discontinue the use of tea, coffee, tobacco, alcoholic liquors, all stimulating and constipating foods, all bread that is used should be made into zwieback, this will be a great help. Do not drink with meals, masticate your food well. The cleansing and nourishing diet as given in this book would be excellent, taken in connection with the herbs given. If the enemas are taken, and the bowels kept thoroughly cleansed, the patient will get over the attacks, and by using a correct diet they would rarely return.

Take the following herbs either singly or in any combination you desire, study them, and use those best suited to your case. Take four cups a day, one an hour before each meal, and one upon retiring. Black cohosh, elder, mistletoe, Peruvian bark, vervain, valerian, lady's-slipper, scullcap. And use antispasmodic tincture.

Eczema

Causes.—Foods that make impure blood, lack of sunshine, fresh air, and constipation.

Symptoms.—A breaking out and itching of the skin, with burning and stinging. Sometimes it comes in the form of little pimples which turn into water blisters. Usually the skin dries up in little scales and itches. There are two kinds of eczema, dry, and moist weeping eczema. The following treatment is beneficial in either case.

Treatment.—Select an alkaline diet. See Table of Contents for alkaline foods. The bowels must move regularly, three times a day. Do not use soap and water for cleansing, use boric acid solution. Take equal parts burdock root, yellow dock, yarrow, and marshmallow, using a heaping teaspoonful of this mixture of granulated herbs, to the cup of boiling water, steep, strain and drink one-half cupful four or five times a day. Also bathe the affected parts freely with this same tea. Healing lotion, as given in this book, applied freely will relieve the itching, and heal the skin.

Look up the following herbs in Table of Contents, select the oes best suited to your case, and take as directed for use of non-poinsonous herbs. Golden seal, willow, poplar, yellow dock, blue violet, strawberry leaves, origanum, cleavers, plantain.

Ear Trouble

Causes.—Earache is usually caused by colds, tonsillitis, la grippe, and sometimes other diseases such as measles, erysipelas, smallpox, diphtheria, scarlet fever, or typhoid fever.

Symptoms.—When the ear becomes red or swollen on the inside it is a sign of inflammation of the head and ears. Sensations of fullness, ringing in the ears. When an infant or young child pulls at his ears, he may have earache.

Treatment.—Whatever the cause, earache can be relieved by the application of heat over the ear and around the neck. A hot foot bath with a tablespoonful of mustard in it often gives relief. Bake a large onion until it becomes soft, and tie it over the eat; this will often give great relief when pain is severe. Lobelia or slippery elm poultice is very effective in allaying the inflammation and pain. (See poultices.) An injection of oil of lobelia or origanum, or a tea made of these herbs, injected warm with a medicine dropper, will often afford relief. If the ear has abcessed and broken, use warm peroxide to wash the ear out; peroxide will loosen all the putrified matter and bring it out of the ear. This should be repeated until the ear is clean. Do this before injecting any medication or applying poultices. A saturate solution of boric acid may be used for a wash.

Erysipelas

Causes.—Erysipelas is a disease caused by a disordered condition of the system.

Symptoms.—Erysipelas appears as an inflammation of the skin, in splotches of deep red and copper color, causing an itching, burning sensation. Affects the face and head more often than other parts of the body. Sometimes starts from a slight wound or abrasion of the skin, although at times it seems to arise spontaneously, at times, as a pimple, then turns into a blister, spreading rapidly (if on the face), covering the face and neck in a short time. Even in cases moderately severe, the face is swollen, the eyes closed, the lips and ears thickened and feverish.

When it begins from a wound of scratch, the spot is slightly reddened, before spreading. Occasionally, the first symptoms begin with a chill or fever, and in a few hours a slight redness over the bridge of the nose and cheeks, in about twenty-four hours blisters begin to appear. An attack of this disease generally leaves the patient particularly susceptible to the disease for a long time.

Treatment.—Do not wash with soap and water. Use saturate solution of boric acid exclusively. Make a solution of the following herbs: one-half teaspoonful golden seal, one teaspoonful lobelia, one teaspoonful each of burdock, and teaspoonful lobelia, one teaspoonful of burdock, and half teaspoonful yellow dock root, one tablespoonful boric acid, and one-fourth teaspoon of myrrh. Dissolve in a quart of boiling water. Dip a piece of cotton in this and lightly touch all the affected parts. A piece of gauze may be wet with this solution and left on the sores with good effects, as it is very cleansing and healing. It will greatly allay the pain. Do not wipe the skin. Chickweed tea made as follows is excellent used in the same way. One heaping tablespoon of the granulated herb to a pint of boiling water.

A poultice of raw cranberries, applied cold, will allay intense burning in erysipelas. Also lemon juice, diluted half with boiled water.

Keep the colon clean, having at least three complete movements a day, by using herb laxative. Take internally a tea of pleurisy root, burdock root, sage, or ginger. These herbs affect the skin and keep it moist, also aiding in keeping the pores open. It is good to take a heaping tablespoonful of pleurisy root, a tablespoonful of sage, and one teaspoonful of ginger, steep in a pint of boiling water. Drink a half cup of this every two hours.

Healing lotion, as given in this book, will give splendid results when applied to the affected parts.

Another excellent wash. Mix equal parts of gum myrrh, echinacea, witch hazel, and golden seal, all granulated. After thoroughly mixing, use one tablespoonful to a pint of boiling water, steep one-half hour, strain. Apply gently with cotton.

A very good, but simple remedy is as follows: Cover the affected parts well with grated potatoes, about one-fourth inch thick. When dry remove, and replenish.

Fevers

Causes.—The body is filled with waste matter, and fever is nature's process of burning up impurities.

Treatment.—Take an emetic to cleanse the stomach. See emetics in Table of Contents. Should the temperature be too high and the patient too ill for this, give a cup of golden seal and myrrh. This will kill the poison in the stomach. To make a pint of this tea, steep a heaping teaspoonful of golden seal and one-half teaspoonful of myrrh in a pint of boiling water for twenty minutes. After taking the first cupful, take a tablespoonful every hour thereafter. More can be taken with benefit.

Cool water enemas will bring down the temperature rapidly. Have the water slightly below body temperature. An herb enema is more effective, but castile or ivory soap may be used; have the water slightly sudsy. It is the removal of the poisons from the system that brings the temperature down. Remove the patient's clothes, and put him between cotton blankets. Sponge off all over with tepid water, beginning with the face, sponge downward over the entire body, sponging well around the head and back of neck. Sponge the feet thoroughly, leaving the soles moist. Do this every five minutes in high fevers. Give sips of cold water every five minutes. In case the patient becomes chilly, stop the bath, cover well, and place hot water bottles or hot fomentations over the stomach. This will usually stop the chill. If it does not, apply hot fomentations to the spine, or give a hot foot bath, and a hot drink, which should check the chill at once.

I have again and again broken up very severe cases of various kinds of fever with this treatment. The bowels must be kept open with laxative herbs. In slight fevers, sometimes lemon juice alone will break it up. Take it diluted in water without any sweetening.

I well remember my mother and father breaking up severe cases of fever with herb teas and fruit juices. They used red raspberry leaves, willow bark, and other herbs.

Slippery elm tea is excellent in all cases of fever, as it is powerful to cleanse, and is soothing to the stomach and intestinal tract.

Any one of the following herbs are useful in fevers; make into a tea, and drink copiously until the fever abates.

Yarrow, red sage, catnip, peppermint, wild cherry bark, valerian, black cohosh, tansy, camomile, elder, boneset, willow (bark or leaves), pleurisy root, marigold, nettle, and lobelia. See Table of Contents for use of non-poisonous herbs.

Red raspberry leaf tea is excellent to reduce fever in children.

Diet.—In all cases of fever and prostrating diseases, a few days of liquid diet will lessen their severity, and give the stomach a much-needed rest. The first point to be emphasized is, drink plenty of water as it dilutes and carries away toxins through the kidneys. Remember, it is the greatest solvent known. Special benefit will be derived from using orange juice. Fruit drinks of all kinds are beneficial when taken without cane sugar. The use of cane sugar will increase the fever, and make acid blood. Weak lemonade given freely is very good. Sweeten drinks with malt honey, malt sugar, or honey, if at all. Use fresh fruits whenever possible. When the fever subsides, special care must be taken to eat light, nourishing, easily digested foods. The following list of foods are nourishing, and can be used in convalescence: soybean milk, potassium broth, zwieback, baked Irish potato, natural brown rice, and bananas (very ripe).

Soybean milk is alkaline and very nourishing, also easy to digest. Dissolve whole wheat flakes in the hot milk. This is very strengthening. Well-ripened bananas made into a puree are excellent, especially for under-weight patients.

Foods to be strictly avoided during fevers: meats of all kinds, meat broths, fish, fowl, oysters, pickles, condiments, cheese, mushrooms, and eggs. These foods should be avoided because of the high amount of protein they contain, and when the intake of protein is greater than the requirements of the system, putrefaction results. As a matter of fact, the continual use of these foods always brings on disease in one form or another. Use salt as sparingly as possible.

Two quarts of orange juice and an equal amount of oatmeal water is a daily ration for typhoid fever, and also other fevers. More can be taken with good results, but do not take the orange juice at the same time the oatmeal water is taken. Take at least one hour apart.

Felons

A felon is a painful abcess, usually on the end of a finger, thumb or toe.

Causes.—A blow or injury; when the tissues of the skin are injured the waste matter in the system will seek an outlet there in the form of a felon.

Symptoms.—Great pain and swelling.

Treatment.—Warm some kerosene and immerse the affected part into it four or five times a day, keeping it in the kerosene from ten to fifteen minutes each time (or longer.) This alone will cure a felon or check one which has just started. This treatment is also good for painful ringworm on the end of the finger. An excellent poultice for this is made of equal parts of slippery elm, lady's-slipper, and lobelia herb. See poultices in Table of Contents. Granulated herbs can be used if the powdered are not obtainable.

To relieve pain, if the felon is on the end of the finger, cut a small hole in the end of a lemon and stick the finger in it. If on other parts, slice the lemon and bandage a thick slice on. This will give excellent results, and will often cure a felon.

Female Troubles

There is so much suffering and disease among women in the world that could be saved if they would use remedies which are simple, harmless, and inexpensive as well.

Womb troubles are very often caused because of constipation. The waste matter stays too long in the colon and is absorbed by the delicate organs and the womb becomes aggravated, inflamed, or ulcerated because of it.

Charcoal poultices with smartweed will do much to take out womb inflammation. See charcoal in Table of Contents. A high enema should be taken, and if there is colon trouble take high herb enemas, such as burdock root, yellow dock root, bayberry bark, or witch hazel. If there is any soreness in the rectum or piles, inject a little Healing Lotion, as given in this book; do this with a small glass syringe, warm before using. The foregoing herbs are excellent for either enemas or douches, or both. When there is laceration, ulceration, or tumors, make a strong tea of one of the following; white oak bark, witch-hazel bark, golden seal, myrrh, or wild alum root. Use a heaping teaspoonful of the herb to a pint of boiling water. Use this in a spiral douche. These teas are very disinfectant and healing. An exceptionally fine solution is, a rounding teaspoonful each of golden seal and myrrh, steeped in a quart of boiling water, use in spiral douche.

When there are other womb troubles, as in menstruation, see Menstruation in Table of Contents. There are herbs which will increase or decrease the flow, or will regulate it when it is irregular. Difficulties in menstruation often cause other womb troubles.

Precautions when your monthly period first arrives are well worth their seeming inconvenience. Stay off your feet as much as possible, keep hands out of cold water. During the entire time, keep your limbs and feet warm. In the winter, and during cold weather, do not go to bed with cold feet. Either take a hot foot-bath on retiring, or use a hot water bottle. A gallon jug of hot water at the foot of the bed is excellent.

Fomentations are a great household weapon as they will relieve much suffering, pain, and are very beneficial when a person is suffering with cramps.

Gonorrhea

Cause.—Gonorrhea, like syphilis, is due to a germ and often contracted by sexual relations. It is more common among men than women. A large percentage of women contract it from their husbands, who are untrue to the marriage vows, or who had thought they were cured before marriage.

Symptoms.—The genitals become inflamed. There is a stinging and prickling sensation when urinating. After a few days this becomes exceedingly painful. There is a discharge of pus, greenish yellow in color and it is very infectious. The discharge continues six or eight weeks. Organic nervous diseases many times follow gonorrhea.

Treatment.—It will greatly shorten the course of gonorrhea if the person affected can go to bed at once. Use a diet that is cleansing, immediately. (See cleansing diet in Table of Contents). Take absolutely nothing into the stomach that is the least irritating to the blood or stomach. It is best to go on a fruit juice diet.

Take two high enemas a day, preferably herb enemas. An excellent douche for women is equal parts red raspberry leaves and witch-hazel leaves. Good results will be obtained if a douche of this tea is given each time after urination. Steep a heaping tablespoonful of the mixed leaves to a quart of boiling water for twenty minutes. Use warm. This solution is also a fine wash for the genitals in both men and women.

If there are sores and ulcers make a solution of a small one-fourth teaspoonful powdered aloes, one teaspoonful golden seal, and one teaspoonful powdered myrrh. Steep these in a pint of boiling water for half an hour. Bathe the sores thoroughly with this. Then sprinkle on equal parts of powdered golden seal and myrrh. Healing lotion, as given in this book, is also fine to apply to either sores or ulcers.

Drink at least one quart of slippery elm tea a day, can be mixed with fruit juices or taken plain. Drink at least eight glasses of water a day.

If the patient stays in bed, be sure the room is well ventilated at all times. A warm sitz bath two or three times a day will give relief from pain. For paints in the legs or any part of the body, apply hot fomentations, or rub thoroughly with liniment, as given in this book.

Black willow, saw palmetto berries, and scullcap, are especially beneficial in acute gonorrhea. Steep a heaping teaspoonful in a cup of boiling water, for one half hour. Take two tablespoonfuls six times a day. Use other herbs as given under syphilis.

The three herbs given above are also good to stop involuntary seminal emissions. Use equal parts of the three, or if not all obtainable, use one of two and make according to directions in Table of Contents for use of nonpoisonous herbs. Take a cupful hot upon retiring, and during the night if awake.

Gangrene

Causes.—Gangrene internally or externally is because of extreme waste matter in the system, which causes the soft tissues of the body to decay. Burns, corrosions by acid or frost bites are often followed by gangrene. Any bruise or sore, such as, boils or carbuncles, which are not properly cared for, become stagnant and gangrene may develop. The white blood cells fail to carry off the waste matter, because they are not given proper nourishment with good food. The tissue dies and blood poisoning sets in.

Symptoms.—There are two kinds of gangrene, moist and dry. There is always inflammation before the moist gangrene sets in. The part affected becomes bluish or black. The tissues sometimes are entirely dead. Therefore, there is no feeling at all in the part affected. Dry gangrene usually begins by a spot in various places, often in spots where the circulation is poor. Frequently the toes are affected. The affected part turns yellow or black.

Treatment.—Follow the diet given under purifying the blood. A person who has pure blood and a good circulation will never have gangrene. I have used the following treatment with excellent success in very bad cases of gangrene.

Take one-fourth pound of powdered charcoal, one ounce of water pepper, or smart weed, put these in a pan and pour one pint boiling water over them, let steep twenty minutes. Then mix 2 tablespoons whole wheat flour and enough dry charcoal with this solution to make a poultice. Spread on a piece of gauze, a little larger than the affected part, so that it will be well covered, apply it, and lay another piece of gauze over it, and bandage it on. If the affected part is painful, add a tablespoonful of lobelia when steeping the herbs. You may use a little flaxseed meal or cornmeal to make the poultice stick together. When there is pus and ulceration, warm some peroxide of hydrogen and bathe the affected part thoroughly with this, applying repeatedly and wiping off with a piece of cotton, until it is absolutely clean. Do this before applying the poultice.

Another excellent poultice may be made as follows: Two tablespoonfuls ground flaxseed (or flaxseed meal), a teaspoonful of golden seal, and one half teaspoonful myrrh. Add enough hot water to make a paste. The paste must not be too stiff, it must be soft enough to penetrate. Apply the same as other poultice. Renew every six hours, cleaning each time with peroxide if pus forms.

Take internally: mix equal parts scullcap, valerian, yellow dock, and buckthorn bark. Use a heaping teaspoonful to a cup of boiling water. Let steep one half hour. Take a cupful before each meal (one hour before), and a cupful hot upon retiring.

If constipated, take herbal laxative. The bowels must be kept open.

Gallstones

Cause.—Hearty eaters and high livers suffer mostly from gallstones. The eating of too much starch, sugar, meats, greasy foods, highly seasoned foods, dairy milk, and foods containing too much protein, are the main causes. The use of hard water, bicarbonate of soda, and lack of water drinking are also causes. Generally there is constipation, and liver trouble, before the gallstones form. If the liver is overloaded, it is not able to perform its work and get rid of the waste matter. A fruit diet for a week or ten days is a wonderful medicine for the liver, especially if high enemas are taken every day and enough laxative herbs used to keep the bowels open, so that they move at least three times a day. If you would do this when gallstones are suspicioned it would prevent their formation.

Symptoms.—In advanced cases there is pain in the region of the liver, which is located under the right rib, the pains extending to the right shoulder blade, and violent pains in the abdomen. There is often jaundice because of the obstruction of the gall bladder, cold perspiration, cramps in the feet and hands, or vomiting. It is not always that these symptoms are present.

Treatment.—If possible, and the agony not too great, give an enema, preferably of catnip tea. Apply hot fomentations of lobelia and hops over the region of the liver, but if the patient is in great pain and you do not have the herbs, use hot water fomentations until you get the herbs. Give a hot foot bath. Give a cup of hot tea made of equal parts of the following herbs just as soon as possible: hyssop, gentian root, nerve root, scullcap, and buckthorn bark. Mix thoroughly, and use a heaping teaspoonful to the cup of boiling water. Take a cup of this tea every hour the first day. Then continue to take four times a day, one cup an hour before each meal, and one upon retiring. This will liquify the bile, and improve the liver.

Continue the fomentation. A half hour after taking the tea, follow by taking four ounces of olive oil and four ounces of lemon juice or grapefruit juice beaten thoroughly together. After taking the lemon juice and olive oil, lie on the right side, with the hips elevated by placing two pillows underneath them. This will cause the oil to run up into the mouth of the gall bladder and thus lubricate the gall bladder so the gallstones can pass. Fomentations of lobelia and hops will not only soothe the pains, but they will dilate the gall bladder duct, so the lemon juice and oil may pass. A thorough massage under the right rib, rubbing toward the center of the body will greatly facilitate the passing of the gallstones after the fomentations have been applied and the oil given. I repeat, if the herbs are not available, use hot water fomentations.

(433)

When suffering from gallstones, go on a fruit juice diet of oranges and grapefruit. Unsweetened pineapple juice is especially recommended for gallstones. Be sure your diet contains plenty of alkaline foods. Potassium broth, recipe for which is given in this book, is one of the best things that can be taken. It is highly nourishing and alkaline. (Look in Table of Contents, for alkaline foods.) This same diet is good for gravel in the bladder and stones in the kidneys, and for liver troubles.

Take the lemon juice and olive oil for three days. You may take it in this way also: Take two tablespoonfuls lemon juice, followed by two tablespoonfuls olive oil, or vice versa. Take on an empty stomach.

The following herbs are very valuable in gallstones. Use a rounded teaspoonful of powdered wood betony, or one of milkweed mixed in one-half glass of cold water; follow by drinking a glass of hot water. Take one hour before each meal and upon retiring.

Dr. Lee, one of New York City's great physicians, said that if the people would stop eating acid-forming foods and eat alkaline foods, any case of gallstones could be cured. Dr. Clark, of Chicago, once said to me, that any case of gallstones, appendicitis, tonsillitis, piles, and hemorrhoids could be cured without the knife. That is in harmony with Bible doctrine, that God has a remedy for every ill of man and operations would be rarely needed. This has been my experience for years.

Gout

Causes.—Gout is a form of rheumatism, caused by over-eating and drinking, eating of wrong combinations that fill the system with waste matter.

Symptoms.—Loss of appetite, heartburn, gas, distented bowels, constipation, often palpitation of the heart, scanty urine, sometimes red in color. Pain may be in any part of the body, the ankles swell, as well as the knees. General distress.

Treatment.—The diet is of first importance. In order to help gout, all harmful products, foods, and drinks, must be given up. Use the same diet as for diabetes. Take a high enema of warm, soapy-sudsy water, and if there is any colon trouble or colitis, take herb enemas. See herb enemas in Table of Contents.

Take equal parts of scullcap, yarrow, and valerian, granulated, mix thoroughly together, and use a heaping teaspoonful to the cup of boiling water, steep, and drink a cupful an hour before meals, and one upon retiring. Take laxative herbs to keep the bowels open; this is important. The liniment, as given in this book, if applied freely and thoroughly rubbed in, will greatly allay the pain. The herbs given under chronic rheumatism, may be taken for gout with good effect; study each herb separately, and take the one or combination that suits your case best.

Any one of the following herbs will be found beneficial; take singly, or in any combination you desire, using a teaspoonful to the cup of boiling water, steep twenty minutes, and take four cups a day, one an hour before each meal, and one upon retiring. Blue violet, burdock, gentian root, mugwort, rue, birch, broom, sarsaparilla, buckthorn, ginger, pennyroyal, plantain, wood betony, and balm of Gilead.

Goitre

Goitre is an enlargement of the thyroid gland.

Causes.—It is an affection of the sympathetic nervous system, in the great majority of cases, due to disorders from indigestion. It would be extremely rare for anyone to have a goitre, if they did not have indigestion and bad stomach before. Goitres are usually a long time in developing. It may take years to develop a goitre of any size.

Symptoms.—The first symptom is an enlargement of the thyroid gland. The breathing is interfered with and there is an increased action of the heart. There are two kinds of goitre, inward, and outward. The inward is more serious.

Treatment.—Build up the stomach, eat a plain, nourishing, alkaline diet. See alkaline foods in Table of Contents.

A powerful stomach remedy is composed of the following: a heaping tablespoonful of golden seal, tablespoonful bayberry, teaspoonful myrrh, mix thoroughly and take one-half teaspoonful in a cup of water an hour before each meal and one upon retiring. Use also as a mouth wash and gargle thoroughly with it.

The bowels must be kept loose. Use high herb enemas to cleanse the colon thoroughly. Also take herbal laxative. See Table of Contents. Bathe the neck thoroughly with the liniment given in this book.

A bayberry poultice used at night, and kept on all night is excellent. It must be well covered with a woolen cloth to keep it warm. See poultices in Table of Contents.

Sweat baths and massage to increase the circulation and build up the nervous system are very helpful. Take herbs for nerves.

Gas in Stomach and Bowels

Causes.—Gas in the stomach and bowels is the result of indigestion. The food remains in the stomach too long, and becomes fermented and sour. A small quantity of wrong combinations will cause gas in the stomach and bowels. Drinking with meals causes sour stomach and fermentation, as does hasty eating and poor mastication.

Treatment.—Peppermint and spearmint tea are excellent to overcome gas on the stomach. Equal parts of calamus root, valerian, with peppermint or spearmint, granulated, should be taken. Mix together, use a teaspoonful to a cup of boiling water, steep, strain, and drink one half cupful an hour before meals, and another half cupful after meals. The above herbs can be used in powdered form, as well as in capsules, if desired.

To strengthen the stomach and cleanse it so that this condition will be overcome, take one-fourth teaspoonful powdered golden seal in one-half glass of warm water an hour before each meal. You may take it as follows if you prefer: one heaping teaspoonful golden seal, one-fourth teaspoonful myrrh to a pint of boiling water, steep, and take a swallow just a few minutes before eating.

Rinse the mouth and throat thoroughly with this in the mornings, swallowing a little.

See Table of Contents for herbs in indigestion, gas, and fermentation.

Coughs

Causes.—Deranged stomach. The vitality of the system has become lowered by improper diet, loss of sleep, lack of exercise and fresh air, and improper elimination. The cough is caused by the inflamed throat or bronchial tubes. This inflammation causes mucus, which the cough is trying to expel. If the stomach and system were kept in good condition, there would be but few colds. Improper clothing and bedding at night are often causes of colds. The poisons and waste matter in the body make one more susceptible. If the system were kept in good health and the powers of resistance good, coughs and colds would be rare.

A cold can be treated and overcome in just one day. When the first symptoms of a cold, la grippe, or cough appear, it is an indication that there is waste matter and mucus in the system. Take a pint of soft, warm water and a teaspoonful of salt. Snuff this up the nose; then blow it out. Repeat this until the nose is entirely clean of mucus. Then gargle the throat and rinse the mouth out thoroughly. Take some good herb mentioned later in this article, snuff it up through the nose, and gargle, swallowing some of it. This would ward off the liability of the cold developing into bronchitis, asthma, lung fever, or maybe consumption. Whenever there is a cold, the first precaution is to keep the nose and mouth clean, which will keep it from going down into the lungs and causing further trouble.

When the head is stuffed up and there is tightness in the chest as well as a mean, drowsy, stupid feeling, we hear people say, "My head is all stuffed up," but the fact is that they are aware of it only in the head. The whole system is involved. Anything we can do to relieve this condition in the system will break up the cold.

Treatment.—First take the salt and water treatment for cleaning out the mouth, as directed above.

Colds would not be so prevalent if systems were not filled with mucus and poison, so one should immediately rid the system of this poison. There is no more successful way to do this than to cleanse the colon by high enemas, continuing the enemas until they reach the upper end of the colon and get it clean. If there is any nausea or bad feeling in the stomach, take an emetic. This can be done with just lukewarm water, or water with a little salt added. Drink all the water possible and run the finger down the throat to wash the stomach out. Repeat this until the stomach is clean; then take a hot herb tea. Sage or red sage is excellent. Drink two or three cups in succession while it is hot. Hyssop, yarrow, black cohosh, peppermint, and camomile teas are also excellent remedies. Take a few cups (hot) in the beginning, and in a few hours take more, also a rounding teaspoonful composition powder every hour for five or six hours.

Keep quiet and stay in bed if possible. Take only fruit juices for nourishment. If you do not have fruit juices, drink water, hot or cold, with lemon juice in it; then later, potassium broth, which is nourishing and alkaline. This treatment will break up la grippe as well as a cold.

If there is continued cough, an excellent help is the cough remedy made from the recipe in this book. (See Table of Contents.)

Bronchitis (Chronic)

Causes.—Bronchitis becomes chronic when acute bronchitis is not properly treated and relieved. When a cold is allowed to run, it gets down into the bronchial tubes and lungs and becomes chronic. Often if it is not cured, it will finally go into consumption or tuberculosis of the lungs. Stomach trouble is one great cause.

Symptoms.—Almost continual coughing, the coughing up of quantities of mucus and phlegm, shortness of breath. The symptoms often become very severe.

Treatment.—One of the first and most effective things to do in order to clear the throat and facilitate breathing is to take an emetic, using warm water. Make a weak tea of cubeb berries, using one heaping teaspoonful to a pint of hot water. A pinch of red pepper added is excellent to cut the phlegm loose so that it can be expelled. After doing this, take a drink of the hot tea to wash out the stomach. Good results will be obtained. A very little lobelia (one-fourth teaspoonful) added will relax the throat, stomach, and bronchial tubes at once.

All foods listed under Acid Forming Foods must be stricken from the diet and scrupulously avoided. Do not drink with your meals, as liquid with meals causes fermentation, acid, and gas. Eat alkaline foods, as listed in this book. Fruit juices of all kinds, especially pineapple, lemon, orange, and grapefruit, are best, as they help to loosen and cut the phlegm.

Take equal parts of wild cherry, mullein, coltsfoot, yarrow, horehound, and buckthorn. Mix together, using one teaspoonful to a cup of boiling water. Take a cupful four times a day. It may be taken more often in smaller doses if preferred. If you do not have all these herbs, read the description of the different ones, and then select the one best suited to your case.

I would repeat: If the breathing is very difficult and the cough severe, take two teaspoonfuls of cubeb berries, one teaspoonful of either peppermint or catnip, and one-half teaspoonful herb or seed of lobelia to a quart of boiling water and let steep. When the mixture becomes lukewarm, strain, and drink as much of it as possible; then run your finger down your throat until it causes you to vomit. This will clear the stomach and bronchial tubes of mucus and phlegm. After doing this, relieve the colon and intestines of waste matter with a high enema, as constipation is one of the causes of the trouble. Then take laxative herbs and keep the bowels open.

A full hot bath, steam bath, or vapor bath, followed by a short, cold shower is beneficial. In the absence of a shower, finish patient off with a cold towel rub of short duration. Hot fomentations to the chest and the spine, finishing with cold, will do much to relieve congestion. Hot foot baths with a tablespoonful of mustard in the water often give great relief. A hot fomentation applied around the neck and followed by a cold compress is also beneficial. The cold compress must be thoroughly covered with a woolen cloth to heat it up. If, for any reason, it should get cold, it must be taken off and the neck rubbed thoroughly dry, leaving a dry woolen cloth on. The air in the patient's room should not be too dry. Place a dish of water on the stove or radiator to produce moisture in the air. The room should be kept at an even temperature, but good ventilation is necessary.

Remove the causes and take some herbs. Everyone should keep herbs on hand for colds and la grippe and not let them run into bronchial troubles. Chickweed, coltsfoot, cubeb berries, golden seal, lungwort, mullein, myrrh, white pine, pleurisy root, sanicle, saw palmetto berries, skunk cabbage, slippery elm, white pond lily, yerba santa, bloodroot, ginger, blue violet, bethroot, red root, red sage, and lobelia can be used singly or in any combination you desire.

Everyone should have on hand antispasmodic tincture and the cough medicine made according to the formulas given in this book.

Bronchitis (Acute)

Causes.—Changeable weather, catching cold, exposure, wet feet, chilling when not sufficiently clothed, insufficient ventilation in house, especially in bedrooms. Bronchitis would be rare if people ate the right food and systems were not filled with mucus and poisonous waste matter, and if they were properly clothed. Where there is bronchitis there is invariably stomach trouble and constipation.

(441)

Bronchitis is a disease which first affects the mucous surface or inner lining of the bronchial tubes and causes an extra amount of mucus to form, which is called phlegm.

Symptoms.—Chills and fever, tightness and stuffiness in the chest, difficult breathing. Sometimes there is a severe cough, and the attack comes on like croup. It may be that one or all tubes are affected, but in most cases it is the large tubes. The cough is worse when the patient lies down, and usually the patient has a bad coughing spell the first thing on waking. At first there seems to be but little mucus, which increases and often turns to yellow pus, sometimes becoming frothy. Children sometimes have convulsions and become unconscious.

Treatment.—Same treatment as for chronic bronchitis. Everyone should have on hand antispasmodic tincture and the cough medicine made according to the formulas given in this book and used in acute and chronic bronchitis and asthma.

Bed Wetting

Causes.—Kidney and bladder trouble caused by wrong diet. Weak and undernourished children are most likely to have this habit. Other causes are late suppers, constipation, worms, gas in bowels, and general nervousness.

Treatment.—Do not let the child eat late at night or eat any stimulating foods, such as tea, coffee, soft drinks, white bread products, or cane sugar products. No food of any kind should be given after four or five o'clock. Liquids of any kind should not be given after four o'clock p.m. Do not allow the child to lie on his back; he should lie on his side or face. It sometimes helps to elevate the foot of the bed a little. Cold morning baths, with massage, if possible, and plenty outdoor exercise will be a great help. A special effort must be made to find out about what time the child wets the bed. Usually it is about an hour and a half after retiring and again about three in the morning. They should be taken up about this time until the habit is broken. Sometimes, when the kidneys or bladder are very much irritated, fomentations to the bladder and the entire length of the spine will relieve the situation.

Make a tea of plantain and St.-John's-wort, equal parts, mixed together. Use a small teaspoonful to a cup of boiling water. Steep. Give the child one to two cups a day in doses of one-fourth cup at a time. The tea may be sweetened with a little honey so that the child will not object to taking it. Either one of the above herbs is effective alone, but it is well to use both. The bowels must be kept loose. High herb enemas are very helpful, given at a temperature a little above body heat. It is often the putrified matter in the colon which irritates the bladder. Good elimination is very necessary. It is absolutely no use to scold a child, as scolding makes him nervous and then it is harder for him to overcome the habit. Make special efforts to help him overcome this distressing habit, which he himself dislikes but cannot help unless his parents help him.

Burns and Scalds

Treatment.—If the clothes should catch fire, a blanket or some large piece of wet cloth, if possible, should be quickly wrapped around a person to smother the fire. The one who is on fire should never start to run or walk, but throw himself immediately on the ground and roll, or grab a blanket and roll up in it. The clothes should be quickly removed. Do not even wait to undress, but cut the clothes to get them off the quickest way possible. The patient should be taken to a quiet place where the burn may be dressed. The first thing to be considered is the nature of the scald or burn, where it is, and to what degree the skin is burned. Dip a cloth in kerosene and cover the burn. This will quickly allay the pain. If there are any blisters, prick them on the edge with a steel needle, and press out the water. The writer has healed large burns with very little pain by the kerosene method. A hot water burn should be treated in the same way. Call your family physician if the burn is bad.

Large burns may be bathed with the following lotion: Take one teaspoonful of golden seal, one of myrrh, and one of boracic acid and add to a pint of boiling water. Let the mixture stand for one-half hour; then pour off the clear liquid, and apply with absorbent cotton. This solution is very soothing and healing, and is an excellent remedy for deep burns. Healing Lotion and liniment, as found in this book, are very excellent for this also. If the sore is deep, it will heal more quickly if just the powdered myrrh, golden seal, and boracic acid is sprinkled on the sore in dry form, thus keeping the burn dry so that it will heal more quickly. Cover with gauze. If there is any proud flesh, sprinkle with burnt alum.

The following tea, taken internally, will bring about a powerful circulation and will greatly aid the healing of burns: Take one teaspoonful each of valerian, scullcap, and peppermint. Mix together and use one teaspoonful to a cup of boiling water. It is very quieting and soothing to the nerves.

Bright's Disease

Causes.—Among the causes are alcoholic drinks, tea, coffee, and spices. The use of patent medicines is often a cause. Food cooked in aluminum utensils is very injurious to the liver, spleen, pancreas, and kidneys. Food cooked in aluminum vessels should never be eaten, but especially not when anyone is suffering from Bright's disease, either acute or chronic. Bright's disease sometimes follows various other diseases, such as typhoid fever, influenza, diphtheria, pneumonia, smallpox, and scarlet fever.

Symptoms.—One of the most common symptoms is loss of appetite. At other times there is a great desire for food; then, when it is set before you, you loathe the sight of it. In some cases the skin will be dry and there will be fever or shortness of breath and palpitation of the heart. There is swelling of the ankles and under the eyes, which is a sign of a dropsical condition developing, and pain in the kidneys. The patient is usually pale, especially after the condition has advanced to some extent. At first there may be scantiness of urine, and alter the urine greatly increases, with albumin in it. Often there is frequent urination at night, accompanied with a burning sensation. Have your family physician test your urine.

Treatment.—Take a high enema. If there is any colon trouble, use the white oak bark, bayberry bark, or wild alum root bark enemas. In the absence of the herbs, use very warm water made slightly sudsy with Ivory soap. Give a daily hot bath. While the patient is in the tub, give two or three cups of pleurisy tea or sage tea. This treatment will open the pores and encourage perspiration. It is good to stay in the bath one-half hour and as much longer as you can. Finish off with a short cold shower, or a short cold towel rub, and rub thoroughly dry. Be sure to keep the patient from chilling. A salt glow will greatly help the activity of the skin. An excellent thing to do after the bath is to wrap the patient in a blanket, put him to bed, and continue giving the pleurisy tea or sage tea to encourage perspiration. Fomentations to the spine, sponging the spine with cold water after each and rubbing the skin thoroughly dry before applying another, are excellent to allay pain. Also give the same treatment over stomach, liver, and spleen.

A tea of broom top and marshmallow leaves, equal parts, is very good. The bowels must be kept open. Take enough laxative herbs so that the bowels will move three or four times a day.

Diet.—The diet should be light and nourishing. All stimulating and heavy foods should be strictly forbidden. (See Nourishing Foods.) All the food eaten should be low in protein. Sprouted soybeans and lentils may be eaten. The soybean recipes as given in this book, cauliflower, asparagus, eggplant, and vegetable broths are good. The free use of fruit juices, or a fruit juice diet for a few days before starting to partake of other foods, is excellent. Soybean milk, with whole wheat flakes dissolved in it, is extremely nourishing and very easily digested. Avoid the use of salt as much as possible, and do not mix fruits and vegetables at the same meal.

Blood Pressure (High)

Causes.—High blood pressure is caused by waste matter in the system, wrong diet, overeating, use of tobacco, liquors, meat, devitaminized foods, and wrong combinations. It would be a rare thing to occur if the liver and kidneys were not overburdened with too much food, and irritating foods. Most of the people who die because of high blood pressure, have liver, pancreas, spleen, or heart trouble.

Symptoms.—A flushed complexion, uncomfortable feelings, usually over-weight, and sometimes pallor of skin with weakness.

Treatment.—Read article, "Impure Blood and How to Cleanse." High herb enemas should be given, for there is always putrid waste matter in the colon. (See Herb Enemas.) Put one teaspoonful of golden seal in a pint of boiling water. Take a swallow of this at least six times a day. Take plenty of red clover tea, as this will purify the blood; it is good to drink this in place of water. The following herbs are useful for high blood pressure. Study each one, under Herbs, and take those best suited to your case; wild cherry bark, vervain, rue, broom, black cohosh, boneset, peppermint, blue cohosh, red pepper, valerian, hyssop, sanicle, and scullcap. (Use Herbal Laxative as given in the Table of Contents.)

Diet and rest.—All stimulating foods and drinks are very harmful, such as tobacco, alcohol, all soft drinks, white-flour products, cane-sugar products, meat, tea, coffee, pepper, vinegar, and mustard. A fruit diet for a few days is one of the best things you can take. Then use a simple, nourishing diet, with plenty of outdoor exercise, and practice deep breathing. Most people with high blood pressure do not get enough rest. They worry about business affairs, have too many social duties, visitors, and keep too late hours. We mention these things because too much excitement and being overtired will always cause the blood pressure to go higher. Rest is imperative. A warm bath at night and plenty of sleep in a well-ventilated room will do a great deal to lower the blood pressure. If troubled with sleeplessness, take some herb teas that will produce sleep, because these are harmless and will leave no bad after effects. If you follow the above treatment and instructions, your blood pressure will surely go down.

The following treatment will greatly aid recovery: Hot and cold applications to the spine, liver, spleen, and stomach; cold towel rubs in the morning upon arising; warm baths at night and salt glows; hot and cold showers. A general massage is excellent, as it will help to work the waste matter out of the system, equalize the circulation, and greatly relieve the heart and nerves.

Blood pressure shows the contractile powers of the heart and the resistance of the blood vessels. The blood pressure increases every two years about one degree. The normal blood at thirty is approximately 125, and at sixty, it is 140. Persons who are weak physically have a slightly lower pressure. When exercise is taken, there will be a higher degree.

When the blood pressure is too high or when it is too low—this indicates that there is something wrong with the circulation of the blood, therefore, a course must be taken to equalize the circulation. When this is done it aids in causing the blood pressure to become nearer normal.

Blood Pressure (Low)

Causes.—Lack of proper nourishment, rest, and exercise; lack of vitality and red blood corpuscles.

Treatment.—Deep bretahing is a great means of restoring the normal temperature of the body. Increase the circulation by means of hot baths and cold morning baths, thoroughly rubbing with a coarse towel when drying. (See Baths.) Any one of the following list of herbs mixed with a very little red pepper, will greatly increase the vitality (See directions in Table of Contents). Hyssop, golden seal, vervain, prickly ash, blue cohosh, gentian, wood betony, burnet, and scullcap.

Diet.—Eat plenty of nourishing food. Potassium Broth and mashed potatoes, as given in this book, baked potatoes, (Eat skin and all.), soybean milk, soy cottage cheese, plenty of leafy vegetables, and vegetables of all kinds. Do not eat any devitaminized or stimulating foods. If you are troubled with indigestion, drink peppermint or spearmint tea, but you will not have indigestion if you eat proper food, and eat it dry. Drinking water and other liquids with meals causes fermentation and indigestion. If you thoroughly cleanse your system and follow the above instructions, your blood pressure will soon become normal.

Plenty of exercise outdoors is very necessary. Take tonic herbs.

Bed Sores and Chafing

Causes.—Infrequent bathing, pressure, or lying too long in one position. The position of a bedridden patient should be changed frequently. If good care is taken of such patients, they will rarely get bedsores.

Treatment.—Hot and cold applications and thorough rubbings will bring about a good circulation, which will prevent bedsores, or will greatly relieve them. Make a tea of witch hazel and bathe the sores at least three or four times a day. Healing lotion, as given in this book, is excellent to heal sores of any kind. If there is any proud flesh, destroy it by sprinkling powdered burnt alum on the sore. The best wash for this purpose is one made of one teaspoonful each of golden seal, myrrh, and boric acid to a pint of boiling water. After washing the sore, it should be sprinkled with equal parts of dry golden seal and myrrh. This will kill the poison and infection, and is very healing. Cover with a little cotton and oiled cloth.

Blood Poisoning and Infections

Causes.—Uncleanliness, improper dressing of sores, and chronic constipation.

Symptoms.—In the beginning there is a decided chill and a feeling of depression. Shivering sensations, followed by profuse perspiration, may be frequent. The pulse becomes very rapid, and the region around the wound looks red and angry. The breathing grows rapid, and there is an anxious expression on the countenance.

Treatment.—Echinacea is a very good herb to correct blood conditions, especially where there is a tendency to gangrene. It is used for an internal bath in acute appendicitis to prevent gangrene and peritonitis, and is a remedy for scarlet fever, malaria, puerperal septicemia, tonsillitis, diphtheria, and typhoid conditions.

Take a high enema. Take as many cups of echinacea tea a day as possible, using a teaspoonful to the cup; or if taken in powdered form in capsules, take two No. 00 capsules every two hours.

Take nothing but fruit juices for a number of days, especially grapefruit, orange, lemon, and pineapple. Do not mix the juices. Take one at a time, but drink plenty of them. Keep the temperature even, and have an abundance of fresh air.

When the patient feels chilly, give a cup of hot water in which a little cayenne pepper has been dissolved. This can be given often. Charcoal taken thus, one heaping teaspoonful put in a cup, with hot water added to make a paste, diluted, and drunk at once, is very good. Charcoal can also be used to advantage as a poultice. (See Poultices in Table of Contents.)

Wash the wounds thoroughly with boric solution, and if the discharge is thin and unhealthy looking, apply powdered myrrh and golden seal (equal parts) directly to the sore, just sprinkling it on. (See herbs given under Blood Poisoning in this book.)

Breast (*Caked or Inflamed*)

Symptoms.—Hard and painful swelling in the breast, throbbing, burning pain, restlessness, fever.

Treatment.—The following treatment is excellent when the breast is inflamed, swollen, caked, or when the nipples are sore. Mix well together one pint of linseed oil and four ounces of spirits of camphor. Soak a cloth in this solution and be sure to cover all the affected part. Apply as often as required. Dry hot and cold applications to relieve the soreness and inflammation are very good. These should be given continuously until relieved. Then apply the above solution. When the breast is swollen, a poultice of slippery elm, with a little lobelia added, will give great relief. (See Poultices.) Drink three or four cups of tea a day made of equal parts of ginger, golden seal, and black cohosh. Often just bathing an inflamed breast with alder tea will relieve the inflammation and pain. Clean out the system and build up the health. If there is any danger of cancer of the breast, take the treatment given under Cancer, externally and internally. A poultice of grated poke root and cornmeal, applied warm, is very good.

Boils and Carbuncles

Causes.—Inactivity of the skin, bad blood from putrefaction in the system, constipation. The fact that one has boils or carbuncles shows that the body is full of poisons and waste matter and is in a low state of resistance. Some of the minute glands die; sometimes the root of a hair dies; then a little pimple appears, which, if treated immediately, would soon disappear. The red spot or pimple is followed by tenderness and great pain. Boils seldom come singly. Often, one is followed by several others.

Treatment.—When the carbuncle or boil is at the root of a hair, it is a good thing to pull out the hair and apply a little liniment, for which a recipe is given in this book. If taken in time and if the liniment is applied repeatedly, the boil should soon disappear. In case of a pimple, it should

(451)

be opened, the pus squeezed out, and liniment applied. It is very necessary that the system be cleansed from waste matter. The bowels must be kept open, moving at least three or four times a day. Take a high enema at night before retiring. (See High Enemas.) Take some of the laxative herbs. Also, a cleansing diet is excellent to rid the system of poisons. (See Cleansing Diet.) A cleansing diet for a week or more, with proper elimination, will be found a very effective means of ridding the system of boils and carbuncles. A hot bath followed by a vigorous salt glow is a very successful measure for preventing the increase of boils or carbuncles. Cold baths are excellent to increase the circulation and build up the system. (See Cold Baths in Table of Contents.) The general health must be built up.

Oranges are practically a specific when a person is afflicted with boils and carbuncles. They assist in putting the system in shape so that the cause of boils and carbuncles is removed. Eat them freely, a dozen or more a day. Eat them alone or combined with grapefruit. Use also plenty of fresh vegetables, especially the leafy ones, as turnip greens, spinach, etc. Eat tomatoes, preferably fresh ones, or canned, without seasoning. It is better to make a meal of them than to combine with other foods.

Cancer

Causes.—Although cancer is increasing at an alarming rate, it can be prevented. Through chronic auto-intoxication, constipation, and the inactivity of all the organs of elimination—lungs, liver, kidneys, skin, and bowels—the system becomes poisoned, and the poisons accumulate around the weakest organs or where the body has been injured by a blow, fall, or bruise. The poisoning of the body has been caused by the use of improper foods; the use of tea, coffee, coca cola, meat, etc.; liquor of all kinds; and tobacco in all forms.

Among the improper foods are meats of all kinds, especially pork; cane sugar and cane-sugar products; white-flour products; white rice; and all denatured foods, which cause waste matter in the system. Cancer would be rare if no devitalized foods and meats are eaten. The life-giving properties and minerals are removed from much of the food which is eaten. The life-giving properties keep the blood stream pure, and cancer will not develop where there is a pure blood stream.

SYMPTOMS: Skin cancers often begin on the face, close to the nose, sometimes in the middle of the cheek, behind the ear, or below the ear, and maybe on other parts of the face or neck. The skin becomes rough and develops into an open sore, which gets worse and worse. Lip cancer is caused usually from smoking a pipe, cigars, cigarettes, or from tea drinking. Sometimes cancer comes inside the mouth.

Many cancers start in the stomach. The victim thinks it is merely indigestion. As it progresses, there is experienced sharp, cutting pains. After eating there is great pain and nausea, followed by vomiting. Often a brown, colored matter is vomited up. Constipation, sleeplessness, and a feverish condition are usual. There is a general wasting away, and finally death. Frequently the cancer is in the rectum, causing great distress at the stool. Sometimes the liver is cancerous, causing pain in that region and general debility. Cancer of the female organs is very prevalent, manifesting itself in the form of a fibrous tumor, sometimes as a tumor on the side of the uterus, as a sore on the mouth of the uterus, or as a cyst in the ovaries. Frequently cancer begins in the bowels, or it may appear in any part of the body. Cancer of the breast is very common, and there is often cancer of the female organs when there is cancer of the breast. There are other causes and manifestations of cancer.

Treatment.—The first step is to cleanse the blood stream by thoroughly relieving constipation and making all the organs of elimination active—skin, lungs, liver, kidneys, and bowels —and keeping them active. For constipation, take Herbal Laxative, as given in this book. It is very good. Use high enemas to cleanse and cure the colon of any bad condition there. It is necessary to take a fruit diet of oranges, grape-fruit, lemons, apples, cranberries, unsweetened blueberries, red raspberries, cherries, peaches, pears, ripe strawberries, avocados, pineapples, and tomatoes. All fruit should be well ripened on the tree or vine to be fully beneficial.

Tomatoes should be eaten by themselves—not with other foods. Make a meal of them. For the first ten days (or a longer or shorter period, depending upon the condition of the patient) it is advisable to take nothing but unsweetened fruit juices, preferably orange, grapefruit, pineapple, lemon, or grape. Do not mix the juices, but take different ones at different times.

Vegetable juices are very useful also—celery, cucum-bers, parsley, lettuce, and carrot. Carrot juice is especially valuable in cancer trouble.

Drink six glasses of fruit juices a day and six glasses of herbs a day. If you can take more, so much the better. If the herbs are taken in capsules, take No. 00 size capsules for a dose (Fill capsules full.), followed by a glass of hot water, as hot as can be taken readily. Take the herbs one hour before taking any fruit juice.

If the patient is thin, after a few days of fruit diet give an alkaline, nourishing diet—vegetable broth (recipe for which is given in this book); mashed potatoes, prepared as described in this book; natural, brown rice, soy-bean cheese; carrots; greens of all kinds; red cabbage (especially valu-able); the green leaves of cabbage; parsley; eggplant (es-pecially valuable); okra; tender corn on the cob, or canned; tender peas, fresh or canned; naturally cured ripe olives;

celery; green lima beans; onions; garlic; cauliflower; baked Irish potatoes; lentils; cucumbers; garden-grown lettuce; radishes; watercress; spinach; squash; kale; asparagus; young beets; dandelion greens; endive; collards; Swiss chard; Chinese cabbage; soybeans, sprouted; wheat, sprouted; salsify; wild rice; yellow corn meal; watermelon; and tomatoes. Watermelon should be eaten alone, and not with any other foods. Likewise, tomatoes should be eaten alone. Make a separate meal of them. Tomatoes are high in vitamin content. Use fresh ripe tomatoes or the best canned ones, but fresh, vine-ripened tomatoes are better. Eaten with whole wheat zwieback, they make an excellent meal. Never cook food in aluminum cooking utensils. Never eat fruit and vegetables at the same meal, nor drink fruit and vegetable juices at the same time.

Get plenty of fresh air and exercise—outdoors in the sunshine, if possible—to cleanse the lungs and increase the circulation. If the patient is unable to be outdoors, he must be in a sunshiny room, well ventilated at all times. He should take deep breathing exercises and all the exercise he can stand in the house.

Give frequent sweat baths to keep the skin active, followed by good salt glows, so that the skin will eliminate the poisons. Keep the head cool by placing a cold towel wrung out of very cold water around the neck, changing often to keep it cold. While giving sweat baths, put an ice bag over the heart if the patient has any heart trouble. If the patient is strong enough, give a cold towel rub every morning. This increases the circulation. Apply alternating hot and cold applications to the liver, stomach, spleen, and spine. (See Poultices in the Table of Contents for cancer poultices.)

Thorough massage is very necessary in the treatment of cancer to assist in eliminating the poisons from the body.

When I was a child, I gathered red clover blossoms for the postmaster in our town, who used them to make a tea for cancer. I do not remember the particulars of his case, but I do remember he lived to be an old man. Use plenty of red clover bossom tea. Drink it instead of water. The tea may be prepared by using a handful of dried blossoms to a quart of cold water. Let it come to a boil, and simmer for fifteen minutes. Let it sit covered up until cool enough to drink; then strain, and drink as many glasses a day as you possibly can. Look under the list of herbs given in this book for herbs suitable for use in treating cancer.

One of the greatest aims of this book is prevention of disease. One of the great causes of cancer is the food we eat. Statistics show that many of the cancers today are of the stomach, caused directly by the improper foods and improper eating habits. A faulty diet irritates the stomach, and develops an ulcer, which, if not cured, develops into cancer without the victim ever realizing what is taking place until the cancer has developed.

There are foods in which cancer germs cannot develop— food that is very nourishing and palatable—and there are non-poisonous herbs that will heal cancerous sores, inside and outside of the body.

Violet leaves (or you may use the whole plant) have been known to cure cancer when the diet and other habits were corrected. Make a tea of the leaves by using one-half ounce of leaves to a pint of boiling water. Steep one-half hour, and drink a cupful every two hours. Dip a piece of cloth into some of this tea and apply warm over the affected part. Leave on until dry. A poultice is made of fresh violet leaves, chopped and steeped in boiling water for thirty minutes, adding some linseed meal to make the poultice. As an enema, use one-half ounce to the pint of water. Inject night and morning.

Agrimony and ground ivy are also excellent. They will dry up and heal cancers.

Herbs for Cancer.—Red clover blossoms, burdock root,

yellow dock root, blue violet (the whole plant), golden seal root, gum myrrh, echinacea, aloes, blue flag, gravel root, bloodroot, dandelion root, African cayenne, chickweed, rock rose, agrimony, and Oregon grape.

Experience in a Small Sanitarium

Some years ago much was said about the wonderful cures effected by operations and the use of electricity. Much expensive electrical apparatus was manufactured, and it was advertised extensively.

I, like thousands of others, thought there might be something to it; so I equipped a small sanitarium in the best location in a beautiful little town, near a lovely park. I furnished this sanitarium with bathrooms for both men and women, so that we could give Turkish, Russian, electric, and tub baths, showers, and sprays.

I had a fine, well-equipped operating room and an electrical room equipped with one of the best X-ray machines, static and high frequency current, galvanic and sinusoidal current, German and ultra-violet rays, sun-rays, and others. I had taken a medical electrial course in one of the best medical electrical colleges.

Then I hired by the year one of the best medical doctors that I could find. He had been graduated as a nurse before taking his medical course. After being graduated from his medical course he studied in Europe, taking several postgraduate courses. I hired graduate nurses from recognized institutions. Then I invited all the doctors in that city to bring their cases to this institution. They did so. I gave the anesthetics for several years for the different doctors, prepared the patients for the operations, and took care of them after the operation, assisted by my corps of workers.

Here, in my own institution, with a well-trained physician and graduate nurses, together with all the necessary equipment, I obtained much valuable experience.

Many years ago, before I attempted to treat cancer and

(457)

had taken it for granted that there was no cure, I made up my mind I would find out the cause of cancer; so I looked up the records to find out in which countries of the earth cancer was most prevalent. When I learned this, I looked to find out what food the peoples of these countries ate. I found that in the civilized nations of earth where a large amount of meat and rich and luxurious foods were consumed, cancer was more prevalent. In the uncivilized nations where they ate plain, natural foods, cancer was very rare. In some instances where cancer was rare, when the people there learned of the diet used by the civilized peoples and used it, cancer increased.

People used to think meat was the great cause of cancer, but in my research I found thta people who did not eat meat at all had cancer, and I also found that people who did not eat meat at all, with whom I was well acquainted with their habits of diet, had cancer. They were eating denatured food and bad combinations of foods of such a nature that these caused much waste matter to accumulate in the system, which caused the different organs to become diseased, and cancer many times resulted.

After learning this, I felt quite sure that I was on the right road to find out the cause of cancer, and since then I have known it. Denatured foods have been robbed of their minerals and vitamins, which are the life-giving properties, the very parts which God put in the different foods to keep the blood pure and to sustain the nervous system.

After deciding that the food people eat and the things they drink were primarily the cause of cancer, I started to search for a cure. While taking a course in one of the best dietetics schools, I learned the water cure, and took a medical electrical course. I also made a study of the body and foods and the effects of food uponthe various organs of the body. I recalled how, during my youth when in my parents home, I learned something of the value of herbs from my parents and from the Indians, who were numerous in those days in northern Wisconsin.

As stated before, I gathered herbs for my parents and the herb doctors, thus learning of the value of herbs which I have never forgotten. I very distinctly remember gathering red clover blossoms, witch hazel bark, white pine bark, white willow bark, white popular bark, bloodroot, mandrake root, hemlock bark, golden seal root, sarsaparilla, and many other herbs which grew all around us in abundance.

After learning the water cure and taking a course in medical electricity, I wanted to know more about herbs; so I took a medical herb course. Also, I have procured from different parts of the world the best books I could learn of and have subscribed for the best magazines dealing with the medicinal value of herbs.

By experience I learned how herbs will cure bad sores and ulcers. I determined to try them on cancer, and I have seen the most malignant cancer sores heal on various parts of the body externally. The herbs have the same healing qualities, too, when taken internally.

I have been asked many times what my cancer cure is. Here it is in a nutshell: correct food, herbs, water, fresh air, massage, sunshine, exercise, and rest.

If herbs are used that would heal the most malignant cancerous ulcer externally, and herbs used internally, that will kill the malignancy of internal cancers, then there must be an elimination of waste matter, to clean the entire system and blood stream, if you want the patient to live. Now, how is the waste matter to be eliminated, and the blood stream purified? First, the five eliminating organs must be made active, the lungs, skin, liver, kidneys, and bowels. Then there must be enough fluid taken into the body so that this waste material will be eliminated. This is done by the copious drinking of herb teas, fruit juices, vegetable juices, and pure water—also hot baths to open the pores, massage, rest, fresh air, and the remainder of the prescribed treatment.

Not long ago a woman came to me who had cancer involving the liver, lungs, and stomach. She lived only a few weeks after I saw her. A post-mortem was held, and we found that her liver was almost entirely gone. Parts of both lungs were hardened, and the throat and stomach had growths in them. She had not been able to retain anything in her stomach for some time. Portions of her intestines were very much shrunken. Upon inquiring into what had been her diet, we found that it had been white bread, jellies, jams, soda crackers, and denatured foods.

Many times I have removed hard swellings in the breast, bowels, rectum, and vagina with hot applications, massage, and herbs.

In different parts of the earth people are searching for cures for cancer and other so-called incurable diseases. The treatment for them is found in this book.

Cancer is a treacherous disease. When there is any suspicion of cancer, take a cleansing diet—fruit and vegetable juices, taken separately. Cancer cannot live in a system where all the mineral elements are present which God put there in the beginning.

If cancer is suspected, clean out the system, and get a new supply of pure blood. There are non-poisonous herbs that will purify the blood and kill malignant growths internally or externally, leaving no bad after effects. Cancer will not live in a system when the blood stream is pure.

While it may be all right to treat symptoms, the cause of a disease must be ascertained and removed before there can be a permanent cure. Practitioners, will you not try it?

Since I have been asked many times about my experiences with cancer cases, I will give a few.

Many years ago I was asked to go to see a man who was in a charity hospital. His trouble had not been pronounced cancer. In fact, he had no outward sign of cancer—just a little swelling on the under side of his jaw which was not painful, but he complained of pain in the region of the navel. There was no outside swelling on or near the navel, but a bunch could be felt there. Something gave way in this region which caused his death. A post-mortem was held, and it was found that the cancer had eaten through the bowels. It had not only spread through all the bowels, but had also affected all his organs. From the crown of his head to the soles of his feet the tissues of his body were full of cancerous growths.

Another man—quite fleshy—who had been sick for some time and whom I had nursed for nearly a year, died suddenly. The attending physician, who was a prominent surgeon, said to me, "We will have a post-mortem of this man." We found this man's bowels to be full of cancerous growths. His liver was very much enlarged and full of tumors, large and small. His heart was much enlarged, and upon opening it we found a large bunch of fat in each lobe. There were no growths in the stomach, but it was full of mucous and the walls were a very dark color. This man was a big eater of pie, ice cream, iced tea and coffee, white bread, peeled potatoes, denatured foods, coffee, tea, liquor, tobacco, and other harmful things. Many times when I talked to him about his eating and drinking, he would reply, "I am going to have what I want while I live."

Another man had a cancer on his cheek. It was in the form of a bunch about the size of a fist and was extremely painful. The cancer had eaten clear through the cheek, had spread on the inside of the cheek to his gums on both upper and lower jaws, and had started to eat his tongue. Pus ran out of his mouth, and he was kept alive by inserting a tube in the other side of his mouth, through which he took liquid nourishment. This sore was so painful that it could not be touched with a little cotton without excruciating pain. In about seven weeks I caused this cancer to heal so that he could sit at the table and eat with his family. The last I heard from him he was doing some work. To heal this cancer, I used some of the herbs which I have enumerated in this article.

Another case to which I was called was a woman who had trouble which had been pronounced cancer of the female organs and stomach. She had a doctor and a trained nurse. I asked the nurse to give her a high enema. She did not succeed very well, so I got a four quart enema can and then we succeeded in giving her the enema, which brought lots of corruption, hard balls, etc., showing that she had pockets in the colon. This treatment greatly relieved her. She had been treated with radium and X-ray over the lower bowels. Soon her bowels turned black. She could retain no food, was full of pus, and soon died.

Another woman, who had cancer of the breast, had had one breast removed and had been treated with radium and X-ray. She was burned from it so that the flesh came off her ribs and she could not eat or drink anything—even water. I did not try to do anything for her except to make her as comfortable as possible.

A man who had cancer of the rectum had his folks come for me. I injected some of the herbs given in this article, and the terrible pain stopped about the fourth day. In about seven days a lot of slush came from the rectum, including a big chunk which looked like a crab. In seven or eight weeks after I began to treat him, he said he felt as well as he ever did in his life, and began to do some light work.

A woman who also had cancer of the rectum, which was about the size of an egg, causing her constant pain, came to see me. When I had treated this woman five weeks, the tumor was gone and every symptom of it. Her health was very much improved generally. However, she continued taking the herbs and some of the treatment to be sure her blood stream was purified. I heard from this woman some years later, and her health was good.

Another woman had a painful, swollen breast, which she had removed. In a short time she developed a large tumor in her bowels. This also she had removed. Then she developed another tumor larger than the first one. When the surgeon operated in order to remove it, finding that the cancer had spread through the entire bowels, he simply closed up the incision without removing anything, stating that she could not live more than from three to ten days. She was taken home to die, and her nurse instructed to give her plenty of medicine to relieve her pains.

Her husband was advised to get in touch with me. He came for me and took me to see his wife. When I arrived at their home and saw her, I found that nothing would go through her bowels. She had a tube in one side of her colon, through which the waste matter came out. In the other side of her abdomen there was an opening through which the urine passed. There was another opening through which pus oozed all the time. She had to lie flat on her back and could retain nothing on her stomach—not even water.

Her husband and family wanted me to try to help her. I gave them no hope whatever, but I said I would try. It indeed took some courage to undertake to help one in that condition.

We did not give her any more hypodermics to quiet her, but tried to soothe her pains with fomentations, liniment, massage, etc. We gave her herbal enemas, which took out the slush and swelling from the colon until she had a natural bowel movement through the rectum. Then I removed the tube from her colon and healed the opening. I worked hard to heal the side where the urine passed, but this was harder to heal, as a little urine oozed away all the time. However, it finally healed. Just as soon as her side was healed, we gave her hot tub baths, so she would sweat freely.

At first she was so weak that it took four persons to put her in the tub and take her out again. There was improvement from the first day we put her in the bath. She perspired freely. We gave her a hot sweat bath every day until she got well, followed by a salt glow, cold towel rub, and a massage. She also had fomentations every day over the stomach, liver, spleen, spine, and over the entire abdomen, after which her abdomen and back were thoroughly saturated with the liniment (recipe for which is given in this book). Her abdomen was thoroughly massaged several times a day for quite a while to work out the poisons and cancerous growths.

This treatment was followed for about four months. In the meantime she went to Florida in a touring car, stayed there for a while, and came home on the bus. She stood the trip by bus fine, and went every day after returning home to visit some of her many friends. Soon she began to do her own housework and has done it ever since, besides raising beautiful flowers and helping materially to raise the family garden.

She took the herbs and diet as given in this article and she made many meals of fresh, vine-ripened tomatoes for some time. She also ate freely of leafy greens.

This was six years ago and she is the picture of health. My wife and I were invited to her home some time ago, and such a dinner which she had prepared! It was delicious, and all the dishes were healthful dishes. We enjoyed this dinner immensely for two reasons; seeing this woman enjoying life in the nice new home which her husband had built for her, and partaking with them of the fine dinner she herself had prepared.

Right here I must say that part of the credit for the recovery of this outstanding case I give to my wife and youngest daughter, Naomi, who were the faithful nurses on this case.

I write this for the benefit of others.

During the summer of 1933 I was taken seriously ill, and was taken to a large institution in the vicinity of Washington, D.C. They found that I had cancer of the breast, so they removed the entire breast. A little later it was discovered I had a large tumor in my abdomen. They then operated and removed it, and then another tumor developed in the bowels which was larger than the first one, so much so that it completely shut off any movement from passing through the bowels to the rectum. They then made an opening in the colon and put a tube in to eliminate the waste matter. My suffering was so intense that they kept me under heavy opiates all the time. I was failing fast and they told me there was no chance for any recovery. I was taken home in an ambulance, and my family was told I could not live more than three to ten days. My husband purchased a burial plot, and about that time we learned of a man by the name of Jethro Kloss, that could cure Cancer, so we looked him up, and my husband brought him to our house. He made no promises as the case was very hopeless, nothing would go through my bowels, could keep nothing on my stomach, and was paralyzed with opiates. But he said that he would try to help me, but would not make any promises.

He treated me with natural remedies, herbs, proper diet, water treatments, massage, sunshine, fresh air, and rest. I was treated by him for four months, when I made a trip to Florida with Mr. Kloss in an auto and stayed there under his care for one month. I then left Miami, and went to visit relatives elsewhere in Florida, returning home to Washington from there by bus. This was five years ago and I am a well woman today, doing my own housework, working in my garden, etc.

I write this so that others suffering from the dread disease of cancer may know that there is help for them.

Mrs. John Rhine

Another case was that of a woman who had large breasts. One was very much enlarged and inflamed, and there were sharp, cutting pains shooting in all directions and into her arm. She had been advised to have her breast removed at once, as that seemed to be the only help.

She came to see me in that condition, and in about three days I had the excruciating pains allayed. However, I continued the treatment for about four weeks. I instructed her what to do, and she took the herbs for some time. About three years later I saw her, and she said she never felt any further trouble in her breast and that her health was good.

To allay the inflammation in the breast, I applied hot and cold applications alternately twice a day, and thoroughly saturated the breast with the liniment (given in this book). As soon as the inflammation was all gone, we thoroughly massaged the breast twice a day and gave her heavy sweat baths in the bath tub daily, followed by salt glows and cold towel rubs to assist in cleansing her system and build up her general health. She took the diet and herbs as given in this article.

Now I feel sure that a good many who read this are going to come to me for help, and right here I want to say that I am not practicing, nor do I want any practice. The only way I can help anyone is through their family physician or some other practitioner.

My ambition is to give my findings to the practitioners so the people may receive the benefit of them. I have written the American Medical Association in Chicago, Illinois, and they have asked me to come to Chicago and give it to their clinic. I wrote the following letter to the National Cancer Research Institute in Washington, D.C.:

WASHINGTON, D.C., 712 18th St., N.W.
March 27, 1939

DOCTORS OF THE NATIONAL CANCER RESEARCH INSTITUTE
WASHINGTON, D.C.
DEAR GENTLEMEN:

Knowing that you are vitally interested in the work to which our government has called you and in which it has shown a deep interest by the large appropriation it has allowed, and realizing that the people generally are looking and watching for the National Cancer Research Institute to accomplish great things for the benefit of the many, many rapidly increasing sufferers from cancer, I am constrained to write you and tell you that I absolutely have a cancer cure that will cure any cancer which has not gone too far.

I know the cause, prevention, and cure of cancer, also of heart diseases, pneumonia, asthma, infantile paralysis, gonorrhea, syphilis, and tuberculosis. I use no poisonous drugs, What I use would harm no one, no matter what his trouble, but would benefit him. I have spent a great deal of money, much labor, and deep research in finding out these things.

I am getting along in years and do not myself want any practice. I wish to give what I have discovered to practitioners who have a license to practice. This is what I would like to do for the benefit of the Cancer Research Institute that the people of the world may have the benefit of what I have found to be a real cure.

Will you permit one or more of your research doctors who know of a cancer patient who has not been treated by radium or X-ray to let me treat this patient under their special observation by the methods which I have found successful? Thus they will see everything done for this patient and will know that a cure really can be effected by the means which I use. You may provide the patient and the patient may be kept anywhere where there are the necessary facilities for treatment.

Not a few prominent citizens of this city who know of my work are urging that I write you thus. They feel sure that you will be pleased to give me this opportunity, for we all know that the government has appointed you to make every effort to find a remedy for cancer. I feel condemned that I have not done more to make public my findings. I must make them public and I would like to do it through you.

If the above terms do not meet with your approval, please advise me.

Most respectfully yours,

JETHRO KLOSS

The Cancer Research Institute doctor who answered my letter said they were not in position to accept my offer, but they suggested that I go to some hospital which takes cancer patients or to some regular practitioner.

They asked me to write out my treatment. To do this means a great deal. Other physicians have asked me again and again to put my findings on paper, not only on cancer but on other diseases as well. One army surgeon asked if I were going to take all this knowledge with me into the grave. Because I am willing to help any physician or group of physicians in helping humanity, I am now presenting the treatments which I have found to be highly successful.

No animal experimentation is required. Nothing poisonous is used. What I use would benefit anyone.

I have been asked many times by physicians and others how I knew that certain cases were cancer. My reply was that I knew only what their physician said it was, and what the laboratory test showed.

In advanced cases of cancer and in other serious cases, it is necessary to have a nurse who is very thorough and persevering in her work and who understands the value of the treatment, diet, water, massage, herbs, sunshine, fresh air, exercise, and rest.

It is very hard to write out all my findings and practical experiences, but I trust I have said enough and made it plain enough so that somebody will be benefited by them.

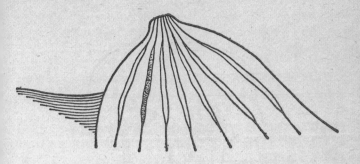

1. BEGINNING OF CANCER IN THE BREAST.

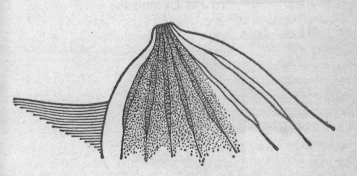

2. PROGRESSED CANCER IN THE BREAST.

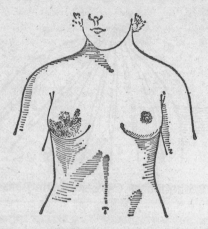

3. Cancer Further Progressed Until It Had Eaten
to the Outside.

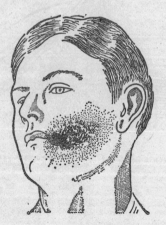

4. Smoker's Cancer. Showing how after it had eaten a
hole through the cheek, affecting both the upper and lower

In another patient the cancer had spread from the gums to the throat; it then progressed to the stomach. Pus was exuding freely on the outside and also from the throat. The patient was kept alive by pouring fluid into his throat through a tube. In seven weeks this man was able to sit with his family again, and to eat at the table. He was enabled to do this only by the use of natural remedies. The last I heard from him he was again able to do some light work.

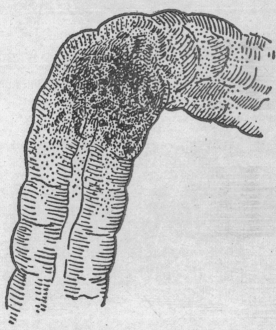

5. Fast Growing Cancer in the Colon.

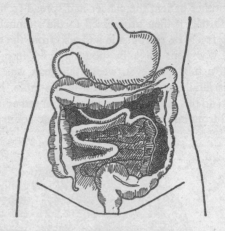

6. CANCER OF THE BOWELS. The small intestine has shrunk to the size of a pencil, with a hard growth on the outside an inch thick.

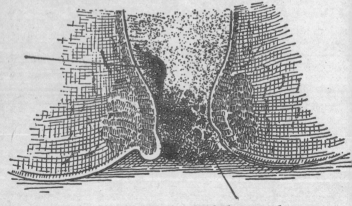

7. CANCER IN THE RECTUM. With the natural treatments I use, this patient was enabled to pass the cancerous growth, part of which was in crab-like form, the size of an egg.

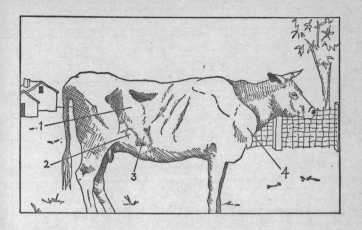

8. CANCEROUS COW IN ADVANCED STAGE. Lumps show cancerous swellings.

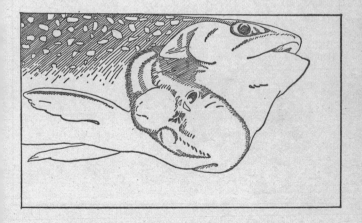

9. CANCEROUS FISH. Many fish are found with cancerous growths, the growth generally being under the gill.

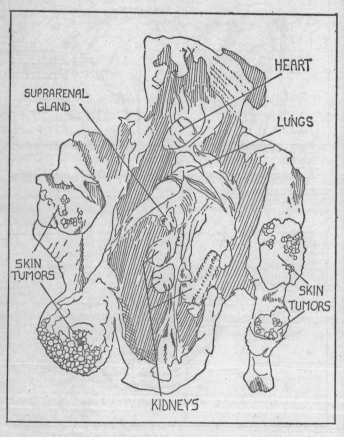

SUPRARENAL
GLAND

HEART

LUNGS

SKIN
TUMORS

SKIN
TUMORS

KIDNEYS

10. CANCEROUS GROWTHS IN VARIOUS PARTS OF A
DISSECTED CHICKEN.

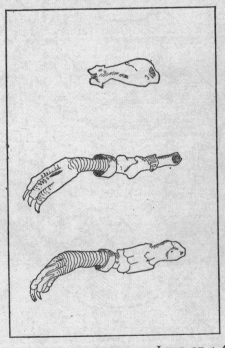

11. CANCEROUS GROWTHS ON THE LEGS OF A CHICKEN.

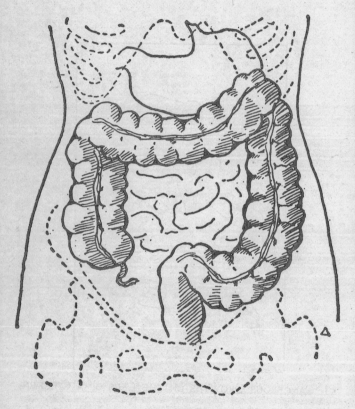

12. NORMAL COLON.

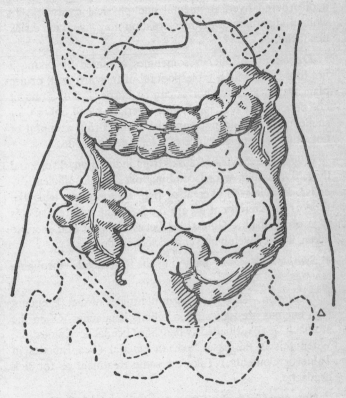

13. CANCEROUS COLON. A piece of this colon was taken
out of either side. The vagina was also cancerous, and the
rectum. The woman is living today and doing her own work.

Headaches

There are three specific kinds of headaches.

Sick Headache.—Is caused from a bad stomach when undigested food is lying in the stomach, or sometimes from a disordered liver, or mental and physical overwork. In women, disorders of the menstruation may give them a sick headache.

Treatment.—Relief is sometimes obtained by taking a hot foot bath, with a tablespoonful of mustard in it, or use plain water. Have as hot as can be borne. Drink a cup of hot peppermint tea, spearmint, valerian, black cohosh, or scullcap. If you do not have the herbs, drink a cupful of hot water, adding the juice of a lemon, take sour.

Bilious Headache.—Caused from indigestion, disordered liver, overeating, wrong combinations, and insufficient exercise. People who overeat of rich, heavy foods, and take little or no exercise at all are the frequent sufferers of this type of headache. Unless the diet is changed and exercise taken, it will develop into chronic headache.

Symptoms.—Dull pain in the forehead, throbbing temples.

Treatment.—Avoid all harmful articles of diet. Frequent high enemas are indicated in bilious headaches. Often the stomach is overloaded when the headache comes on. When this is the case, take an emetic. (See Emetics in Table of Contents.) Take the same treatment as for sick headache.

Nervous Headache.—Nervous people, and those whose work is sedentary, usually suffer from this form of headache. Mental strain and worry will cause nervous headache. Bright lights or noises of any kind usually make the headache worse. Lie down and rest where it is quiet with plenty of fresh air. Take a cupful or two of hot peppermint, catnip, red sage, or spearmint tea. Upon retiring take a cupful of hot hops tea, or if possible to retire when the headache comes on, take then; it will soothe the nerves and produce sleep. Red sage is one of the best herbs for headache.

Liniment (recipe for which is given in this book), when thoroughly applied to the forehead, temples, and back of the neck, will give prompt relief. If the headache continues, use an injection of catnip, blue cohosh or black cohosh tea. The injection should be retained as long as possible, using a pint or more. Use very warm.

Hiccough

Causes.—Irritation of the phrenic nerve, which causes contraction of the diaphragm. Excessive food or drink in the stomach.

Treatment.—A woman was once brought to me that was nearly dead with hiccough. I got an orange, cut it in half, gave her the juice of half, and the hiccoughs stopped immediately. The juice of an orange will usually stop hiccough. The eating of chalk that is used for writing on blackboards will often stop it. Sometimes a swallow of very hot water or very cold water will stop it. A bad case can be stopped sometimes by taking onion juice in teaspoonful doses. Another helpful thing is to make a tea of wild carrot seed, using a heaping teaspoonful to a cup of boiling water; let steep one half hour. Invariably a half cupful will stop hiccough. The blossoms are also good, used in the same way.

A poultice of one-half teaspoonful cayenne pepper to a pint of vinegar thickened with cornmeal, whole wheat flour, or linseed meal, applied to the diaphragm, is excellent.

One-fourth teaspoonful antispasmodic tincture taken in a half glass of water every fifteen minutes until relief is secured is also very good.

A tea made of blue cohosh, black cohosh, taken separately or mixed, equal parts, is good.

Hay Fever

Causes.—We hear all kinds of theories about the causes of hay fever, but the general belief is that it comes from the pollen of various plants and weeds. It usually occurs from June until October and depends somewhat upon the section of the country and the climate where one lives. I have known men to get hay fever every summer while making hay and loading it. Many believe the ragweed is at fault, and is the cause of this disease. This may all be true, as far as I know, but it is also true that it would be a rare thing for anyone to have hay fever who had good digestive organs and whose nose membrane was in a healthy condition. Wrong eating habits have much to do with it.

Symptoms.—Hay fever usually comes on suddenly, and at about the same time every year with many people. There is a tickling in the nose, sneezing, and irritation down into the bronchial tubes. The mucous membrane is swollen in the nose and mouth, and there is coughing. At times there may be distress in breathing, with smothered feelings, much the same as in asthma. The eyes are filled with tears, and the nose runs continually. These conditions exist as a rule until colder weather returns.

Treatment.—You may greatly relieve the irritation in the nose at once, by snuffing salt water up the nose. For this purpose, dissolve one heaping teaspoonful of salt in a pint of warm water. Gargle with this solution, and blow the nose entirely clear of mucus, before snuffing this up.

In addition to this, make a solution, using a rounding teaspoonful of golden seal and a heaping teaspoonful of borax in a pint of boiling soft water. Shake well. Let stand an hour or two, shaking occasionally; it is then ready for use. Pour some into the hand and snuff up the nose. Repeat this a number of times until the nose is entirely clean. This is very healing and soothing to the membrane and should be repeated four or more times a day.

I have had good success in treating hay fever with rag-weed and golden rod. Use one teaspoonful of each, and one teaspoon each of skunk cabbage, and calamus root. Mix thoroughly, and take a teaspoonful in a glass of warm water an hour before each meal and one upon retiring.

Put one tablespoonful of ephedra in one pint of boiling water. Let steep one-half hour, strain through a cloth, then snuff up the nostrils, drawing it through into the throat. Repeat this several times until relieved, using the same treatment three or four times a day. This treatment is also excellent for other nasal troubles.

Take one heaping teaspoonful of powdered bayberry bark and pour over it one pint of boiling water. Steep twenty minutes. Let settle and snuff up the nostrils four to six times a day. This is also good to take internally, one half glassful three or more times a day.

Hemorrhoids or Piles

Causes.—Wrong diet, overeating, intoxicating liquors, tobacco, spices of various kinds, white bread, sugar, fried foods, and all acid forming foods which cause fermentation. This wrong, devitalized diet causes constipation, clogs the liver, causes an impure blood stream, and irritates the stomach and intestines. Taking of ordinary purgatives that are on the market is also a cause, as they irritate the membranous lining of the bowels and intestines.

Symptoms.—Swollen tissue at mouth of the rectum or inside, also swollen blood vessels, swelling sometimes, so much that they burst, and are called bleeding piles. Sometimes on the outside little tumors are formed around the anus. Both internal and external piles are very painful. At times they are so swollen on the inside that when the stool passes they are pushed outside. Then some oil should be used and they should be pushed back inside. Often there is extreme itching.

Treatments.—First, take a high hot enema, temperature from 102° F. to 108° F. Use either white oak bark or bayberry bark, or white alum root tea. This will cleanse the entire length of the colon.

Make a strong tea of witch hazel bark, and one teaspoonful of catnip, one-half teaspoonful bloodroot, and one teaspoonful yellow dock root. If you do not have the other herbs, you may use just the witch hazel bark and catnip. Use a tablespoonful of witch hazel and a teaspoonful of catnip to a cup of boiling water, steep twenty minutes. If the trouble is external, dip a small piece of cotton in this tea and bathe the affected part. If they are internal, get a baby syringe, and inject two tablespoonfuls at a time, or you may use a glass syringe. You will find that this will give relief in a short time.

In taking the herb enemas, you will find that it is less painful and the piles will go back inside easier if you take the knee-chest position, as this causes the intestines to drop forward.

Another herb tea injection that is very effective is white oak bark, or alum root tea. Use a teaspoon of either to a cup of boiling water, steep twenty minutes, strain, bathe the affected parts, and inject a little. This will give relief.

This sometimes will cure them alone, if the enemas and diet are taken as recommended.

I have cured bad cases with kerosene alone. Apply to the affected parts either inside or out. If inside, inject a little. Kerosene gives instant relief. Lemon juice is also excellent used in the same way.

Take the following internally: Equal parts mullein, yarrow, wild alum root, and pilewort. Mix thoroughly, and use one teaspoonful to a pint of boiling water. Boil, then let steep one-half hour. Take half a cup three or four times a day.

For a suppository, the following is a very excellent remedy for healing.

> 2 oz. Powdered Hemlock Bark
> 1 oz. Golden Seal
> 1 oz. Powdered wheat flour
> 1 oz. Boric acid
> 1 oz. Bayberry bark

Mix with glycerine, stiff enough to form suppositories, inserting one into the rectum at night and leaving it.

Diet.—All heavy and stimulating food should be avoided. Tobacco, tea, coffee, vinegar, alcoholic drinks, and meats of all kind. The diet should be simple and light. Potassium broth is very excellent, as given in this book. (See Table of Contents.) Soybean milk, soybean zwieback, thoroughly ripe bananas, vegetable broths of any kind. To go on a fruit diet for a few days is a very helpful measure.

In all these treatments judgment must be exercised. There are perhaps other things that could be eaten, but a simple alkaline diet will hasten a speedy cure.

A hot sitz bath, as hot as can be borne, should be taken. Sit in this bath for fifteen minutes or longer until the body is thoroughly heated through. Have another tub containing cold water, and after being heated, sit in this for a second or two. Return to the hot water, and repeat. If you use a bathtub, have the water well over the hips. Place the other tub alongside the bathtub, tilting it by using a piece of wood or some solid article under one side. Continue this for one hour.

Hysteria

Causes.—Those who have hysterics are very nervous as a rule. There is a large list of causes, but to mention a few will suffice. Anxiety, sudden fear, indigestion, extreme nervousness, fit of rage, and menstruation in young girls. In some cases, it is simply perverseness and nothing else. The cause should, of course, be ascertained in order to deal with it successfully.

Symptoms.—An attack of hysterics never comes on when a person is asleep, as it is usually a desire for sympathy, or to frighten and disturb others, and it is always managed when others are around. The beginning is usually a sob or sigh, then there may be a twitching of the limbs, or perhaps violent convulsions, the person throwing himself about. After the attack, there is usually a free discharge of urine.

Treatment.—Always be firm with a person like this. They should not have excitement or sympathy, but be kind. Do not make fun of them after the attack, but take as little notice as possible.

Any one of the following herbs is useful: Black cohosh, blue cohosh, valerian, vervain, scullcap, or catnip. Use a heaping teaspoonful to a cup of boiling water, steep thirty minutes, and take a cupful four or five times a day. It is good to take a cupful hot upon retiring.

For quick relief take one-fourth teaspoonful antispasmodic tincture, every fifteen minutes. (See Table of Contents for Antispasmodic Tincture.)

Hemorrhages

Causes.—Wherever a blood vessel, artery, or vein, large or small, is severed or cut, hemorrhage or bleeding will start at once. It may be from the lungs, stomach, rectum, or any other part of the body. If an artery is cut, the blood spurts and flows fast, and will usually be bright red in color. If a vein, the blood will be dark and flow more constantly and slowly. When the wound is small, the blood usually coagulates and stops flowing.

Hemorrhage of the stomach.—Quiet and rest are required. Put an application of ice over the stomach for a short time, and have the patient swallow small bits of ice rapidly for a short time. Shepherd's purse made into a tea is very reliable in hemorrhage. One cupful has been known to stop a hemorrhage. Witch hazel leaves, wild alum root, bistort root, red raspberry, and sumach are also good. Make any one into a tea by steeping a teaspoonful in a cupful of boiling water thirty minutes, strain, and take.

Hemorrhage of the lungs.—Give a hot foot bath, and have patient refrain from coughing as much as possible. Hemlock spruce with a pinch of cayenne added has been known to stop bleeding from the lungs almost immediately. Also use same herbs as for stomach hemorrhage.

Hemorrhage from the uterus.—Have patient lie down, and elevate the foot of the bed. Give a hot douche made of bayberry bark or bistort root. Use either in powdered or granulated form. Steep one tablespoonful in a quart of boiling water for a few minutes. Use a spiral douche if possible; if not, use an ordinary douche tube.

Red raspberry leaves, white oak bark, witch hazel bark and leaves, wild alum root, are also good; make a tea from them. If used in the granulated form, use two tablespoonfuls to a quart of boiling water, steep twenty minutes, let settle, strain, and use as hot as possible.

Hemmorrhage of the bowels.—Keep the patient lying down. Inject warm wild alum root tea. White oak bark, or red raspberry tea may be used. Inject two or three ounces of the tea with a small syringe, and retain as long as possible. Repeat. Take internally, shepherd's purse, raspberry leaves, bistort root, witch hazel, bayberry or sumach. Use one or a mixture of two or three. Make and take according to directions for use of non-poisonous herbs.

Hemorrhage of the nose.—Make a tea of golden seal, using one teaspoonful to a pint of boiling water. Steep a few minutes, let settle, and when cold pour a little into the palm of the hand and snuff it up the nostrils. Sometimes cold or pressure applied to the back of the neck helps to prevent the free flow of blood to the head. Use the golden seal a number of times during the day. If this is done thoroughly, it would be rare for there to be a recurrence. Tea made from wild alum root, witch hazel leaves and white oak bark is also very useful to check nose bleed as these herbs are astringent.

Heart Trouble

There is a large list of heart troubles and various causes. The greatest cause of all heart trouble is a wrong diet, which causes impure blood and weakens the heart. Often palpitations of the heart are due to gas and fermentation in the stomach. Some years ago an elderly woman, who had complained for years of heart trouble, came to see me. I advised her to take a sweat bath, a thorough salt glow, with vigorous rubbing of the body, also cold morning baths, and to correct her diet. Before a week had passed that woman had forgotten all about her heart trouble. I knew this woman for years, and she never had a recurrence of the attack, as far as I know.

Not so long ago, shortly after a dinner that I attended, a woman complained of severe heart trouble. I told her that there was not anything wrong with her heart; she simply had gas on her stomach that was pressing against the heart. I told her to lie down on her face, roll on her left side, then the right, then drink a cup of hot water, and her heart trouble was gone.

Much of the so-called heart trouble is not organic, but the heart is weakened by impure blood, caused by a wrong diet, also lack of exercise, and poor circulation. Thus the blood that should be on the outside of the system is on the inside and consequently overburdens the digestive organs and heart. There is also real organic heart disease. I knew a middle-aged man who suffered from heart trouble for a number of years, and one day while reaching up for a drinking glass from a high shelf, dropped dead. His physician held a post-mortem. His liver was very much enlarged, and full of little tumors which were very hard and inactive. His gall bladder was much enlarged and also his heart. The spleen and pancreas were very large and flabby, also the kidneys. When the heart was opened there were large clots of fat in each corner of the heart, just as they are sometimes found in fat chickens. This man was a large eater, and lover of cakes and pies. I had warned him a year before this and told him what would happen if he would not give up his wrong diet and habits of eating, but he said he wanted something good to eat and he had it until he died.

Many heart troubles are caused by tea, coffee, tobacco, and alcoholic liquors. Sometimes heart trouble is caused by too much food made of white-flour products, and cane-sugar products. When so much food is eaten that has been robbed of its life-giving properties, and since the real health-giving properties that have been refined out of the foods are the properties that strengthen our bodies and heart, the heart gets weaker and weaker.

Most heart trouble can be overcome. My heart was so weak many years ago that in my weakened condition I could scarcely walk across the floor. I am now above seventy-six years of age, and only a short time ago I ran five miles, and then took a deep breath and sang, "Nearer My God to Thee," in a full voice. There was not the slightest sign of a flutter of the heart or palpitation. Those who witnessed this said it was too good to believe, when they felt my pulse and listened to my heart. I only mention this to show what right habits of living and correct food will do for a weakened body.

Diet in heart trouble.—See cleansing and nourishing diet in Table of Contents. This is very good in any kind of heart trouble.

Herbs.—There are a number of herbs that are a great help in any kind of heart trouble. Tansy is very good in palpitation of the heart. Make into a tea by using one heaping teaspoonful to a cup of boiling water, take three or four cups a day. Or it may be taken in half cup doses, an hour before meals, and upon retiring.

When the heart is irregular in its beating, or there is weakness of the heart, the following may be used with excellent results. Take one teaspoonful each of black cohosh, scullcap, valerian, lobelia, and a pinch of cayenne. Mix thoroughly, and use a heaping teaspoonful to a cup of boiling water. Steep one half hour. Drink four cups a day, one an hour before each meal, and one upon retiring, or you may take a swallow every two hours, or a half cupful as needed. This is very beneficial.

Look up the following herbs, read the description of each herb, and use the one that best suits your condition. Any one may be combined with others.

Lily of the valley is excellent in palpitation, and for quieting the heart. Angelica, blue cohosh, borage, cayenne, golden seal, wood betony, valerian, vervain.

In all severe heart troubles, call your physician.

Hair and Scalp

Any disease that impairs the vitality of the body has an effect upon the hair. When the circulation is diminished by a general nervous condition, the scalp cannot be properly nourished. Diseases of the scalp and loss of hair, are expressions of bodily ailments. A poisoned or impure blood stream, carries little or no nourishment to the hair. The color, luster, dryness, or oiliness, and brittle condition of the hair is all due to the condition of the system. The real treatment for diseases of the hair and scalp lies not in the many tonics that are used, but in the attention to the foods which are eaten, many of which cause diseases of the body, thereby affecting the hair and scalp. The blood which nourishes the hair must be purified by using wholesome, nourishing foods, which will build a healthy body.

Loss of hair may be caused by catarrh, nervous diseases, fevers, worry, mental disorders, skin diseases, excessive shampooing, injurious tonics, eczema and anesthetics. Curling and crimping with metal curlers and hot irons dry the hair and break it.

Since the analysis of the hair shows it to be composed of iron, oxygen, hydrogen, nitrogen, carbon, and sulphur, the blood must be supplied with these minerals so that nourishment will be carried to the scalp. Raw foods carry the highest percentage of minerals obtainable. Many of the best foods are prepared in such a way that most of the minerals are boiled and drained off.

Proper nourishment and good health will do more to make beautiful hair than any external treatment it is possible to give.

A thorough brushing of the hair every day keeps it free from lint and makes it silky and lustrous. To manipulate the scalp lightly with the tips of the fingers, always using a rotary movement, is good. It should be done very thoroughly.

The leaves and bark of the willow tree, made into a tea, will cure dandruff. A tea made of marshmallow leaves and thoroughly applied to the scalp will do much to prevent falling hair.

Anyone of the following herbs are useful to nourish and brighten the hair, and make it grow: nettle, pepper grass, sage, henna leaves, burdock. Steep a tablespoonful in a pint of boiling water for one half hour and add a level tablespoonful boric acid. Massage the scalp with this solution. May be used before shampoo, or between shampoos.

Hydrophobia

Causes.—Bites of rabid dogs, rats, wolves, and maybe other animals.

Symptoms.—The early symptoms are restlessness, melancholy, loss of sleep, and a sense of tightness about the throat. Soon difficulty in swallowing follows. Hydrophobia patients dread water. There is great thirst with an inability to swallow. The more violent symptoms now appear. They are convulsions, struggling for breath and strangling on the saliva. During the time between spasms the victims warn people around them of their danger, realizing their dreadful condition.

Treatment.—Obtain a physician at once if possible. Immediately after being bitten, tie a tight bandage above the wound, and apply warm water and vinegar. Let it dry, then apply a few drops of hydrochloric acid. This will neutralize and destroy the poison of the saliva from the dog's mouth. After this apply a poultice made of granulated slippery elm, with a teaspoonful each of powdered golden seal, myrrh, and lobelia added. (See poultices, how to make.) Make the poultice large enough to cover the entire wound, and change every four hours. A poultice of burdock is good for mad dog bites.

Take an emetic to cleanse the stomach and a high enema to cleanse the colon. After the enema, take an injection of lobelia tea, using one teaspoonful to a cup of boiling water, steep twenty minutes, strain, and use warm. Inject a half cupful at a time. Retain as long as possible.

· For an internal tonic take a compound of the following: one teaspoonful each of golden seal, gentian, myrrh, lobelia, and one-eighth teaspoon cayenne. Steep in one quart of water (boiling), for one half hour. Take a swallow every hour. It is better to take the herbs in compound as given, but in case you cannot get them all, use any one, two or three, you can obtain. I recommend this compound very highly. This treatment has been very successful in mad dog bite, snake bite, or insect bites, when the treatment was strictly followed.

If the patient becomes nauseated, or weakened, give the following herbs: scullcap, black cohosh, valerian, gentian, and angelica. Use equal parts, mix thoroughly together, adding a little cayenne. If you do not have all, use the ones you have. Take according to directions for use of non-poisonous herbs.

All poisonous insect bites and snake bites should be lanced. If this is not possible, they should be sucked by someone who does not have any sores of any nature in the mouth.

A tea made of plantain leaves is very effective and cleansing for a wash, or a poultice made of the plantain leaves is very good.

"DOG AND SNAKE BITES—HYDROPHOBIA"

"This terrible, always to be dreaded, affliction exists in both the human and animal species; it is produced by a specific virus, and is taken up by the absorbents, and carried through the medium of the saliva into the circulation, when, after a certain period, the wound becomes red and inflamed, accompanied by pain and spasms.

"They have always a dread of liquids, particularly of water, even the sight of it causing spasms.

"There is a frothy saliva ejected, and often a desire for biting anyone near them is manifested, and if not speedily attended to alarming convulsions are experienced. Most people know that hydrophobia is madness caused by the bite of a mad dog, or other rabid animal, while labouring under the disease.

"M. Buisson read an interesting paper on the subject before the French Academy of Arts and Sciences, as a discovery and remedy for hydrophobia, in which he gives the particulars of his own case. He was called to attend a woman who was suffering from hydrophobia, and some of the poisonous saliva coming in contact with an ulcerated sore on one of his fingers, he contracted the disease himself. He says: 'The ninth day after the accident I suddenly felt a pain in my throat and a still greater pain in my eyes. My body seemed to have become so light that I fancied I could leap an immense height; and the skin of my ulcerated hand became so acute in feeling that I thought I could have counted every hair on my head with it, without seeing. The saliva was constantly rising in my mouth, and not only the sight of shining objects but the very contact of the atmosphere became painful to me. I felt a desire to run about and bite every animate and inanimate object but my fellow creatures. In time I experienced a great difficulty of breathing, and the sight of water was more distressing to me than the pain in my throat. The effects returned at intervals of five minutes after each other, and it appeared to me that it originated in the diseased finger, and extended as high as the shoulder blade.' M. Buisson's account is thus concluded in a London Medical journal.

"Concluding from these various symptoms that he was suffering with hydrophobia, he resolved to make an end of himself by suffocating himself in a vapour bath. With this view he raised the heat to 140 degrees F. but was delighted, no less than surprised, to find that all his pains disappeared. He went out of the bath completely cured, ate a hearty dinner, and drank more freely than was usual with him.' He adds that he has treated more than fourscore persons who have been bitten by mad dogs in a similar manner, and they all recovered, with the exception of a child seven years old, who died in a vapour bath he was administering.

"Dr. Buisson mentions several other curious facts: 'An American had been bitten by a snake away from home. Wishing to die with his family, he ran all the way home, and going to bed perspired profusely, and the wound healed as a simple cut.' Mr. Hubbard of Illinois, in a letter, says:

'Eighteen years ago, my brother and myself were bitten by a mad dog; a sheep was also bitten at the same time; we were then ten or twelve years old. A friend suggested the following, which he said would cure the bite of a rattlesnake: Take the bark from the root of common ash, and boil it into a strong decoction, and of this drink freely. Whilst my father was preparing the above, the sheep spoken of began to be afflicted with hydrophobia; when it had become so fatigued from its distracted states as to be no longer able to stand, my father drenched it with a quantity of the ash bark tea, hoping to ascertain whether he could depend on it as a cure for his sons; four hours after the drenching had been given, to the astonishment of all, the animal got up and went quietly with the flock to graze.

" 'My brother and myself continued to take the medicine for eight or ten days, a teacupful three times a day. No effects of the dread poison were ever discovered on either of us. It has been used successfully in snake bites. To our knowledge the author has used the seeds or keys of ash for more than twenty years, and they are an old English remedy, but we have no hesitation in saying that the bark of the roots is much better.'

"A Saxon forester named Gastell, at the age of 82, unwilling to take to the grave with him a secret of so much importance, has made public in the *Leipsic Journal* the means which he used for fifty years, and he affirms he has rescued many human beings and cattle from the fearful death of hydrophobia. Wash the wound immediately with warm water and vinegar; let it dry, and then pour upon the wound a few drops of hydrochloric acid, and that will neutralize and destroy the poison of the saliva.

"*Treatment:*—These are remedies we also recommend; the vapour or hot water bath is an invaluable auxiliary in the treatment of hydrophobia. And give the following to all above ten years of age: half a teaspoonful tincture of lobelia, with a teaspoonful anti-spasmodic drops, while in the vapour bath, and repeat this every twenty minutes, till it operates. Then give an injection of lobelia, cayenne, scull-cap and rhubarb, half a teaspoonful each in a half pint of warm water, with a tablespoonful of tincture of gum myrrh added if the symptoms are violent. Repeat this every six hours. Wash the wound with acid tincture of lobelia, oil tincture, or tincture of gum myrrh; keep the part constantly wet with it. At night apply a poultice of bloodroot and lobelia powder, equal parts, mixed with yeast.' " Taken from *"The Model Botanic Guide to Health,"* pp. 189, 190, 191, 192.

Itch

Causes.—There are various kinds of itch, seven years itch, barber's itch, bricklayer's itch and others. The itch that went by the name of seven years itch for a great many years, is caused by a very small insect, called "itch mite." They bore beneath the skin where it is thin, or warm and moist, usually between the fingers, wrists, forearm etc. On the children they attack the feet and buttocks, the itching being greater at night when the body is warm. The irritation and scratching causes pimples and then scabs. The following treatment is good in case of chiggers or anything of that nature.

Treatment.—Before each application of the following, thoroughly wash the affected parts with tar soap. All clothing must be washed with boiling water, or boiled if possible. When they cannot be washed or boiled, press with a hot iron to destroy any insects which may be on them.

Take one tablespoonful of each of the following, burdock root, yellow dock root, and yarrow. Steep in a pint of boiling water a half hour. Strain through a cloth, put in a granite cooking pan (do not use aluminum), add one pound of cocoa fat, or crisco. Boil this slowly, stirring frequently, until it has boiled down to the consistency of salve. This is an excellent salve for itch or eczema of any kind. Healing lotion, as given in this book, is very useful in itch and eczema, it is healing and soothing. If you do not wish to make the salve, bathe the affected parts with the tea, as directed above.

Infantile Paralysis

Causes.—Is caused by poisonous toxins in the system, under-nourishment, and denatured foods.

Symptoms.—It may manifest itself in any part of the body, drawing the affected part out of shape, usually the limbs, shoulders, and back. The affected part becomes rigid and out of shape. Read my experiences in treating and curing cases of infantile paralysis on page fourteen.

Treatment.—See Cleansing and Nourishing diets. If the cleansing diet is used, followed by the nourishing diet, and proper water treatments given, the colon cleansed twice a day, and a similar course followed as given in my experiences, this dread disease can be cured.

The following herbs are used with excellent results. See their descriptions (See directions for use of non-poisonous herbs.): prickly ash berries, wild cherry bark, English or American valerian root, poplar bark, dandelion root, scullcap, golden seal, black cohosh, catnip, red clover, yellow dock. Select the one or several best suited to the case, mix equal parts.

For a small child, give the tea in tablespoonful doses, several times a day, sweetened with a little honey or malt sugar. Select the herbs best suited to the case. An excellent compound is made of the following: one tablespoon of each, valerian, catnip, and calamus root. Mix together, steep a teaspoonful in a cup of boiling water. Give one-fourth cupful every two hours. Considerable may be taken, as it is harmless.

Anti-spasmodic tincture given in doses of eight to fifteen drops in one-fourth glass of water (hot) is very good. Dose; according to age.

Inflammation of the Bladder

Causes.—Inflammation of the bladder occurs very frequently with people who have excess acid, caused by excess of starch and sugar. Those who suffer with gout and rheumatism often have this trouble, also those suffering from piles and extreme nervousness. One of the immediate causes may be exposure to cold after perspiring. It may also be caused by injury, blows or falls, as well as infectious diseases. One of the common causes among men is infection caused by venereal diseases. Another cause is the waste matter that is absorbed by the putrefaction in the colon.

Symptoms.—There is a burning pain in the region of the bladder, frequent urination, and a desire to pass urine when unable to do so, even when the bladder is empty. There may be slight fever, or even high fever, little or no appetite, great thirst, and a distressed countenance. The urine is cloudy, acid, contains mucus and sometimes red sediment. Pus and blood pass.

Treatment.—The very first thing to do is to take a high enema of catnip tea, as catnip is very soothing. Make the catnip into a tea, using a tablespoonful to a quart of water. Take the enema as hot as can be borne, 105° to 110°F. Then take some laxative herbs, equal parts of senna, buckthorn bark, spearmint, cubeb berries, and marshmallow being an excellent combination. After mixing these together, make the tea by using a teaspoonful to a cup of boiling water. Drink one to four cups per day, more or less, to suit your case, but keep the bowels loose.

A most effective remedy is to take one heaping teaspoonful of golden seal, one of cubeb berries, and one of marshmallow herb, mix them, and dissolve in a quart of boiling water. Steep for twenty minutes, stirring well. After it has settled, pour the tea off carefully, so that it will not have sediment in it. Use a soft rubber catheter and an enema can, put the herb tea, a little more than lukewarm, in the enema can, attach the catheter to the rubber tip of the enema tube, and insert the catheter. Permit the tea to flow into the bladder slowly, until there is a feeling of fulness. One or two ounces will usually give this feeling, but repeat until several ounces are used. Retain the liquid as long as possible. This process should be repeated two or three times a day and you will have good results. This should be done by a graduate nurse, or one who is competent to teach you. An injection of slippery elm water into the bladder in this way is excellent also, for it is soothing and healing.

Give thorough fomentations over the bladder and the whole length of the spine. A hot sitz-bath is very beneficial. (See Sitz Baths). In severe cases the sitz bath must be repeated two or three times a day until relief is obtained.

Diet.—The diet should be light and nourishing. (See Nourishing Diet). All irritating and stimulating foods are strictly forbidden. Avoid foods high in protein. Mashed potatoes, as given in this book, are very good, as they are unlike the ordinary mashed potatoes because of the addition of soybean milk, which is highly alkaline, and because the potatoes are not peeled before cooking. It must be the whole potato, for when you remove the peeling, the mineral salts are gone. Use Potassium Broth as given in this book.

It is very good. Also, soybean cottage cheese, soybean milk with zwieback, all leafy vegetables, carrots, okra, cauliflower, and eggplant are very good.

To go on a fruit diet is the best means of cleansing the system and getting rid of the uric acid, which is causing this trouble. Fruits are always good, as they are rich in alkaline salts and help to overcome acidity. Drink two or three quarts of water daily, so that the urine will be bland and non-irritating. This same treatment is excellent for any kind of bladder trouble.

Infant Feeding

The natural food for infants is mother's milk, which is by far the best. Unless the mother is in a weakened condition, or suffering from disease, she should nurse her child, and nine times out of ten would be able to do so, by using the right diet. Diet for nursing mothers is given in article on Pregnancy; see Table of Contents.

Regularity in infant feeding is essential. The child should not stay at the breast more than thirty minutes. All infants should be weaned by the end of the first year. Weaning should be gradual. Give a bottle once a day with the breast feeding, increasing the number of bottles each day until the child is entirely weaned. Mother's milk is much richer in iron than any supplementary feeding that can be given.

Cane sugar, in any form, should never be given to infants, under any circumstances. Many times cane sugar is the cause of fever and a number of other ailments. Malt sugar, malt honey, or honey, should always be used in place of cane sugar.

Diarrhea in infants can be checked by the use of thin rice, or barley water. For an older child, use oatmeal gruel. This should be given until the looseness is checked.

Soybean milk is a good food for infants and children, and can be given from the first day. In using soybean milk, you eliminate the danger of contaminated milk, and disease is not encountered. Note soybean milk analysis. See Table of Contents. Soybean milk can be improved by the addition of a little powdered oatmeal, powdered wheat malt, barley malt, or Avenex.

For infants, soybean milk should be diluted by using one-fourth water to three-fourths soybean milk. Discretion must be used in diluting soybean milk as in other infant's food, depending upon the needs of the infant. When the infant has a weak stomach, or is not strong constitutionally, dilute the milk more. The milk can be given full strength at the age of five or six months. When the baby is six months old, dilute four tablespoonfuls of whole wheat flakes in boiling water until completely dissolved, put through a fine sieve, and add to the baby's bottle. This will give added nourishment, in an excellent form. A smaller amount of wheat flakes may be added earlier with benefit.

Begin feeding wholesome simple foods in puree form, such as greens, vegetables, also fruit juices and gruels, when the first teeth appear. Orange juice and tomato juice, should be given from the beginning, starting with a half teaspoonful at about the age of one month.

When a child is given meats, white flour products, cane sugar products, candies, etc., they lose their taste and relish for wholesome natural foods. The eating of these detrimental things by children is responsible for night terrors, anemia, convulsions, rickets, scurvy, inflammation of the tonsils, and many other diseases.

Never allow children to eat between meals. Irregularities in eating ruin the digestive organs by keeping them overworked, causing indigestion and nervousness.

Insomnia

Causes.—One great cause is overeating, eating late at night, worry, fear of something that might happen, etc. Cold feet, poor circulation, nervousness, and poor ventilation are also causes. Constant loss of sleep, whatever the cause, is always injurious.

Treatment.—A full warm bath, or hot foot bath, taken with a cup of hot tea, as given below, will oftentimes bring sleep immediately. If the person is very tired, nervous and worn out, a fomentation given to the spine, liver and stomach will produce sleep, if the extremities are warm. Use a hot water bottle. People have been put to sleep by brushing their hair, and sometimes rubbing their feet, gently.

The following herbs are very effective in producing sleep: Lady's-slipper, valerian, catnip, scullcap and hops, especially hops. Use a teaspoonful of any one of the above, steep in a cup of boiling water twenty minutes, and drink hot. These herbs will not only produce sleep, but have many other good qualities: they tone up the stomach and nerves, never leave any bad after effects. Instead, they act as a tonic to the entire system. Aspirin, bromides, etc., taken for this purpose may seem to help for a time, but, as their effect is to deaden the nerves, every dose taken makes the condition decidedly worse and finally they lose their effect altogether.

If you do not have herbs on hand, hot lemonade (sour), or hot grapefruit juice is excellent. Hops and catnip may be purchased at nearly every drugstore.

Impure Blood (*How to Cleanse*)

Causes.—A wrong diet, constipation, overeating, eating a combination of food at the same meal which causes fermentation, devitalized foods. From many foods the very elements that would keep the blood pure are removed, as, for example, the heart and the outside of the wheat, the eyes and peelings of potatoes, the outside of rice, and the heart of corn, which is taken out of the meal. These are wonderful medicines, alkaline, and do a great deal toward keeping the blood pure.

One great cause of impure blood is improper breathing, improper ventilation, dark rooms, sleeping in rooms that are not properly ventilated, lack of exercise. Often the muscles are poisoned and feel tired because of the waste matter and insufficient exercise.

Drinking impure water and other harmful drinks as tea, coffee, liquor, all kinds of soft drinks, are other causes. These confuse the mind and cause wrong thoughts and ideas. The brain is made up of about ninety per cent water, and when we drink these unwholesome drinks, many of which are stimulating, the blood is made impure and the mind is very much affected.

Worry, fear, anger, unhappiness, and hate generally hinder the circulation of blood and thus the impurities are not carried off as they should be. The stagnated condition of the skin is one cause of impure blood. Many times the blood that should be on the outside of the body is in a congested form on the inside of the body, overloading the various organs, thereby causing congestion and various diseases.

Symptoms.—The symptoms cover a large list of diseases and complaints: Pimples, boils; discolorations of the skin; jaundice; headaches; drowsiness; wrinkles; old age when young; insanity; nervousness; getting angry at best friends; frowning when we ought to smile; thinking evil thoughts when we should think evil of no man; seeing darkness where there is light; gray hair; loss of hair; loss of eyesight; loss of hearing; stiff joints; pain in various parts of the body. All of these symptoms will vanish to a great extent when the blood stream is purified.

Treatment.—To make the blood stream pure, the first thing to do is to eliminate all harmful articles of food and drink, such as tea, coffee, all alcoholic drinks, soft drinks, all white-flour products, all cane-sugar products, and the liberal use of free fat or grease. The bowels must be kept active by proper diet and use of Herbal Laxative when needed. Take high herb enemas to clean out the colon and make it active and strong. Drink plenty of fresh, pure water; take plenty of outdoor exercise with deep-breathing; and get plenty of sleep in a well-ventilated room. Keep the skin active by cold morning baths and vigorous rubbing with a coarse, Turkish towel. Take hot baths at least two or three times a week. Wash the body thoroughly with some good soap, as Ivory. A thorough salt glow is good after a hot bath. This will stimulate the skin, make it active, and open the pores. A massage from head to foot is beneficial. Give it thoroughly on the neck and upper part of the spine and especially on the feet. Go on a fruit diet for one week. In the absence of abundance of fruit, eat vegetables, prepared as given in this book, as, for example, the green part of leafy vegetables, carrots—either raw, grated, or baked until tender—carrot juice, and potatoes.

Reader, if you want to see wonderful results, live on the food that God gave to man before he sinned. There is an abundance of it. Just live on fruit for a while, and follow the sanitary habits as mentioned above. Make use of the herbs which God let grow for the healing of the nations, and you will say with many whom the writer has heard say, "Truly the day of miracles has not passed." "The fruit of the tree is for man's meat, and the leaves for his medicine." (Ezekiel 47:12)

Influenza or La Grippe

Causes.—Exposure to cold and dampness when the system is not in good condition and is full of waste matter, and toxins.

Symptoms.—The first symptom, usually a distinct chill, or chilly feeling all the time, backache, head stopped up, no appetite, ringing in the ears, dizziness, incessant sneezing, sometimes sore throat, hoarseness and irritable cough. Coughing usually causes a splitting headache. Fever rises in the evening. Small children sink into a stupor. The real danger of influenza is, if it is not checked by proper treatment, complications may set in and the patient will have pneumonia. When not properly attended to, many times it causes other troubles which are difficult to overcome, such as, weakness of the heart and lungs, as influenza tears down the system greatly. After an attack, the system should be built up with good, nourishing foods.

Treatment.—When first taken influenza can be overcome in twenty-four hours. Stop eating. Take a high herb enema (see high enemas in Table of Contents.) Use either white oak bark, bayberry bark, wild alum root, or red raspberry leaf tea.

Use the following internally: one tablespoonful yarrow, one teaspoonful pleurisy root, a small pinch of cayenne. Steep in a pint of boiling water for twenty minutes, and take a cupful every hour.

Go to bed between cotton blankets. The blankets, and drinking of the tea will cause profuse perspiration; when the blanket become damp, change. If there is fever, bathe the entire body with tepid water thoroughly, have the towel very wet, exposing only part of the body at a time. Alternate the herbs with fruit juices, orange and grapefruit preferably. Lemon juice is excellent to reduce fever. Do not use sugar in any of the juices. Orange juice is very strengthening. If you follow the treatment outlined, being sure you thoroughly cleanse the colon, and follow with some laxative herbs, you will find your influenza practically gone the next day.

If the case has advanced, take the herbs given above and also orange juice and other fruit juices. Take sweat baths, also some tonic herbs, such as wild cherry bark, scullcap, valerian, lady's-slipper, feverfew. Plenty of fresh air in the patient's room is essential.

Dr. Zalabak gave me this formula many years ago, saying that it would cure a cold in twenty-four hours. Equal parts of cinnamon, sage, and bay leaves. Use a heaping teaspoonful of this mixture to a cup of boiling water, steep and drink freely.

A very effective remedy which works like a charm is the following: equal parts of the following herbs: agrimony, vervain, boneset, and culvers root. Use a heaping teaspoonful of this mixture to a cup of boiling water. Take a cupful every hour.

Herbs for influenza: Indian hemp, peppermint, white pine, poplar, butternut bark, lungwort, nettle, pleurisy root, saffron, sweet balm, tansy, ginger, golden seal, saw palmetto berries, wild cherry bark, wood betony, angelica, hyssop, boneset, vervain, culver's root, agrimony, scullcap, feverfew, lady's-slipper, and valerian. Use singly or in combination. Read their descriptions. Use those best suited to your condition.

Jaundice

Causes.—Obstruction of the bile. When the bile gets into the blood or circulation it causes the skin all over the body to become yellow, as well as the whites of the eyes. The bile does several important things: It neutralizes the gastric juice which would otherwise interfere with intestinal digestion; it alkalinizes the food and enables the system to take care of it; and it has a special effect on fatty foods. Deficient bile is a cause of constipation. Derangement of the stomach, liver and bowels is the cause of this ailment, and, of course, these troubles arise from errors in diet.

Symptoms.—Yellow skin, whites of eyes are yellow, bitter taste in mouth, constipation, urine is dark, slight fever, headache, and dizziness.

Treatment.—Give a high herb enema twice a day, as hot as can be borne. Use either white oak bark, bayberry bark, wild alum, root, or red raspberry leaves. (See high enemas in Table of Contents). Take one-fourth teaspoonful of golden seal in a glass of water one hour before meals, three times a day. At first, use nothing but fruit juices, especially lemon and grapefruit. These will help to alkalinize the system, and wash out the poisonous toxins. Potassium broth may then be given; it is very nourishing, and would keep the patient's strength up if nothing else were given, except the fruit juices. The patient should drink a glass of water with lemon juice in it every hour as long as there is fever, and continue drinking freely after the fever is down. During the acute stage it would allay the pain to give fomentations to the liver and stomach.

In infectious jaundice, there is usually itching of the skin. Washing with very hot boric acid water will allay this. Also see herb washes given under treatment for itch.

The following herbs are excellent for overcoming jaundice: Dandelion, agrimony, yarrow, and self-heal. Make the herb tea and take according to directions given for use of non-poisonous herbs. Self-heal and dandelion are especially beneficial. Self-heal alone is very good. Use the herbal laxative, as given in this book. The bowels must move three times a day.

Another good remedy is: Take a handful of peach pits, grind or crush them. Make a tea by putting them in two cups of water and let simmer slowly for thirty minutes. Take one-fourth cupful of this tea upon arising every morning, the same dose before each meal, and at bed time. If the pits cannot be secured, use a handful of the bruised leaves or twigs, with enough cold water to cover them. Simmer the twigs a little longer than you would the leaves. Take the same as directed for tea made from the pits.

Lemonade, unsweetened, may be beneficially taken in place of water. The same treatment as given for gallstones is good in jaundice, also.

Kidney Stones

Causes.—Wrong diet, acid-forming foods, white flour products, cane sugar products, meat, tea, coffee, condiments and spices, mustard, vinegar, etc. Excess of rich foods. Overeating is one of the main causes. By doing the forementioned things, the liver becomes overloaded and congested, and what it cannot take care of it passes on to the kidneys, and there is causes inflammation and gravel, and kidney stones. The kidneys pass as much as they can to the bladder, which will eventually result in inflammation or other troubles of the bladder, sometimes causing ulcers or tumors.

Symptoms.—Pains in the back, or below the waist line on either side of the spine. Dust sediment passes in the urine. Vomiting. Great desire to urinate, but efforts fail. If urination stops, a catheter must be used.

Treatment.—Give a large, high hot enema. Follow by a hot bath, starting with a temperature of one hundred degrees and increase to 112°F. Keep the head and neck cool with cold applications. If the patient becomes very weak, have him stand, and sponge off with cool water, getting immediately back into the hot water. This should be given for at least thirty minutes. Give the enema before the bath, using catnip tea if possible; it will give great relief. It soothes the kidneys and warms up the bladder. Use a tablespoonful catnip herb to every quart of water used. Use a four-quart enema for adults, children less proportionately to age. See high enemas in Table of Contents.

Hot fomentations applied across the back in the region of the kidneys will relieve the pain. A poultice made of hops, with a little lobelia added, and applied just below the waist line on the back, will relieve the pain. Give as hot as can be borne. Liniment, as given in this book (See Tables of Contents) if freely and thoroughly applied, rubbing in well, is excellent for relieving the pain.

Internally take a tea of the following: equal parts, wild carrot seeds, valerian, peppermint. Mix together and use a teaspoonful to a cup of boiling water, steep one half hour. Take one half cupful every hour until relieved. Queen of the meadow, peach leaves, or cleavers may also be used with good results.

In case of hemorrhage from the kidneys or bladder, use shepherd's purse. It will stop the hemorrhage immediately. Use a heaping teaspoonful to a cup of boiling water, steep thirty minutes, strain, and drink a half cupful five or six times a day, more if needed.

For tumors, or inflammation of the bladder use a teaspoonful of golden seal, one-half teaspoonful myrrh, one-half teaspoonful boric acid, in a pint of water, and inject with a soft catheter into the bladder. This should be done by a graduate nurse, or someone with experience. I do not recommend that anynone do this for themselves, unless they have been shown by a physician or graduate nurse how to do it.

Follow the same diet as given under gallstones. This same diet should be used in all kidney and bladder troubles.

Leprosy

Causes.—Leprosy is a very ancient disease, more common in the tropics and along the seashoes where people live largely upon fish and meats, using very few fruits and vegetables.

Symptoms.—The skin becomes spotted, and there is a breaking out which continues to grow and become ulcerated and decayed. Even the bones decay. Loss of feeling in the affected parts. The fingers and toes drop off from decomposition.

Treatment.—Fresh air, and a nourishing diet is absolutely essential. Fish and meats of all kinds strictly forbidden. Eat plenty of fresh fruits and vegetables.

Take a heaping teaspoonful of golden seal, one-half teaspoonful of myrrh. Steep in a pint of boiling water. Take one cupful of this solution, one half hour before each meal, and upon retiring.

An excellent herb composition in leprosy is: Take one heaping teaspoonful red clover blossoms, one teaspoonful yellow dock root, one teaspoonful calamus, one teaspoonful burdock, and one-half teaspoonful mandrake. Mix together, and use a heaping teaspoonful to a cup of boiling water, take four cups a day, one an hour before each meal, and one hot upon retiring.

The following herbs are also good; look up their descriptions and take those best suited to your case: Bittersweet, dandelion, and myrrh.

Lungs (Or Lung Fever)

Inflammation of the lungs, or lung fever is sometimes known as croup, pneumonia, or congestion of the lungs.

Causes.—Exposure to cold and dampness. If promptly treated at the first signs of cold or chilliness, it will prevent a severe attack, and prevent in all probability an attack at all.

Treatment.—Keep the nose and throat clean by snuffing salt water up the nose, and then blowing the nose, holding one side shut while blowing the other. Use one teaspoonful of salt to the pint of water. Do this several times a day. Gargle and rinse out the mouth with salt water. Take a rounded teaspoonful of golden seal, and one-fourth teaspoonful myrrh. Steep in a pint of boiling water and use in the same way as above. Be sure to gargle deeply and thoroughly with this, as it will clean all the germs and impurities out of the mouth and throat. If this is repeated often enough the cold or grippe will not go down into the lungs. Take internally, one tablespoonful of this same solution of golden seal and myrrh, six times a day.

If the lungs are not already seriously affected, take the above treatment, giving hot foot baths, and a high herb enema at least once a day to cleanse the colon. Take laxative herbs to clear the intestinal tract; the bowels must be kept loose. Drink quantites of water. Give the patient short, hot fomentations, with short cold applied between each hot fomentation, to the chest and back of the lungs.

Only liquids should be given the first few days. The best ones are, lemonade without sugar, grapefruit juice, orange juice, pineapple juice (unsweetened), and other fruit juices may be used. When there is high fever this diet should be followed until the fever abates. When it is advisable to administer more nourishment, give vegetable broths, but strain it. Soybean milk with whole wheat flakes or whole wheat zwieback are very good.

Herbs that are lung tonics: comfrey, cudweed, elecampane, hoarhound, ground ivy, ginger. A small amount of cayenne added to any of these herbs when making the tea is beneficial. Take as directed for use of non-poisonous herbs. See Table of Contents.

Any one of the following herbs may be taken. Look up the descriptions, and take the ones best suited to your case. Plantain, lungwort, pleurisy root, slippery elm, wild alum root, coltsfoot, mustard, vervain, flaxseed, hops, hyssop, white pine, spikenard, wahoo, mullein, yerba santa, yarrow, skunk cabbage, hoarhound, myrrh. Also see article on "Fevers" in Table of Contents.

Lumbago

This is a form of rheumatism and is usually brought on by becoming very warm and suddenly cooling off, or getting in a draft.

Symptoms.—Pain and tenderness in the muscles, sometimes affecting one and then another muscle. At times it comes on suddenly and feels as though there was a kink in the back. Adults are the most frequent victims, but children are sometimes attacked.

Treatment.—The bowels must be kept open. Use herbal laxative (see Table of Contents) when a laxative is needed. When having an attack, take high herb enemas. Those who suffer from lumbago should not use tea, coffee, liquors, tobacco, or any stimulating, or unwholesome foods.

Rubbing the affected parts thoroughly with herb liniment (see Table of Contents), after fomentations have been applied to the affected parts, will greatly relieve. Patient should be kept warm. Use same herbs as for Rheumatism.

The taking of alcohol into the system always produces unnatural conditions. Habitual users of alcohol often have ulcerated stomach, because alcohol injures the lining of the stomach.

The continual use of alcohol makes a total wreck of the person and often leads to insanity. The heart becomes weak and the blood vessels are affected. It hardens the arteries, sometimes causes hemorrhages in the brain or paralysis. It ruins the nervous system, and weakens the mental powers. It makes one coarse and unrefined. Alcohol is certainly a snake in the grass, it is stimulating to the senses, makes a person feel happy when he is miserable, makes him feel strong for a while, but weakness follows. Alcohol numbs the nerves to such an extent that a man feels warm when he is cold. It makes him quite active while he is under its hellish influence, but there is great collapse as the effects wear off. It surely mocks a man and makes a fool of him. The wisest man that ever lived said that "wine is a mocker."

While in Minnesota many years ago, the foreman of the red marble works, who was not a drinking man, had stomach trouble and the doctor prescribed brandy in tablespoonful doses, and in order to quiet his misery, he kept taking more and more, until he became a wreck, and was afflicted with what is known as the "snakes." It took two men to control him, for when he imagined he saw the snakes coming, he would try to get away from them and go through any door or window near at hand, using all the power that was in his body to get away. Often he looked for a gun to kill the snakes. Two men brought this man to me, when I had a sanitarium. The first thing I did was to put him in a warm bath. These two men placed him in the tub.

When he could not be kept in the bath tub any longer, we would put him under a shower. I went in the shower with him, keeping him under it as long as possible, using cold water. Then we had him drink all the quieting herbs we could make him drink, or force down him. An enema was given to clean out his bowels, and he slept for two hours the first night. When he woke up he said, "Oh! how good I feel." The men who brought him to me, told me that previous to the treatment he had absolutely not slept for three weeks or more. They said that he would doze off, then wake up all excited and try to get out of the way of the snakes.

The next day we went through quite a program. We gave him several warm baths, and he was made to stay in for quite long periods. He was given hot and cold fomentations to the spine, and over the stomach, liver, and spleen, as well as cold fomentations to the spine, and over the stomach, liver, spleen, and pancreas. He was given nourishing food, which was easy to digest. The second night he slept six hours. After this we went through a course of treatments again, and the third night he slept all night. In three days he got so that he could be left alone. In three weeks this man who was a wreck, physically very weak, went back and took his former position.

The happy part of it all was that this man who was separated from his family through drink, was restored to them, and there was great rejoicing. The beauty of it was that he quit drinking and could not be hired to touch it under any consideration. Many a family which was torn apart through the cursed alcohol, have been brought together again through the loving service and simple remedies God has given to man. We could cite many such cases but space does not permit.

To help anyone to get over the drink habit, he must be willing to quit. When he decides to give it up, it is very easy and simple to help him quit.

Treatment.—A fruit diet is very effective, and following, a light nourishing diet. Give daily high herb enemas to help the system get rid of the poison. Heavy sweat baths every day should be given and take some of the laxative herbs to keep the bowels real loose.

Give hot baths, with thorough rubbing while in the tub. This helps the waste matter to be eliminated from the system. A massage every day is very valuable. Have him take or give him a vigorous cold towel rub every morning upon rising, followed by brisk rubbing with a rough turkish towel.

To help destroy the taste for liquor, the following is very beneficial.

Quassia chips are very effective. Use one teaspoonful to a cup of boiling water, steep one half hour, covered. Take a swallow every two hours. In very bad cases, the patient should have a daily attendant, so he will not get more liquor.

Never taper off, QUIT and NEVER taste the stuff again. That is the way I did. I was a very heavy drinker, when I made up my mind one day that I would give this damnable stuff up which was ruining my health and my life, and I never tasted it again, and that was about forty years ago. I was also a heavy tobacco user, both chewing and smoking. That was also given up and I never tasted it again.

Menstruation

Tardy or suppressed.—When a young girl does not menstruate at the natural time, it is usually because the girl is undernourished, lacks fresh air, sunshine, and proper exercise. Improper food, constipation, and other wrong habits which make a child nervous are causes of tardy menstruation. When these causes are removed, the menses usually appear. The following herbs can be taken with confidence that there will not be any harmful after-effects. Select one, after looking up the description, and take according to directions in Table of Contents: tansy, black cohosh, wild yam, mugwort, camomile and gentian. Take a hot bath when retiring. It is very necessary that the bowels be kept loose. Hot sitz baths are very beneficial. The legs and feet must be clothed so as to be warm all the time. The same treatment applies to all women troubled with suppressed or scant menstruation.

Profuse.—The main cause is general debility. It is most common in women suffering with diseases of the kidneys and liver. A common cause with married women is marital excesses. If excessive menstruation is not checked it will lead to other diseases such as, leucorrhea, displacement of the womb, unpleasant symptoms in connection with urination. The legs and feet should be well clothed for warmth.

Treatment.—Eat plain, simple food. All stimulating foods, drinks, and narcotics are harmful. Keep the colon clean with high enemas, and keep the bowels loose. Keep off the feet as much as possible when menstruating. The body must be kept warm and well clothed. A warm douche of white oak bark, wild alum root, or bayberry bark is very helpful. This of course, is taken after the menses have ceased. Use a heaping tablespoonful of one of the herbs to a quart of boiling water, steep covered, and use four or five times a day if needed, using a bulb syringe. Also take bayberry, white oak bark, or wild alum root internally.

(515)

If the menses are extremely profuse, make small balls or tampons of absorbent cotton, immerse them in a tea made of wild alum root and white oak bark, equal parts, with a little lobelia added. Tie a strong cord around the middle of the cotton ball, leaving it long enough so that the ends remain outside. The balls should be large enough to be pressed in the vagina against the womb. Remove them every twelve hours, and wash the womb out with a herb douche.

Painful menstruation.—Constipation is the one common cause of painful menstruation. Relieve the bowels and colon with high enemas. Keep the body warm at all times, using a hot water bottle at night, if necessary. Keep off the feet as much as possible, especially the first day. A douche made as follows will give relief: one tablespoonful lady's-slipper, one-half teaspoonful lobelia, steeped in one quart of water. Use warm. For internal use, make a tea, using equal parts of black cohosh, penneyroyal, and bayberry, adding a little lobelia. If you do not have all these herbs use what you have. A hot sitz bath or hot fomentations to the spine and abdomen often afford relief at once. Fomentations will always relieve the pain. Give as long as necessary and repeat.

When the period first comes on, keep off your feet as much as possible. During the entire time of menstruation keep your limbs and feet warm. In the winter never have wet or cold feet. Keep them warm at night by the use of a hot water bottle or soapstone. Keep the hands out of cold water, if possible.

Mumps

This is a child's disease, although adults sometimes have it.

Symptoms.—Chilliness. Sometimes fever. Loss of appetite, headache, jaws swell, swallowing is painful and difficult.

Treatment.—Give the child a light, nourishing diet, such as fruit juices, potassium broth, soybean milk, and zwieback.

If constipated, give to enemas of catnip tea every day, if catnip is not available, use Ivory soap in the water. The bowels should move at least three times a day.

If there is fever, give a hot bath, twice a day, leaving them in the tub about twenty minutes. If the fever is too high, sponge them off thoroughly with a real wet towel, wrung out of tepid water.

Liniment as given in this book is most excellent to lessen the pain of the affected part. Apply freely.

A poultice of the following will give relief: Use a small handful of mullein, add one tablespoonful lobelia. Mix together, and pour enough boiling water on them to make a poultice. A little flaxseed meal, or cornmeal may be mixed with these to make them stick together. Apply hot between pieces of gauze, and cover with a woolen cloth to keep it warm, remove when it cools, and replace.

Internally.—Take equal parts ginger and scullcap, mix, steep a small teaspoonful in one cup boiling water. Have the child take a swallow of this every hour. You may sweeten it with a little honey or malt sugar.

Measles

Causes.—Few children escape having measles in childhood. Adults sometimes have them. Measles are caused by unhygienic living and are a contagious disease. Measles are merely the system's attempt to cleanse itself of impurities and purify the blood.

Symptoms.—Loss of appetite, complaint of feeling cold. In a day or two the nose runs, sneezing, the sick one has a slight cough, and about the fourth day starts breaking out. The breaking out, which is red in color, usually begins on the forehead, then all over the face, chest, and back. Fever increases with the eruption. When it begins to scale the fever abates. Mothers should guard the patient against earache, sore eyes, and bronchial troubles.

Treatment.—Give the patient a warm catnip enema. Put him to bed, and immediately give a tea, made as follows: one teaspoonful of pleurisy root, one-fourth teaspoon ginger, steep in a pint of boiling water. You may sweeten the tea a little for children; if you do, use honey or malt sugar. For a nervous person add a teaspoon of lady's-slipper or catnip to the above. Two tablespoonfuls of the tea should be given every hour, more or less according to age. Catnip or peppermint tea used separate is excellent.

The patient must be kept in a room of even temperature, but with good ventilation. Keep the room dark so that the eyes will not become irritated. Drink plenty of water and give hot foot baths.

If the patient is slow in breaking out, give a good hot bath.

In the event the patient's eyes become sore, make a solution of one-fourth teaspoon golden seal, steeped in a pint of boiling water (soft or distilled), for thirty minutes, then add enough boric acid to make a saturate solution. Strain through a cloth and bathe the eyes, two or three times a day or oftener. The same diet as is given for fevers, is excellent after the fever has broken.

A simple, nourishing diet is essential, such as soybean milk with wheat flakes and whole wheat crackers. If cow's milk is used, in the absence of soybean milk, boil a little oatmeal in it, or use half cow's milk and half oatmeal and barley water. Look under oatmeal and barley water, in Table of Contents. Very ripe bananas with soybean milk and whole wheat toast are good. Potassium broth, as given in this book, is nourishing, cleansing and tasty, and would be fine. Ripe fruits of all kinds may be used.

Given any of the following herbs: catnip, peppermint, camomile, vervain, yarrow, or lady's-slipper. Steep a teaspoonful in a cup of boiling water, covered. Give one-fourth cupful every two hours.

Nervousness

Causes.—A large variety of circumstances and conditions cause nervousness. The stomach and nervous system are very closely connected. Many times a woman is extremely nervous because of overwork, worry, care of children, improper food, lack of sleep, and in many instances it is true that a woman's work is never done. Many time the husband finds fault and makes unpleasant remarks, which make her more nervous, and which would be unnecessary if he would understand the situation and lend a helping hand.

Waste matter in the system gets into the blood and comes into contact with the nervous system, and especially affects the nerves of the brain, causing irritability, headaches, etc. We must never forget that the food in the stomach affects all the nervous system, because what we eat and drink is what feeds and nourishes the nerves.

Novel reading and dissipating habits, sedentary habits, and lack of exercise and fresh air, are causes, as well as constipation.

Treatment.—Hot and cold fomentations to the spine, stomach, liver and spleen, are very beneficial to nervous people. A prolonged warm bath of an hour's duration or longer if agreeable, finishing with a cool bath or spray, and vigorous rubbing, is excellent. Gentle massages after

(519)

baths or any time when possible to have them will help greatly.

A nervous person must always get the system cleaned out. Use high enemas, and herb laxative. The bowels must move three times a day for good health. Plenty of rest in a well-ventilated room is essential. Scullcap is one of the best herbs for nerves. Red sage is excellent for nervous headaches. Take a cup of the tea, strong, as often as necessary.

The following list of herbs are excellent for strengthening the nerves, or for any nervous disorder: Horehound, lady's-slipper, motherwort, mugwort, marshmallow, poplar bark, catnip, spearmint, camomile, ginger, peach leaves, vervain, blue and black cohosh. Make and take according to directions for use of herbs.

Night Sweats

Anyone suffering from night sweat will be greatly benefited by taking a hot salt water sponge before retiring. Use two tablespoonfuls of salt to a quart of water, or a hot bath followed by a salt glow is good. Wild alum root, or white oak bark tea is excellent used in the same way. Use a tablespoonful of the herb to a quarter of boiling water, steep twenty minutes.

Make a tea of golden seal, one teaspoonful steeped in a pint of boiling water, drink two cups upon retiring. This will do much to prevent night sweats. Sage, coral, or strawberry leaves may be used in the same way with good effect. The bowels must be kept loose and the colon clean; use herbal laxative, and herb enemas.

Nightmare

Anyone who eats a heavy evening meal, or midnight supper, is susceptible to nightmares. They are caused from overloaded stomachs and sleeping on the back. Anyone who is apt to have a nightmare should sleep on the right side or stomach.

Children troubled with bad dreams, sometimes termed night terrors, are usually constipated, or have stomach trouble in some form. Relieve their constipation with catnip enemas, and give them catnip to drink. Give them proper diet, keep their bowels loose, and they will not have them.

Neuralgia

Causes.—Neuralgia is a form of nerve irritation. Decayed teeth are sometimes the cause. Exposure to dampness and cold, eye strain, diseases of the nose are also causes.

Symptoms.—One side of the face is usually affected. Pain in the temples and neck.

Treatment.—Give a high herb enema of catnip. Have it as hot as can be borne. Prolonged hot and cold compresses to the side affected are very effective. The cold must be very short. The bowels must be kept loose and any stomach or liver trouble corrected.

A hot fomentation wrung out of tea made of mullein and lobelia, applied to the affected parts will do much to relieve the pain. Liniment as given in this book, applied freely, and rubbed in thoroughly will relieve the pain in a short time.

Placing the opposite hand and arm in very hot water for twenty minute will frequently give relief.

Look up the description of the following herbs, and choose those best suited to your case. (Make and take according to directions given for the use of non-poisonous herbs.) Valerian, origanum, scullcap, queen of the meadow, nettle, poplar bark, peppermint, Solomon's seal, hops, lady's-slipper, twin leaf, motherswort, and wood betony.

Nosebleed

Causes.—Injury to nose, excessive heat, occasionally high altitude, acute congestion in the head.

Treatment.—Application of very cold water or ice above the nose and on the back of the neck will sometimes stop the bleeding. Pressure on the back of the neck hinders the free flow of blood to the head.

Take a heaping teaspoon of golden seal, steep in a pint of soft or distilled water, which is boiling, add enough boric acid to make a saturate solution, put in all the boric acid the water will dissolve; if some is left undissolved in the bottom of the bottle, there is no harm. Shake it thoroughly and let stand until it settles, and it is ready for use. After this solution is cold, snuff some up the nose; do this several times a day, or often, until the bleeding stops.

Wild alum root, white oak bark, or bayberry bark is very good. Use one heaping teaspoon to the cup of boiling water, steep thirty minutes, strain or let settle, then snuff up the nose. Gargle with it also, as no harm is done if you swallow some.

The above things are all good remedies for nosebleed, also adenoids, colds in the head, and sinus trouble.

Another most effective herb for running nose or nosebleed is Ephedra Valgaris. Use one heaping teaspoonful to a cup of boiling water, steep thirty minutes, let settle or strain all the sediment out, snuff up the nose, repeat until relief is obtained.

In all the above solutions use the best water obtainable, preferably soft or distilled.

Nausea and Vomiting

If the nausea is because of undigested food in the stomach, or fermentation, take an emetic and clean the stomach out. (See Emetics).

A cup of hot peppermint or spearmint tea, taken after the stomach is clean, will strength and settle it.

A hot fomentation applied over the stomach or a hot water bottle with a moist towel under it will often prove beneficial.

The following herbs are excellent for nausea and vomiting: spearmint, peppermint, catnip, sweet balm.

To stop vomiting in cholera morbus, use origanum, peppermint, spearmint or peach leaves. Sweet balm settles the stomach. Use one teaspoon of the herbs to a cup of boiling water and steep. Lobelia is also good. Use a teaspoon to a pint of boiling water, steep, take a teaspoonful of this tea every fifteen minutes until relief is obtained.

Antispasmodic tincture given in small doses is very good —ten drops in a glass of warm water.

Obesity

Causes.—Obesity is occasionally hereditary, but can be overcome to a great extent by proper living. It is increased by wrong habits of eating, excessive starch and fatty foods, sugar, and lack of exercise. Some cases are due to a disturbance in the functioning of the thyroid and pituitary glands.

Symptoms.—Excessive fat, shortness of breath, palpitation of the heart upon slight exertion.

Treatment.—Reduce the diet to a minimum, eating only nourishing and non-fattening foods. Start exercising moderately, increasing in vigor, always in the open air if possible. Oxygen burns up fat and waste matter in the system; therefore, deep breathing and exercise are essential.

Chickweed is especially helpful to those suffering from obesity, as it thoroughly cleanses the system, and will reduce fat. Steep a heaping teaspoonful to a cup of boiling water, drink at least four cups a day, one an hour before each meal, and one on retiring. If there are other troubles, clear them up with the herbs indicated. Seawrack, burdock, and nettle can also be used with good results.

Paralysis
(General or Paraylsis of any part of the body)

Often in cases of paralysis half of the body will be paralyzed from head to foot, so that the patient is entirely helpless, unable to talk, and there is no sign of life, even when pricked with a needle. I have cured such cases. (Read personal experience in front of book.)

Treatment.—The following treatment can be used with benefit, no matter what part or parts of the body are affected. I have restored feeling in a single day to the affected part by using hot and cold fomentations, massage, liniments, and herbs, when the attack first came on. A stimulating liniment used on the part affected is always beneficial. Liniment as given in this book should be thoroughly rubbed in, and the part well saturated. Use the treatment described under My Experiences. Use the same herbs as given for infantile paralysis. Give a cleansing and nourishing diet. (See Table of Contents.)

Pancreas (Inflamed)

Causes.—Denatured foods, combinations that form fermentation in the stomach, such as, fruit and vegetables used together, white flour products, cane sugar, unpolished rice. These things should never be used. Cow's milk is highly mucus-forming. When the pancreas becomes inflamed or hardened, it does not secrete enough juice to properly digest the food in the intestines, which is its work. Disease of the pancreas leads to other serious diseases such as diabetes, etc.

Symptoms.—Gas and disturbance in the lower bowels and colon.

Treatment.—Give hot fomentations to the spine, stomach, liver, and pancreas. In bad cases, follow the treatment and diet given under diabetes. Give slippery elm enemas. Cut the slippery elm bark into pieces the size of a match. Put a large handful of these in four quarts of cold water, put on stove and simmer for ten to fifteen minutes, stirring frequently, cover tightly, and let set thirty minutes. This will draw the wonderfully healing jelly out of the bark. Strain, and use warm. Drink the slippery elm tea made in the same way. Steep a heaping teaspoonful of lobelia in a cup of boiling water for one half hour, and add a tablespoonful of this lobelia tea to every cup of slippery elm tea that you drink. Take a cup one hour before each meal, and one upon retiring. Alternate one of the following herbs, made into tea, with the slippery elm as given above. Bitterroot, Indian hemp, vervain, wahoo, buchu, dandelion, yarrow, and blueberry.

Pleurisy

Causes.—There are a variety of causes of pleurisy, among which may be mentioned diseases of the lungs, rheumatism, pneumonia, consumption, scarlet fever, blood poisoning, etc. Pleurisy occurs when the housing of the lungs—the pleura, becomes filled with water. When the cause of the diseases that cause pleurisy is considered, it is simmered down to waste matter in the system.

Symptoms.—In acute pleurisy the symptoms are fever, sharp pain in the affected side, nervousness, high colored and scanty urine, difficulty in breathing, etc. The pain is increased by coughing, lying on the affected side, or pressure. In chronic pleurisy, the symptoms are slight pain, rapid pulse, hacking cough, shortness of breath, increased debility, phlegm expectoration.

Treatment.—When acute, confine the patient to bed. Relieve the bowels immediately with a high enema. When there is a great deal of pain use catnip of valerian herb enemas. Apply hot fomentations to both chest and back. Have the fomentation large enough to cover the lungs. Keep this up for an hour or two, then let the patient rest, and repeat. Keep this up until the pain has ceased. Change the fomentations often as cold or chilliness will increase the pain. The fomentations given hot and very thoroughly will disperse the water in the lungs.

Give a hot herb tea of equal parts of the following: pleurisy root, yarrow, buckthorn bark, and valerian. Steep a heaping teaspoonful in a cup of boiling water for twenty minutes, drink a half cupful every two hours. If the tea is not laxative enough, add more buckthorn bark.

If the pain is severe and does not subside quickly, mix together equal parts of lady's-slipper, scullcap, and calamus root. Steep a heaping teaspoonful in a cup of boiling water for twenty minutes, and take a large swallow every hour. A specific cure for pleurisy can be made by steeping one tablespoonful yarrow, one tablespoonful pleurisy root, and a pinch of cayenne in a quart of boiling water, let steep, take warm—a large swallow every hour. This has been known to cure many cases.

A slippery elm poultice is very effective. Use three heaping tablespoonfuls of granulated slippery elm, one tablespoonful lobelia, one-half teaspoon cayenne. (See poultices for directions.) If both lungs are affected a larger quantity will have to be used to make the poultice large enough to cover both lungs. Put poultices on the chest and the back over the lungs. If you do not have slippery elm use flaxseed or cornmeal with the lobelia and cayenne. Pleurisy root alone is very effective if taken freely.

The diet should be restricted to oatmeal water, fruits, vegetables, and grains. Positively no meat, milk, or stimulating foods, such as condiments, or intoxicating drinks of any kind should be given.

If these directions are faithfully followed, and the treatment thoroughly given, the pain will soon cease, and the fluid which has gathered in the lungs will be dispersed.

Pyorrhea

Causes.—Toxins in the system caused from wrong diet and poor elimination.

Symptoms.—Bleeding and swelling of the gums. In bad cases the teeth become loose.

Treatment.—Correct the diet, using alkaline foods, and see that the bowels move three or four times a day. Go on a fruit diet for a time, as this is always good in overcoming an acid condition in the body.

Take one teaspoon of golden seal, one teaspoon of myrrh, steep in a pint of boiling water. Rinse out the mouth with this and gargle with it freely. Also brush the gums thoroughly with this solution at least three or four times a day. You will be pleased with what this one measure will do to overcome pyorrhea.

The liniment (see Table of Contents) is also very effective. Apply it to the gums with a small swab, or rinse out the mouth with it. The golden seal and myrrh can be used as a powder on the toothbrush, instead of making the tea.

Palsy

Causes.—Palsy is a nervous or physical condition due to fatigue, or the use of alcohol, tea, coffee, liquor, and stimulating foods. All refined food products, white flour, cane sugar, etc., are contributing factors, as they all lack the properties that sustain and strengthen the nerves. Collapse in one form or another is always the result of living on a diet composed mainly of such foods.

Symptoms.—Trembling and shaking of the limbs, arms, hands, and sometimes the head. A peculiar manner of walking.

Treatment.—Tea, coffee, liquor, and ALL stimulating foods must not be used if a person wants to be cured. Use the Cleansing and Nourishing diets, see page 159.

Hot and cold applications to the affected parts, with vigorous massage following, are very beneficial; this increases the circulation. A warm bath and salt glow can also be given with good results. The pores of the skin must be opened, and a good circulation started. Take laxative herbs enough, so you will have three or four good bowel movements a day, then take a high enema once a day.

Steep one tablespoonful prickly ash bark or berries, a pinch of cayenne, and one teaspoon of lobelia in a pint of boiling water. Take a tablespoonful every two hours.

Take any one of the following list of herbs internally, see descriptions and take the one or ones best suited to your case. (See use of non-poisonous herbs.) Masterwort, scullcap, vervain, lady's-slepper, and black cohosh.

Prostate Gland (Inflammation of)

Causes.—Usually caused by sexual excesses, weakness of the muscles, impurities in the blood stream, taking of strong cathartics. Improper diet which causes a diseased liver, kidney and bladder, thereby causing inflammation of the prostate gland.

Symptoms.—Pain and tenderness in the fork of thighs, painful urination.

Treatment.—Diet is of first importance. Alcoholic liquors, tea, coffee, and the use of all stimulating foods and drinks are strictly forbidden. A person suffering from this disease must have a diet consisting mainly of fruits, vegetables and grains. Several of the recipes in this book are good, such as soybean milk, zwieback, potassium broth, etc.

Constipation is nearly always present in this condition, and great benefit will be derived from the frequent use of hot enemas, as often as three times a day. A high enema as hot as can be borne of either catnip or valerian gives great relief when there is much pain.

A slippery elm poultice is extremely beneficial; apply between the legs, in the fork of the thighs.

Equal parts of gravel root, and cleavers, or peach leaves, or either one used alone, using a teaspoon to a cup of boiling water. Drink one to four cups a day, more or less as needed.

For an injection in any bladder trouble, take a teaspoon of golden seal, one-half teaspoon of myrrh, one-half teaspoon boric acid, pour on one quart of boiling water, and steep thirty minutes. Inject with a catheter, connecting the catheter to a nozzle of a fountain syringe and hang up high, so the water will flow in freely. Everyone should learn to use a catheter. This solution is wonderful to heal bladder trouble when the causes are removed. It is very powerful to destroy poisonous mucus or inflammation in the bladder.

Prostate Gland (Enlargement of)

Causes.—Enlargement usually results if inflammation is not properly treated.

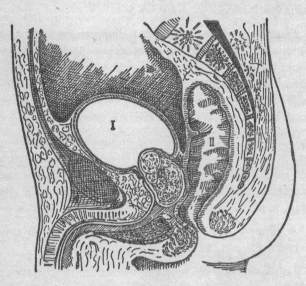

No. 1, Bladder; No. 2, Enlarged Colon;
No. 3, Enlarged Prostate Gland.

Symptoms.—Hard lump is present in the fork of the thighs, or rectum, which becomes very painful when pressed. Difficult and painful urination.

Treatment.—Follow the same treatment as for inflammation of the bladder.

A sitz-bath at temperature of 105° to 115° F. is excellent in relieving the enlargement when due to congestion. Remain in the sitz bath from twenty minutes to an hour.

The diet as given for inflammation of the prostate must be strictly adhered to. Massage is beneficial, also electrical vibrator.

Pregnancy

The first sign of pregnancy is the ceasing of the monthly periods. Occasionally this period continues, but this is rare. An early symptom is morning sickness. Some do not suffer this at all, but some suffer severely. In about six or eight weeks the breasts enlarge and the nipple becomes prominent with a dark ring around it. Movements of the child are felt between four and five months.

Regular, but not strenuous exercise must be taken during the entire nine months to keep the muscles in good condition, as child-birth is chiefly a muscular action. The habit that a large majority of women have of lying or sitting most of the time, is a most injurious one to the child and mother, as it causes the muscles to become weak and the health generally run down.

I have seen many instances where women were obliged to do their own housework, as well as work in the garden, right up to the time of confinement and they had an almost painless delivery. Care should be taken, nevertheless, not to exercise to the point of exhaustion.

All bad habits must be abandoned. Due to the fact, that nowadays so many women smoke and drink, *it cannot be overemphasized* that this will have an extremely damaging effect on the child, mentally, morally, and physically. The mother should have plenty of rest, fresh air, and moderate exercise. A simple, nourishing, non-stimulating diet is necessary if you would have a happy, healthy, normal child. Meats of all kinds should be eaten very sparingly, if at all.

Inflammation of the kidneys is a frequent occurrence during pregnancy, and is greatly encouraged by the use of meats. The diet should consist largely of fresh fruits and vegetables. It is an erroneous idea that the infant will be marked if the craving for some particular article of food is not satisfied.

Special attention must be given to the bowels. They should move thoroughly at least three times a day. If necessary, use laxative herbs to keep them regular, but it is much preferable to keep the bowels regular as far as possible with the diet. Figs, raisins, prunes, etc., are good for this.

Dress.—The wearing of tight girdles or corsets is extremely detrimental to the child. They should not be worn. The dress should be loose and suitable for the different seasons. When the abdomen becomes greatly enlarged, it will be found beneficial and comfortable to wear a wide band to support the abdomen, but do not have it tight. Tight clothing should not be worn around the breasts.

Baths.—Frequent sitz-baths will relieve many of the local ailments which women suffer during this period. They should be taken at least two or three times a week. During the last few weeks of pregnancy they should be taken daily. A full bath should be taken at least twice a week to keep the skin and circulation in good condition.

Mental attitude.—If you want a cheerful, happy child with a sunny disposition, that is just what you yourself will have to be during pregnancy. Special effort should be made by the mother to avoid as much unpleasantness as possible. A fit of anger, or great fright, novel reading, etc., have a very bad effect on the child. The surroundings should be made as pleasant as possible, and it is positively the husband's duty to bring this about, as far as lies in his power. By proper living, care and treatment, pain can be almost entirely banished at childbirth.

There are special herbs that will help to make childbirth painless and save a great deal of suffering. Lobelia is quieting to the nerves and causes them to relax. Red raspberry leaves made into a tea is good to relieve nausea and vomiting. It is also used as an aid to labor, and has been efficacious in promoting uterine contractions when ergot has failed. If red raspberry tea were taken continuously during pregnancy and drank in place of ordinary tea, then a cupful taken every hour during labour, hemorrhages would seldom occur and the use of instruments would rarely be required.

Spikenard is an old Indian remedy to promote easy and painless childbirth. Indian women were noted for their painless childbirths.

I have stopped a very profuse hemorrhage with a hot douche of around 120°F. after childbirth. Using a tea made of wild alum root, or white oak bark combined with it will increase its efficiency. The hot water coagulates the blood and stops the flow. In the absence of the herbs a solution may be made of alum crystals, which can be obtained in nearly every drugstore.

After the birth, rest is essential. The mother should stay flat on her back for at least ten days, better fourteen, so that the organs can all get back into place and rested.

Diet of nursing mothers: Tea, coffee, rich and heavy foods, fish, oysters, condiments of all kinds, all stimulating foods and drinks, should be strictly avoided. Very little, if any, meat should be eaten as meat is full of bacteria, which causes poisons in the intestines and the infant as well as the mother may become poisoned by it.

Eat as many bulky foods as possible to keep free from constipation, such as lettuce, carrots, spinach, beets, prunes, figs, apples, apricots, zwieback, shredded wheat biscuits, wheat flakes, ripe olives, grapes, raspberries, and berries of all kinds. Orange juice is especially excellent and fruit juices of all kinds.

Foods to increase the milk.—Potassium broth and mashed potatoes as given in this book, are both very strengthening and nutritious, and will increase the milk. Whole grain cereals, especially oatmeal, and oatmeal water. Always drink six to eight glasses of water a day. Insufficient water will always cause insufficient milk.

When a mother gives way to a fit of anger, or rage, the milk becomes poisonous and unfit for food, and the infant may be made very ill. It is a known fact that if a mother becomes extremely angry just before nursing an infant, it has caused the infant to have violent convulsions. Dill herb tea will help to increase the milk.

To decrease flow of milk.—The drinking of sage tea will dry up the milk. Do not take much liquid, eat dry foods.

Two of the most important things when nursing a child is to keep the bowels regular and the mother should be calm at all times. Sexual intercourse, during this time, often causes children to have colic and stomach trouble, as it has a damaging effect on the milk because of the excitement.

During the entire nine months it is an excellent thing to thoroughly massage the entire area of the stomach and abdomen every evening before retiring with cocoa butter, or some good oil, as this will prevent or help to prevent the marks left on the skin from childbirth, to a great extent. It lubricates the skin and makes it more elastic.

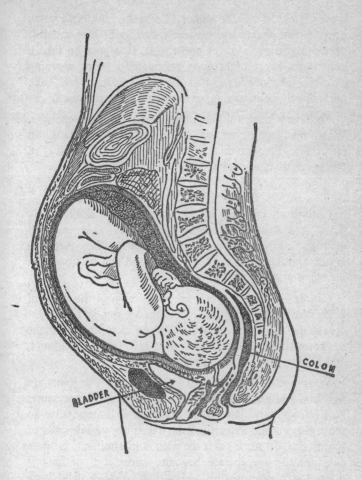

BLADDER

COLON

KNOWN FACTS ABOUT SEX DETERMINING. When pregnancy occurs within four days after menstruation, it is likely to be a girl; when it occurs after a period of twenty days after menstruation, it is likely to be a boy; if between these times, it may be either. To make childbirth easy, drink red raspberry leaf tea freely during the nine months, preferably in place of tea and coffee. It is good to take a cup warm, every night upon retiring. To lessen morning sickness, take lobelia in small doses, or spearmint tea. Take immediately upon arising, or whenever there is nausea.

To have a beautiful baby, take plenty of gentle exercise. When sleeping, or resting, lie in different positions, on either side, then stomach, then on back. Brisk walking in the open air is one of the best of exercises.

Rheumatism and Arthritis

Chronic rheumatism and chronic gout, are similar, only manifested a little differently. Frequently what is called arthritis follows an acute attack of rheumatism. Arthritis is just another form of rheumatism, and can be treated in the same way.

Causes.—Rheumatism is an obstruction in the body of acids and waste material. Exposure to wet and cold increase the pains and suffering. Wrong diet, which fills the system with uric acid and poisons, which the liver, kidneys, and bladder are not able to throw off.

Symptoms.—Enlarged and painful joints. The joints are red, hot, and very tender upon any movement or pressure. Not infrequently they get so stiff that it is impossible to move them at all. Sometimes the hands draw backwards or to one side. In some cases the pain is intermittent, in some constant. As the disease becomes chronic, if nothing is done, the muscles shrink and wither away. A child born of parents or even one parent that has had an attack of rheumatism or is rheumatic, will have a predisposition to rickets, hip joint disease, and may be inferior mentally. A woman having a child before six months or so, after an attack of rheumatism, will suffer untold agonies at birth, and the child will be likely to be inferior.

Treatment.—All unwholesome devitaminized food must be strictly avoided. Tea, coffee, liquors, white flour products, cane sugar products, soda biscuits, fried potatoes, meats, pork and bacon especially. The blood corpuscles in the body when fed on the foregoing foods, will not be able to rid the system of impurities. See cleansing and nourishing foods in Table of Contents. All food should be eaten as dry as possible, well masticated, so that it is thoroughly mixed with saliva to help digestion. This will alkalinize the system as much as any other one thing you can do. Wonderful results would be obtained from a prolonged fruit diet. After taking the fruit diet two or three weeks, use potassium broth, French toast, and mashed potatoes as given in this book. Drink slippery elm tea; it is very nourishing, cleansing and strengthening. Solid food must, of course, be taken sparingly at first, after the fruit diet.

A high enema must be taken every evening for some time. Herb enemas are preferable as they cleanse and heal. Use either white oak bark, red raspberry, or alum root. See high enemas in Table of Contents. Take a good sweat bath every day, and drink two or three cups of pleurisy tea, using a teaspoon to a cup of boiling water, steep twenty minutes. Drink this while in the tub. Thorough massage after the bath is very beneficial. If there is inflammation of the joints do not massage those parts.

Mix equal parts of the following herbs: Black cohosh, gentian root, angelica, columbo, scullcap, valerian, rue, and buckthorn bark. Use a heaping teaspoon to the cup of boiling water, steep, and drink three or more cups per day, as the case may require; take in half cup doses.

(537)

An excellent poultice for swollen joints is as follows: two tablespoonfuls mullein, three tablespoonfuls granulated slippery elm bark, one tablespoonful lobelia, a small teaspoon cayenne; mix thoroughly together, then mix with enough boiling water to make a stiff paste, spread on a cloth about one-fourth of an inch thick, and cover the swollen joints with this poultice. This will give great relief.

Another excellent thing to relieve the pain is to take equal parts of oil of origanum, oil of lobelia, then add a few drops oil of capsicum, or extract of capsicum (red pepper). This can be applied full strength, or mixed with cocoanut oil. Massage thoroughly with this.

The following herbs are very beneficial in rheumatism; look up their descriptions and take those best suited to your case. Use singly or in combination. Bitterroot, buckthorn bark, burdock, saw palmetto berries, black cohosh, wintergreen, yellow dock, sassafras, scullcap, bearsfoot.

Ringworm

Ringworm usually appears first on the face or upper part of the body. The scalp and the fingers are likely to be affected. It begins as a small red patch, which causes itching. The patch enlarges and forms a ring, usually covered with small blisters. When the scalp is affected the hair falls out in circular spots.

Treatment.—Ringworm of the scalp is difficult to cure. Shampoo the hair with tar soap and borax. Every morning and evening moisten the spots with the following solution: 1 teaspoon golden seal, one-half teaspoon myrrh; steep in a pint of boiling water.

For internal use, adults should take a level teaspoon of golden seal to a cup of water twice a day: make it weaker for children, according to age. Hops, boneset, and plantain may also be taken internally with good results. Blood-root tea made strong, and applied externally is excellent.

Rickets

Causes.—Children would not have rickets if they were properly fed. Insufficient nourishing food, and the use of devitaminized foods and refined products, such as, white flours, polished rice, cane sugar, etc. These are especially detrimental.

Symptoms.—The abdomen becomes enlarged and the teeth do not develop. Fretfulness, restlessness at night, the head perspires, stomach trouble and possible diarrhea. Very susceptible to colds. Children afflicted with rickets are very apt to get spinal meningitis, bowlegs, knock-knees, enlarged head, and the lungs may become affected and even enlargement of the heart and dropsy of the brain.

Treatment.—If a child does not develop it is usually a sign of rickets, especially if they are slow in teething. Children suffering from rickets should be given plenty of fresh air, frequent warm baths with friction to increase the circulation. Keep them off their feet until they gain strength and show definite signs of improvement.

The diet is of main importane. The diet as given in the book for infants is very good. If cow's milk is used add a tablespoonful of lime water to every bottle of milk given the child, or add a little strained oatmeal gruel to the milk before feeding. This keeps the milk from fermenting and adds to the food value. For older children, give all the fresh vegetables simply prepared. Fruits of all kinds. Mashed potatoes, soybean cottage cheese, potassium broth, as given in this book. Do not let them combine fruits and vegetables at the same meal. Do not allow the child to drink with meals as this hinders digestion.

Steep a heaping teaspoon of scullcap in a cup of boiling water, strain, and give a tablespoonful six or seven times a day. Catnip tea is very excellent in all children's diseases and may be taken freely. Sweeten the tea a little with honey or malt sugar.

The bowels must be kept open. Use injections of catnip, tea, or just plain warm water with a little Ivory soap dissolved in it. Senna tea taken internally is good. If possible, keep the bowels open with fruits and vegetables. Give plenty of fruit juices of all kinds between meals.

Spleen (Inflammation of)

Cause.—Inflammation of the spleen may follow inflammation of the stomach, lungs, or other organs.

Symptoms.—There is severe pain in the left side, extending up to the shoulder. Sometimes the person is taken with a chill, followed by high fever and the skin becomes dry and hot. Constipation is always present. In some cases the urine is suppressed and very dark in color. The person is very thirsty.

Treatment.—A light nourishing diet must always be provided. A fruit diet for a few days is excellent. The bowels must be kept open by the use of some laxative herbs as given in this book under laxatives.

Hot fomentations applied to the left side, followed by short cold will do much to relieve the inflammation and pain. Repeat this two or three times a day, until the pain is relieved, and then given once a day.

The liniment (see Table of Contents) rubbed in well over the spleen, will also do a great deal to relieve the pain.

Use the same herbs and in the same way as given under, Pancreas (inflamed).

(540)

This treatment applies to acute and chronic enlargement of the spleen as well.

Sinus Trouble

Cause.—Sinus trouble is directly caused by wrong eating habits that can be controlled by the one afflicted. There is little use to treat for a cure unless the causes are removed. Wrong diet causes the catarrhal condition which oftentimes affects the sinuses, consequently you have sinus trouble. Auto-intoxication, which is caused by constipation, is one great cause of sinus trouble. Lack of exercise, bathing, fresh air, all tend to bring on a catarrhal condition of the system.

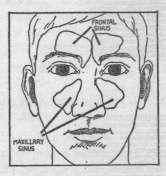

LOCATION OF SINUSES

Symptoms.—Pain in the sinuses, sometimes becoming very severe, eyes ache, a watery discharge from the nose in the acute stage. Symptoms are akin to hay fever which is brought on by the same causes.

Treatment.—Remove the causes, regulate the bowel eliminations, so as to have three good eliminations a day. Thoroughly cleanse the colon with a high enema, you may

(541)

have to take a high enema every day for several weeks to help rid the system of mucus and poisons.

Take a fruit juice diet for four of five days, drinking all the juice you can of oranges, grapefruit, lemon, pineapple, and grape (all unsweetened). Do not mix the juices, drink one at a time, alternating them. Then go on a vegetable diet, using all kinds of greens, red cabbage, and eggplant being especially useful as they are very rich in potassium, but use all kinds of vegetables. Continue the fruit juices, but drink them between meals. Never use fruits and vegetables at the same meal.

At times cold applications over the sinus will give great relief; at other times alternate hot and cold applications, use which ever give you most relief. Have a pan of both hot and cold water, bathe the whole face with hot water, as hot as you can stand, then apply short cold.

The liniment (as given in this book) thoroughly applied and well rubbed in over the sinus often gives relief. Inhale it also. But, the only cure is to thoroughly cleanse the body of all poisons, then there will be no sinus trouble.

To cleanse and heal the nose, make a tea of bayberry bark, use a teaspoon to a cup of boiling water, let it simmer for thirty minutes, strain, when cool, or just warm, snuff it up the nose, getting it up both sides, one side at a time thoroughly; this will cleanse and heal at the same time.

Sprains and Strain of Muscles

Sprains generally occur in the ankles, wrist, elbows, shoulders, back or hips.

Causes.—The causes are numerous. Result of a sudden or unexpected movement, or missing a step in going downstairs, stumbling, falling, etc. When ligaments are torn there is extreme pain and puffiness around the joint. If the sprain is bad get a good bone physician at once.

Treatment.—If the strain or sprain is in the wrist, elbow, or ankles, put the affected part in very hot water, and keep it there at least twenty minutes or thirty is better. Keep the water hot. Every few minutes take it out of the hot water and plunge it into cold water for about one minute, then back into the hot. Do this several times. This can be kept up an hour or longer. I have kept it up for two hours with gratifying results, and repeated it two or three times a day. Then gently massage the affected part, 15 or 20 minutes. If it should be the ankle or foot, massage the entire foot and leg well up over the knee. If the hand, massage the entire hand and arm over the elbow. Do not use the affected part for some time. If the ligaments are badly torn, bind with a fairly tight bandage, to hold them in place, after the treatment. If this is repeated for a few days, the results will be most gratifying. Massage at least twice a day. If swelling and fever set in before you have an opportunity to treat the sprain or torn ligaments, use a hot fomentation, followed by short cold applications; usually three fomentations are applied. This will take out the swelling and inflammation. Then use the two dishes of water, hot and cold, as given above. If you do this, the soreness and swelling will leave. After the inflammation and soreness have abated, you can massage directly over the spot, but not at first; simply massage around it.

If the sprain or strain is in the back or shoulder, treat it with the hot fomentations, and short cold, and massage.

Make an herb tea of equal parts of gentian, scullcap, valerian, buckthorn bark, a pinch of red pepper. Mix thoroughly together, use a heaping teaspoon to a cup of boiling water. Take a tablespoonful every hour. More may be taken if needed.

Liniment, as given in this book, which everyone who can should make for themselves, and always have on hand, will take most of the soreness out of a bad sprain in one single day. Apply the liniment freely, and massage gently before the inflammation sets in. Keep this up 15 to 20 minutes at a time, using it three or four times a day. The liniment will also take the soreness out of black and blue spots. Massage the spot gently as you apply the liniment. A bad bruise on any part of the body may be treated the same as a sprain and torn ligaments, or pain in the back. Treat with hot fomentations and short cold, then apply liniment thoroughly. I have taken a bad kink out of the back in one single day with this treatment. Keep up the applications, giving them thoroughly. When there is a kink in the back, take herb enemas to cleanse the bowels.

Sore Mouth

The most common inflammation of the mouth is caused from indigestion and acid forming foods. There is a general redness and it is almost impossible to masticate the food. In infants and children, the mouth should be carefully sponged with the following solution.

Use one teaspoon golden seal, one-half teaspoon myrrh, steep in a pint of boiling water, adding one tablespoonful boric acid. When settled, pour off clear liquid. For adults use this as a mouth wash and gargle several times a day, holding some in the mouth for a few minutes.

White oak bark, wild alum root, or red raspberry leaf tea used as a gargle and mouth wash are also very beneficial.

Undue Sexual Desire

Causes.—Excessive eating of all stimulating foods, such

as, eggs, meats of all kinds, cheese, chocolate, tea, coffee, and all alcoholic drinks.

Treatment.—Avoid all the above mentioned articles. Eat plenty of fresh fruits and vegetables. Use a simple, nourishing diet. Exercise out in the fresh air is most beneficial. Tennis playing, swimming, useful labor, brisk walking, and all forms of healthful exercise are helpful. (Novel reading and impure thoughts are often great causes.)

Herbs.—Sage, scullcap, or black willow. Black willow is especially good. Steep a teaspoonful of either one of these in a cup of boiling water for twenty minutes, and drink four cups a day, one an hour before meals and one on going to bed.

Skin Diseases

All skin diseases are caused by impure blood or infection. Go on a prolonged fruit diet when you have boils, carbuncles, blackheads, pimples, or a skin affection of any kind. Stop using meats of all kinds, do not eat between meals. Do not use cane sugar, white flour, or white flour products. Take plenty of exercise in the fresh air. Eat plenty of fresh fruits, vegetables, and well-cooked grains.

Cold towel rubs are very helpful, rubbing vigorously afterwards to increase the circulation.

Make a strong tea of red clover blossoms, using three or four tablespoonfuls (granulated) to the quart of water. Steep one half hour in boiling water, covered. Drink this tea freely in place of water. Chickweed tea may be used in the same way, the taste being similar to spinach and not at all disagreeable. If you follow this treatment outlined above, using either of the herbs as directed, the skin disease will disappear.

The following herbs are also beneficial in skin diseases: burdock root, yellow dock root, hyssop, sanicle, blue violet, golden seal, plantain, echinacea, beech, bittersweet, buckthorn bark, elder, bloodroot, dandelion, sassafras, sarsaparilla, and spikenard. These can be taken singly or combine two or more in equal parts. Take four cups a day, one an hour before each meal and one upon retiring. Study the description of the herbs listed, and use those best suited to your needs.

A very effective external remedy, is the following; make into a tea, and bathe the affected parts. Equal parts golden seal, echinacea, yellow dock root, burdock root, and witch hazel bark, mixed thoroughly. Use a heaping tablespoonful of this mixture to a pint of boiling water, steep one-half hour, pour off the liquid or strain, add a level tablespoonful of boric acid: this will keep the fluid from souring. Apply a number of times during the day to the affected parts.

Citrus fruits are especially beneficial in all skin troubles.

Smallpox

Smallpox is a contagious, filth disease.

Symptoms.—The skin becomes red, and pustules form.

Treatment.—The patient must be kept clean, the room darkened, and good ventilation and an even temperature kept, of not over 70°F. During the fever stage give plenty of lemonade without sugar. Give high herb enemas, and clean out the bowels thoroughly, using Herbal Laxative (as given in this book). When the skin is hot and dry, take equal parts of pleurisy root and ginger, steep a teaspoonful in a cup of boiling water for twenty minutes, give a cupful every hour or until there is free perspiration. Equal parts of yarrow and valerian taken in the same way will also produce perspiration. Red sage made into a tea or taken in the powdered form in capsules is very good.

If there is great itching of the skin, bathe with a tea made of burdock root, golden seal root, or yellow dock root. The pustules must be opened by pricking with a sterilized needle, about four days after they have come to a head, then bathe them with hydrogen peroxide after pricking. This will prevent pitting. Bathing the pustules with golden seal tea is a specific against pitting.

The diet should be very light. Soybean milk, oatmeal water, also bran and barley water is good. Vegetable broth is very nourishing. Fruit juices are excellent.

When there is exposure to smallpox or any danger of contracting it, cleanse your system by high enemas. Take the Herbal Laxative, as given in this book, or any good Herb Laxative, go on a fruit juice diet for a number of days, then take vegetable broth, or vegetable puree made from leafy vegetables, combined with thick potato peelings, and some oatmeal or natural brown rice added, and after cooking, strain, and use.

Hot baths taken before contracting smallpox or after contracting it will make the skin active and shorten the course of the disease.

Sore Eyes

Causes.—Eye troubles are caused mainly from a deranged stomach, for they receive their nourishment from the food taken into the stomach and, naturally the eating of unhealthful foods and drinks such as tea, coffee, condiments, alcoholic drinks, tobacco, etc., weakens the nerves and hinders the free circulation of blood to the eyes.

Unhealthful foods and drinks cause impure blood and when the circulation carries impure blood to the eyes, it weakens them. The all important thing is to eat food that will give you a pure blood stream.

Inflammation of the eyes from any cause will greatly benefit by the following treatment.

Treatment.—To cure eye trouble or remove it, it will be necessary to correct the diet and leave off all harmful foods and drinks. Get plenty of sleep in a well-ventilated room. Cleanse the system thoroughly with high herb enemas, blood purifying herbs, fruit and fruit juices, and cleansing vegetables such as, cucumbers, carrots, celery and the leafy greens.

Take the juice of a lemon every morning one hour before breakfast in a cup of hot water. Steep one teaspoon of red raspberry leaves, one teaspoon witch hazel leaves in a cup of boiling water, strain through a cloth, saturate a soft cloth with this tea and apply as a wet pack to the eyes or bathe the eyes with it often, using an eye cup. Fennel tea is excellent to take internally. It will benefit the eyes, as it strengthens them. When used in an eye cup, dilute one-third with water.

Charcoal or slippery elm poultices applied (cold) to the eyes will relieve inflammation.

An excellent eye wash for every day use as well as when there is particular difficulty, is the following. One teaspoon golden seal, one level teaspoon boric acid, dissolve in a pint of boiling water, shake well, let settle. You may pour off the liquid, or use just as is.

Stomach Trouble

All stomach troubles arise from the eating and drinking of harmful foods, wrong combinations, eating of fruits and vegetables together, milk and cane sugar together, pies, cakes, white flour products, greasy and fried foods, drinking with meals, and poor mastication. No matter what, or how much you eat, if it is not properly masticated it will not digest properly. Drinking with meals will dilute the digestive juices, so that they cannot do their work properly. Ice cold drinks are especially harmful, as they chill the stomach as well as dilute the digestive juices.

The best thing to do for any kind of stomach trouble is to go on a fruit diet, for at least a week or more. Give the stomach a chance to rest so that the pepsin and gastric juices will be strong enough to digest the food.

When on the fast or fruit diet, do not drink anything but pure water, and the prescribed herbs. Upon arising, drink one-fourth teaspoon of golden seal in a glass of very warm water, before taking anything else into the stomach. This is one of the best remedies. Continue doing this after you have completed taking the fruit diet. If this is taken regularly, good results will follow.

Stomach (Inflammation of)

Causes.—Excessive use of spices, mustard, condiments, alcoholic drinks, and all stimulating foods.

Symptoms.—Severe pain in the stomach, nausea with vomiting, inability to retain food, medicine and drinks.

Treatment.—Give a high enema first. Then hot and cold applications to the stomach, liver, and spine. Give an emetic herb, if the person is strong. (See emetics.) Take oatmeal, bran, or barley water. Oatmeal water with soybean milk is an excellent nourishing drink, half and half. To get the stomach into shape to retain food, take golden seal, steep a teaspoonful in a pint of boiling water. Take six or more large swallows a day.

The following list of herbs are excellent in stomach troubles, see descriptions. Use the one or ones best suited to your condition. They may be taken singly, or two or more combined.

Red raspberry tea is very soothing to the stomach. Excellent results will be obtained from drinking chickweed tea, or red clover tea in place of water, six or eight glasses a day. Sage, wood betony, poplar bark, bitterroot, cayenne, slippery elm (excellent), colombo, pleurisy root, hyssop, plantain, wild yam, sweet flag, yarrow, strawberry leaves, wild alum root, rue, violet leaves.

Slippery elm tea should be used in all stomach trouble. It heals, strengthens, and nourishes.

An excellent stomach remedy is to mix equal parts, golden seal, echinacea, burnet, wood betony, myrrh, and spearmint (use powdered herbs). After thoroughly mixing these together, take one-half teaspoonful in a glass of hot water one hour before meals, and one upon retiring.

Spinal Meningitis

Symptoms.—High fever, sleeplessness, spasms of the muscles in the neck and back, burning pain in spine, extending to the limbs, sometimes partial paralysis of the lower limbs, difficult breathing, suppressed urination, constipation, followed by diarrhea, prostration, occasionally delirium and unconsciousness. In small children a spasm at the beginning.

Treatment.—The patient must be kept very quiet in bed. The bowels must be relieved by high enemas. Keep the patient's room dark, allow no visitors. The room must be well ventilated at all times. Give fomentations to the spine, liver, and abdomen. This is very necessary to bring about a good circulation and relieve the congested organs. Thorough massage will do a great deal to hasten a cure.

The bowels must move two or three times a day. Use the herb laxative as given in this book, when necessary. Any one of the following herbs are beneficial. Make a mixture of two or three of the following: scullcap, catnip, blue and black cohosh, golden seal, prickly ash bark, queen of the meadow. Use one teaspoon of the mixture to a cup of boiling water. Take at least four cups per day, one an hour before each meal, and one upon retiring.

The diet must be non-stimulating and light. A fruit diet at first is advisable. Bran, oatmeal, and barley water are excellent. Use vegetable broth freely, as given in this book. It is very nourishing, alkaline, and cleansing.

Syphilis

Causes.—Syphilis is due to a specific germ and is most frequently contracted by sexual relations. Usually children born of parents who have this disease contract it and they are either born dead or die when only a few days old, or, are sometimes cripples or invalids for life. It can be contracted by kissing, using towels of an infected person, or silverware, dishes, washbowls, and toilet seats. The living germ must come in contact with the mucous membranous surface to be contracted, as the germs die as soon as they become dry. This disease is constitutional. It affects the whole system. The treatment must be continued several months after all the symptoms have disappeared in order to be effectual. It is imperative to lead an active life in the open air as much as possible. Eat simple nourishing foods continuously for years to build up a constitution that has been weakened by the poison of syphilis.

Symptoms.—All the symptoms are too numerous to mention, but there are three distinct stages. The first, a small chancre which usually appears about three or more weeks after infection. Sometimes it is so small as to almost pass unnoticed. The second, usually appears from one to three months after the chancre. This stage is preceded by pain in the bones, weakness, loss of weight, poor digestion, etc. A rash appears which may cover the entire body or only a part. The tonsils become ulcerated. The rash in itself is not painful. The glands of the neck become enlarged, the tongue, palate, and entire mouth become sore. The hair is dry, brittle, and falls out in small or large patches in some cases. If the eyes become infected, temporary or permanent blindness may result. This stage lasts from six to twelve months, occasionally much longer. The third stage: ulcerations in any part of the body, skin eruptions and tumors. These ulcers are very difficult to heal, and are great destroyers of tissue. It is not unusual for several ulcers to start at the same time. Syphilis often causes the bones to decay. Frequently the whole nose, palate, and ribs have been destroyed in syphilitics.

Treatment.—Syphilis can be treated successfully with natural remedies, which leave no bad after effects.

Meats of all kinds, especially pork, also tea, coffee, oysters, shell fish, tobacco, all condiments, stimulating foods and drinks must not be used. These foods tend to irritate and heat the blood; they fill the system with waste material and poisonous toxins.

Mix thoroughly together two tablespoons each of the following herbs: Oregon grape, uva ursi, burdock root, blue flag root, red clover blossoms, prickly ash berries, and buckthorn bark, and one teaspoon of bloodroot. Steep a heaping teaspoonful in a cup of boiling water for one half hour. Drink at least four cups per day, one an hour before each meal, and one upon retiring. Also may be taken in capsules; take two No. 00 four times a day. Continue taking these herbs at least one year.

Bathe the sores with a solution of golden seal and myrrh, using a teaspoon of each to a pint of boiling water. When the eruptions first appear, bathe thoroughly with this tea. Heavy sweats and salt glows will help to eliminate the poisons. Take high enemas every day, using either bayberry bark, burdock root, yellow dock root, or echinacea.

Any of the following list of herbs can be used with good results. Look up the descriptions and use those best suited to your case, in the event you have some other trouble or disease also.

Red clover blossoms, holy thistle, archangel, Oregon grape, parsley, uva ursi, witch hazel, burdock root, bitterroot, red raspberry, yellow dock root, elder, bittersweet, turkey corn, wintergreen, cleavers, poplar, witch hazel, golden seal, prickly ash, rock rose, spikenard, twin leaf, wild elm root.

If the treatment outlined above is started immediately, when the first symptoms appear, you need not suffer greatly at all. The worst cases of syphilis have yielded to the above compound of herbs, when the rest of the treatment, diet and hygiene, was strictly adhered to.

Tuberculosis and Consumption

Causes.—Tuberculosis may affect not only the lungs, but other parts of the body, as liver, spleen, intestines, spine, and bones. Intemperance in eating and drinking, also dressing, exposure to cold, loss of sleep, impure air, lack of proper exercise, and not breathing deeply enough to open up all the lung cells, sedentary life, overwork, lack of properly prepared nourishing food, and an unbalanced diet—all pave the way for tuberculosis to develop. Persons with feeble constitutions are those mostly affected with tuberculosis. Contaminated milk, use of tobacco in any form, liquor of all kinds, tea, coffee, and all harmful drinks are active causes.

Symptoms.—Usually slow in developing. Habitual cough, gradually becoming severe, causing vomiting and profuse expectoration. The victim becomes extremely weak, is subject to night sweats, and bleeding from the lungs.

Treatment.—A moderate temperature should be maintained at all times, never having it excessively warm, and always having good ventilation. Avoid becoming chilled. Patient's room should be sunny, airy, and dry. Get plenty outdoor exercise, and stay outdoors as much as possible. If the patient is not too weak, clean the stomach out thoroughly with an emetic. It will be surprising how much mucus will be brought up that otherwise would have been brought up in paroxyms of coughing.

Steep one teaspoonful of powdered golden seal, one teaspoon of cubeb berries, and one-fourth teaspoon lobelia, in a pint of boiling water for one half hour. Take a swallow every hour. Mix two tablespoonfuls of powdered bugleweed with a pinch of cayenne and use a level teaspoon of this mixture to a cup of boiling water. Take a swallow of this every two hours. A cupful of this tea is also useful to check bleeding from the lungs. Powdered bayberry bark or shepherd's purse is also very good to check hemorrhage of the lungs. Use half a teaspoon to a cup of boiling water, let steep, strain and drink cold.

Drink at least one quart of slippery elm tea daily, drinking one cup an hour before each meal, and one at bed time. It will strengthen, heal and nourish. If the digestion is not good, take one-fourth teaspoon powdered golden seal in a glass of water an hour before each meal.

A nourishing diet is necessary. Soybean milk can be taken freely. Soybean milk with whole wheat flakes is very nourishing. Other good foods to use in the diet are: very ripe bananas, oatmeal with malt honey, and whole wheat or soybean bread, zwiebach, potassium broth (see recipe in this book), tender fresh peas, steamed figs, dates, graham crackers, all kinds of vegetables (seasoned with soybean milk or soybean butter), natural brown rice, and baked Irish potatoes.

When there is fever, look up in this book the diet for fevers and treatment of fevers.

Deep breathing and plenty of fresh air are absolutely necessary in connection with gentle exercise. Sun baths are excellent. Expose the entire body. Take sweat baths to open the pores, drinking two or three cups of tea made from pleurisy root while in the tub.

All sputa and discharges of a patient suffering from tuberculosis or consumption should be burned or buried.

The following herbs may be used to advantage in tuberculosis. Look up their descriptions, and use those best suited to your condition: wild cherry, flaxseed, sanicle, mullein, vervain, hyssop, skunk cabbage, colt's foot, lungwort, and marshmallow root.

In treating this disease one must take into consideration its extent, and the length of time the patient has suffered with it. If we find that tubercles have formed, we must find a preparation of a solvent nature to soften and break up the cheezy particles of the tubercle so it can be eliminated. An agent must be used that will clean away the pus and accumulation, and at the same time be of a healing nature. Such herbs as powdered comfrey, marshmallow, chickweed, and slippery elm are beneficial. Mix together equal parts of the foregoing herbs, and use 4 oz. of this mixture to four quarts of water, and boil down to 2 quarts. Strain and take a half cupful every two hours, either hot or cold. This will ease the irritation or inflammation as well as dissolve and break up the cheezy substances. In addition to healing properties, there must be something having astringent and healing properties, which will cause the cavities to heal and become sound again.

For this, use 1 oz. each of powdered black horehound, bur-marigold, hyssop, lobelia, and ½ oz. ginger, to four quarts of water, boil down to two quarts. Take half cup doses every two hours. Give these two preparations alternately, give a dose of the first preparation, followed in one hour by a dose of the second, etc.

Short hot fomentations, with short cold, alternate, applied to the chest both in the front and back over the lungs, also apply the full length of the spine, and over the stomach, liver, and spleen. These will prove very beneficial.

Warm baths followed by a thorough salt glow and massage is necessary. Judgment must be used in giving these, giving them according to the strength of the patient.

Take cough medicine as given in the book, in teaspoon doses, give freely. Always give after a coughing spell.

A patient must always be kept warm with warm clothing, especially the feet, legs and arms.

Tonsillitis

Causes.—Disordered stomach from wrong diet. I have known cases where I had been sitting at the table with people whose throat was all right the day before, and they ate an abnormal amount of rich food, and developed a case of fever the next day with tonsillitis. They blamed the food, but it was not that but the abnormal amount they had eaten. The stomach was unable to handle it, so it became a poison in the stomach, and inflamed the entire esophagus from the mouth to the stomach. This poisoned and inflamed the tonsils and caused them to become swollen and sore. Most throat troubles, sinus, adenoids, bronchitis, and various coughs, can be traced directly to a bad condition in the stomach.

Symptoms.—Chilly feeling, fever. Throat swollen, sometimes practically closed with the soft palate hanging on to the tongue. The throat and mouth are dry, and then soon lots of poisonous mucus accumulates. The tonsils are swollen and red in color. Small ulcers appear on the tonsils. Often the glands of the neck swell.

Treatment.—First, take a high enema and relieve the bowels. If you have ice, crush some, wrap it in a towel, put it around the neck, pinning securely in the back with safety pins. When this becomes painful, take it off, and apply a hot fomentation, keeping it on three to five minutes. Then put the ice on again. Keep this up for an hour or more, then gargle the throat with a solution made of a teaspoon of golden seal and one teaspoon of myrrh to a pint of boiling water. Let steep one half hour. Gargle thoroughly with this every half hour, swallowing a little. If the tonsils are swollen so large that the tea does not reach the back of the tonsils when gargling, swab the back side of the tonsils with it. Lemon juice may be used in the same way with splendid results.

A hot bath and a good salt glow in the evening before retiring is beneficial.

Take some hot tea made of red raspberry or sage, one teaspoon to the cup of boiling water. Slippery elm is an excellent remedy in sore throat and stomach trouble. This may be taken freely during the day in cup doses. Take five or six times a day. Look under slippery elm to prepare.

Diet.—The diet should be very light for the first few days. A fruit diet is excellent. If fruit is not on hand, make a vegetable broth, as given in this book. It may be used as a hot or cold drink. It is a nourishing soup.

Give hot soybean milk over whole wheat flakes. This may also be taken by a small child or infant; for infants, put it through a fine sieve, and give in the bottle.

Soybean milk does not form curds like cow's milk.

Use plenty of fruit juices during an attack of tonsillitis; pineapple, and other citrus fruit juices are especially valuable.

Another excellent gargle: Steep a teaspoon wild cherry bark and sumach, a small teaspoon lobelia, powdered, in a pint of boiling water, one half hour. Gargle or swab the tonsils with it often, and swallow a little. Do this every hour, until the condition is better, and then as often as needed.

A tea may also be made from red sage, wood betony, or bistort, for an excellent gargle in tonsillitis.

Tobacco Habit

Tobacco is an active cause of stomach diseases. Smoking and chewing weakens and debilitates the digestive organs. Waste of saliva caused by smoking and chewing is one of the ways by which the system sustains loss and injury through the use of tobacco. Many girls smoke to keep thin. If smoking prevents excessive fat, common sense should tell them that it is very destructive to the system. The same can be said of the much advertised reducing pills and medicines. Everyone knows that the first attempt made to smoke usually makes one deathly ill and pale, causing vomiting.

I had the same experiences when first starting to use tobacco. It made me deathly sick, so sick I could hardly stand on my feet. But, gradually, the system becomes accustomed to it, builds up a resistance, and then the evil effects are not so noticeable, but they are still there. All the time I was using tobacco I was confident it was injuring my stomach and digestion, and when giving it up, I was extremely nervous and lonesome in the midst of pleasant surroundings. It took a long time until this feeling wore off. Had I known then what I now know, I could have overcome it in a few weeks, while then it took me half a year to accomplish it.

Tobacco very readily finds its way into the blood stream, and anything that affects the blood affects every organ and tissue of the body. It greatly harms the blood corpuscles and has a very damaging effect on the nervous system which causes poor circulation. Smoking is one of the causes of cancer of the lungs, and other lung diseases.

Tuberculosis, palpitation of the heart, intermittent pulse, cancer, inactivity of the skin, paralysis of the nervous system: persons suffering from any one of the foregoing diseases, who use tobacco in any form, in many cases, it could be directly traced to the use of tobacco.

Due to the fact that a woman's nervous system is more delicate than that of a man, the woman who smokes develops poisons and degenerates much more rapidly than men, thus, one of the last barriers for the protection of children from hereditary taint is fast giving way. Children born of parents who are tobacco users, more especially if the mother is a user, have weak vital organisms, nervous temperaments, and are much more susceptible to disease. The use of tobacco has so many bad effects upon the system that it is impossible to give each and every one in detail. The use of tobacco has a serious effect upon the moral character.

Too much emphasis cannot be placed upon the fact that people who use tobacco in any form will soon find their bodies in a weakened condition and cannot be as mentally alert and have as high ideals as those who do not use these poisons. Do we not see the truth of the above statements lived before our eyes every day?

The following treatment will be found extremely successful in curing anyone of the habit:

Go on a diet of fruit juices and vegetable broths for a period of eight to fifteen days. Vegetable broth is very nourishing and is therefore helpful in keeping up the strength.

Take plenty of hot baths, warm enough so that you perspire freely. At least one a day. Finish with a cold towel rub or spray. Remain in the tub as long as possible, thirty minutes to an hour, or longer if possible, keep continuously adding hot water. Put cold cloths on the head and throat if weak, or faint. Copious drinking of water while in the tub helps one to perspire more. Poisons are given off through the skin by means of perspiration. Rub vigorously while drying off, to increase the circulation. Those who take Turkish baths should have one every day, with thorough rubbing.

Red clover tea is very effective in cleansing the system. Use the blossoms, one teaspoonful to a cup of boiling water. Steep, and drink from five to twelve cups a day.

Magnolia tea is specifically used for the curing of tobacco habit. Also, myrtle leaves and seeds. Make the tea as you do other herbs.

Slippery elm tea is also excellent to drink while curing the tobacco habit.

The following herbs are also good: Scullcap, vervain, peppermint, catnip, nerve root, quassia chips, motherwort, angelica, burdock root (for cleansing the blood), black cohosh, blue cohosh, echinacea.

Typhoid Fever

Causes.—Typhoid is a communicable disease. Impure drinking water is responsible for a large majority of typhoid cases. Contaminated milk is also a great source of this disease. If the body were kept clean, and only pure food and water taken into the system, typhoid fever would be extremely rare.

Symptoms.—Fatigue, loss of appetite, weak digestion and headache. These symptoms increase for about three weeks, then the patient is in a serious condition. Then extreme weakness, tongue usually shrunken, abdomen enlarged, sometimes sharp and constant pain in the right groin, rapid pulse.

Treatment.—Pure air and good ventilation are essential in every case. If patient has a high temperature see fever diet in Table of Contents. Read article on "Fevers." A sponge bath of temperature agreeable to the patient should be given morning and evening, or much more often if patient has high temperature. Give a high herb enema every day using white oak bark, red raspberry leaves, or wild alum root. After giving the high enemas, inject two ounces of the enema tea into the rectum with a small syringe and retain. It will heal the ulcers in the rectum. The high enema and this solution injected will greatly relieve the patient, and will hasten recovery.

Pleurisy root tea is excellent when the skin is dry and hot. Give wild cherry bark tea when there is diarrhea. Cold cloths laid on the right groin will often stop bleeding from the bowels. Injections of cold witch-hazel tea are also helpful in this condition. (See Bowel Hemorrhages.)

Often those who suffer from typhoid fever have ulcers of the stomach and rectum. If such is the case, steep a heaping teaspoon of golden seal and one of wild alum root in a pint of boiling water, take a swallow every hour.

Have the patient drink all the water he possibly can. Orange juice and oatmeal water taken at separate intervals are good nourishment. A vegetable broth made from several vegetables, such as, carrots, celery, a little onion, and spinach, will be nourishing: strain it, and give as a liquid broth.

Tumors

There are many kinds of tumors. They are named according to the tissues involved, such as glandular, muscular, fibrous, fatty, and there are also cancerous tumors.

Any one of these tumors may enlarge rapidly and become ulcerated.

Tumors are invariably caused by impure blood and impurities of the system, unbalanced diet, constipation and a run down condition.

Sage poultices have been known to remove external tumors. Slippery elm poultice is also excellent. See Poultices in Table of Contents.

Take any one of the following teas internally in tumors, or a combination of two or three. Bayberry, slippery elm, mugwort, white pond lily, chick weed, sage, or wild yam. They are good.

When suffering from tumors, use the same treatment as for cancer.

Urine Difficulties

Scalding Urine.—The cause is uric acid in the system. Cleanse the system by taking the following herbs, and scalding urine will be overcome. Use equal parts of fennel, burdock, and slippery elm, or milkweed. Steep a teaspoonful in a cup of boiling water twenty minutes and drink cold one cup before each meal and on retiring. A tea of cubeb berries is excellent, used in the same way.

Drink plenty of pure water to wash out the kidneys and bladder. Go on a fruit diet for a few days to rid the system of uric acid.

Inability to Urinate.—Retention of urine is caused by inflammation, and swelling inside the bladder and neck of the gland causes an obstruction in severe cases. The bladder becomes enlarged. Pain from retention may be so intense that the patient will break out in a cold sweat, the odor of urine being very prominent.

Give a hot sitz bath repeatedly, followed by a short cold bath. If patient is bedridden, apply hot, with short cold, applications over the genitals, bladder, and entire length of spine. Give a high enema of catnip tea; this is very necessary and will cause natural urination when other means fail.

Inject into the bladder with a soft catheter, a tea made as follows: one heaping teaspoonful of golden seal, one-half teaspoonful myrrh, one-half teaspoonful boric acid; steep in a quart of boiling water, strain through a fine cloth. Connect the catheter with a fountain syringe, and inject into bladder. Retain this solution as long as possible. If the patient has not urinated for some time, draw the urine out before making this injection. Moisten the catheter with slippery elm tea. This makes it slip freely, is very healing and will thus help the condition.

(563)

Suppression of Urine.—Suppression is because the kidneys do not secrete the urine into the bladder. In severe cases the urine is almost completely suppressed.

Symptoms.—If the urine has not been secreted for several days, there will be severe symptoms, such as convulsions, extreme pain in the back and bladder. Always a great desire to urinate.

Treatment.—The patient should have perfect quiet. A very warm high enema of catnip tea will give great relief. Hot fomentations wrung out of smartweed tea, applied to the bladder and small of the back, will afford relief. Give two or three hot sitz baths a day.

Yarrow herb is especially recommended. Steep a heaping teaspoonful in a cup of boiling water for twenty minutes. Drink a cup before each meal and upon retiring. *Drink cold.*

This is an unfailing remedy for suppressed urine; use a strong catnip tea, hot as can be borne, as an enema; also drink freely.

Any one of the following herbs may be used to good advantage. See their descriptions and use those best suited to your condition. Make the same as yarrow given above. Hyssop, burdock, broom, cleavers, dandelion root, wild carrot, meadow sweet, gravel root, tansy, wahoo, corn silk, parsley, St. John's-wort, cubeb berries, milkweed, and buchu.

Involuntary Flow of Urine.—When this disorder is not caused by some other disease such as gout, palsy, stones in the kidney, etc., it can be easily remedied by using the following treatment. If caused by some other disease, correct that.

It will be helpful to sleep either on the side or face.

Take equal parts of white pond lily, sumach berries, white poplar bark, bistort root, and valerion. Mix together. Steep a heaping teaspoonful of this mixture in a cup of boiling water, take a cup one hour before each meal and on retiring. Drink at least four cups a day.

Plantain is also very good taken singly. Dose the same as above. It is all right to increase the dose, if you find it necessary.

Ulcers

Ulcers may form where the skin is cut or broken and does not readily heal. When the tissue has been destroyed by a burn, cut, or wound of any kind, pus may form. There are several classes of ulcers.

Treatment.—A light diet is necessary, and the food must be well digested. The bowels must move two or three times a day. Use laxative herbs and high enemas. Steep one teaspoonful of golden seal, and one-half teaspoonful myrrh in a pint of boiling water. This solution cannot be excelled as a cleansing wash and for dressings. Take a tablespoonful of this six times a day, internally. Mix together two teaspoonfuls of powdered golden seal, and one teaspoonful myrrh, sprinkle on the ulcer after it has been thoroughly washed. Bandage loosely with bandaging. See poultices for ulcers in Table of Contents.

Any one of the following herbs may be taken internally with benefit—read their descriptions and take the one or ones best suited to your case. Or use two or three, mixing equal parts thoroughly, and use a heaping teaspoonful to a cup of boiling water, strain, and drink four cups a day, one an hour before each meal, and one upon retiring:

Bayberry, golden seal, ragwort, lady's-slipper, chickweed, sage, wood sanicle, slippery elm, bogbean, ground ivy, bittersweet, agrimony, and raspberry leaves.

Varicose Veins

Causes.—Pregnancy, local obstructions, sluggish circulation, and long standing on feet.

Symptoms.—The blood veins become greatly enlarged and knotted. Dull aching pain. Ulcers may develop.

Treatment.—The diet should be simple and very nourishing. Be careful not to overeat in order that waste matter may not accumulate in the system. Take high herb enemas to cleanse the colon. Keep the bowels carefully regulated; they should move three times a day. Regulate them with food if possible; if not, use laxative herbs.

Cold morning baths should be taken regularly, rubbing the entire body vigorously and thoroughly with a wet cold towel, then a dry one. If cold morning baths were more widely used varicose veins would not be so common. When the veins are very large, use a rubber stocking, such as you can buy in drugstores; they give relief as the result of distribution of pressure. Bathing the limbs with white oak bark tea is very helpful.

I was once called to treat a very fleshy woman who was suffering with varicose veins. Every night in order to sleep she let her limbs hang out over the bed. I made some strong white oak bark tea, and had her bathe her limbs with it two or three times before retiring. It relieved her so much that she was able to sleep all night. I have seen some bad cases of varicose veins get well when this treatment is used. A cleansing diet and thorough cleansing of the system is necessary to make pure blood. It is necessary to have pure blood for a successful recovery.

Steep a heaping teaspoonful of golden seal, and a small half-teaspoonful of myrrh in a pint of boiling water for twenty minutes. Take a swallow six or seven times a day.

If there are open sores, apply healing lotion, recipe for which is given in this book.

Take one teaspoonful each of powdered hyssop, wild cherry bark and yellow dock root. Mix thoroughly and take one-half teaspoonful in a fourth glass of cold water, followed by a glass of water as hot as can be taken readily. Take this four times a day one hour before each meal and upon retiring. Tansy or coral may be used in this way with benefit.

Wounds and Cuts

If the body is in a healthy condition, a wound or cut will heal readily. Tie a banndage on the cut immediately to stop the bleeding. Wash the cut or wound with a solution of powdered golden seal and myrrh, steep a heaping teaspoonful of each in a pint of boiling water for twenty minutes. If the wound bleeds freely, tie it up in its own blood; this will cause it to heal readily. Apply liniment, as given in this book, all over it and around it. After bandaging, moisten it thoroughly with liniment five or six times a day or oftener. This aids healing, and relieves soreness and pain.

If the cut is large and gaps open, place it in the golden seal and myrrh solution, as hot as can be borne. Continue this, keeping the solution hot, until the wound closes. I have kept a wound in as long as two hours. When the wound is practically closed, press it together, sprinkle a little powdered golden seal on the outside, and bandage, using strips of adhesive tape to keep it together. Apply liniment all around it; this will relieve pain and inflammation. If on the hand, wear it in a sling, to prevent tearing the wound open again. If on the foot, it will be necessary to stay off the feet, or use crutches until healed.

I have healed many bad wounds in this way, without stitches, and without leaving a scar, and the patient does not suffer nearly as much. Be sure to apply the liniment freely; it will work like magic. If proud flesh should develop, it can be killed by sprinkling on burnt alum.

Wood sage is an excellent remedy for old wounds, or anywhere where there is inflammation. Use as a poultice.

Wood sage, self-heal, chickweed, golden seal, myrrh, slippery elm. These herbs can be effectively used as poultices and washes. See poultices in Table of Contents.

Whooping Cough

Whooping cough in its first stages appears very similar to an ordinary cough, but later develops into a peculiar cough and is recognized by the sound, very aptly termed a whoop. In most cases, if the cough were treated and the simple herbs taken as described in this book under coughs and colds, the whooping would be prevented. It is contagious.

A splendid remedy for whooping cough is wild cherry bark. Use in a tea. The following is also good: one teaspoonful each, red raspberry, cubeb berries, colt's foot, and a small teaspoonful lobelia herb. Put in a dish and pour on one pint of boiling water, allow to steep one half hour. Give a teaspoonful of this every hour until the cough is better.

Coughs

Coughs of all kinds, bronchial, asthmatic, and croup, are mainly due to a bad stomach. In all kinds of coughs, first, cleanse the system thoroughly. Take high herb enemas, and herbal laxative as given in this book.

Take one teaspoonful each of colt's foot, black cohosh, cubeb berries, mix thoroughly and steep in a pint of boiling water. Take a glassful every hour according to age. You can also make this into a syrup by adding a pound of strained honey or malt sugar, boil down to one-half pint. Take a little of the syrup on the point of a spoon every hour or two. When the cough is violent take every half hour. But it has a better effect without the honey or malt sugar.

When the cough is severe, as in whooping cough and asthma, it is a good thing to drink warm water, one cupful after another, as much as you can, then stick the finger down the throat to produce vomiting. It is more effective if you steep one teaspoonful of cubeb berries, and one-half teaspoonful lobelia in a pint of boiling water, and drink when warm. This will cut the phlegm, clean the throat and stomach of poisonous mucus.

In cases of croup, whooping cough, asthma, etc., it is very good to soak the feet in hot water, to which has been added a little mustard and salt.

One teaspoonful of strong pennyroyal tea taken every fifteen minutes, decreasing to every half hour after the cough is checked, is very beneficial. Make the tea by using a heaping teaspoonful of the granulated herbs or one-half teaspoonful of the powdered herbs to the cup of boiling water. You may sweeten with a little honey.

Thick slippery elm tea is extremely good in whooping cough; drink it freely, you may add lemon juice.

Any one or two of the herbs listed below may be selected to make into a tea, or use those given above. Make the tea by using a teaspoonful of the granulated herbs, or one-half teaspoonful powdered herbs to a cup of boiling water. Drink three cups a day, an hour before meals and one on retiring.

Tansy, wild cherry bark, hyssop, mullein, flaxseed, horehound, pepper weed, water cubeb berries, white pine, spikenard, colt's foot, blue violet, palmetto berries, thyme, golden seal, red clover blossoms, and lobelia.

Worms

Causes.—Diet, hygiene and constipation are usually at fault. Worms are found where the stomach is deranged from eating improper foods.

Symptoms.—Restlessness at night, picking the nose, gritting the teeth during sleep, dry cough. Worms sometimes cause spasms, fits, or convulsions.

Treatment.—The cause must be removed. It is easy to remove the worms, but this does not cure the disease. Do not eat food robbed of its life-giving properties, such as, white flour products, cane sugar products, vegetables cooked in lots of water and the water thrown away, peeled potatoes, candy, cakes, ice cream, etc. Meats of all kinds. Constipation must be overcome. The bowels must move three times a day, every day.

Fast two or three days, and eat raw pumpkin seeds, generously. You can eat as much as one pound a day. After doing this two or three days, drink freely of fennel seed tea; worms do not like this, it is sedative to them and they will pass from the body if the bowels are kept loose. Slippery elm tea taken freely will remove worms from the body and is good for the entire system. White oak barks tea used in an enema will remove pin seat worms.

An onion cut up and soaked for twelve hours in one quart of water, then squeeze the juice out and take for four days, will kill and expel worms. Take as much juice as possible, fasting while taking it.

Any of the following herbs are beneficial to those suffering from any kind of worms. Use them singly or in combination to suit the need. Read their descriptions and take according to directions given for use of non-poisonous herbs.

Wild yam, tansy, wormwood, bogbean, poplar bark, balmony, hyssop, wormseed, American worm root, meadowsweet, white oak bark, golden seal, bitterroot, fennel and slippery elm.

Food Preparations of Various Kinds

If all the refined breakfast foods and baked products on the market would be discarded and people would make their own bread from whole grain flour, their expenses would not only be very much less, but they would save a great deal of suffering and doctor bills. There are some institutions where when treating for Bright's disease, kidney, liver, or bladder trouble, they feed them exclusively on carrots for some time. It is not necessary, of course, to confine them to carrots alone, as there is a list of foods that could be taken to a good advantage for these diseases.

Much of the good food is ruined in its preparation, and more which is not ruined in preparation, becomes detrimental because served in too many varieties and often in too large quantities. Thus acids, gases, and fermentation are set up which spoil the food after it is eaten, and keeps it from making good blood.

White flour bread cannot impart to the system the nourishment that will be found in whole grain bread. The use of fine flour aggravates the difficulties under which those who have inactive livers labor. Most of the cheeses are not good food.

Most of the graham and whole wheat breads purchased in the grocery and other stores are unhealthful, as they contain various percentages of white flour, and are seldom baked enough. Bread is more healthful when eaten at least one day old. It should be baked clear through so that not any part of it is soft or gummy.

Composition of

Graham Flour		White Flour	
Energy	46%	Energy	46%
Protein	60%	Protein	52%
Calcium	26%	Calcium	9%
Phosphorus	126%	Phosphorus	21%
Iron	112%	Iron	21%

Diet Rules

1. Do not eat fruits and vegetables together.
2. Do not eat fruit and milk together.
3. Do not drink any liquid with meals.
4. Do not drink any water within an hour of meals.

Breakfasts

Shredded wheat	All-bran
Wheaties	Hot whole wheat cereals
Figs	Ripe bananas
Whole Grain Rice	Oatmeal
Dates	

When acid fruits are taken with breakfast, use only pure cream. No milk.

Luncheon

Fruit luncheons, eaten with whole wheat zwiebach, are very healthful, or it is better to have this meal at night, if it is possible to have the heavy meal in the middle of the day.

Apple sauce with raisins added

Whole grain rice with dates, or raisins cooked in it.

Apples	Cantaloupes
Peaches	Watermelons
Pears	Cherries
Grapes	Pineapples

Many times when fruit does not agree with one, if when it is taken and thoroughly masticated with whole wheat zwiebach there will not be any difficulty.

Dinner

Potatoes (baked or boiled with skins on)

Sweet Potatoes	Squash
Okra	Eggplant
Spinach	Cauliflower
String Beans	

Do not use tomatoes with a vegetable meal. All vegetables should be cooked plain and with as little water as possible, so that they are dry when done.

Normal Diet for the Average Person

First, observe the rules for eating. Second, this nation needs less spacious hospitals, more vitamins and better cooks. More care must be exercised in the cooking of food every day so as not to destroy in preparation, the vitamins, minerals, and life-giving properties. Third, seventy-five to ninety-five per cent alkaline food should be used in the everyday diet. If you have any ailments, then your diet should be at least ninety per cent alkaline base-forming foods. Eating acid foods brings on diseases, while alkaline foods overcome disease and prevent it.

Fruits

all berries	apricots	apples	pears
grapefruit	cherries	lemons	plums
pineapple	raisins	grapes	figs
quinces	bananas	prunes	dates
peaches	oranges	melons	limes

Do not use cane sugar on fruits. Do not eat bananas unless they have dark spots on them, and the ends are not green. Dried fruits are good if they are not sulphured. Do not mix more than two kinds of fruit at a meal. It is best to eat fruits raw. Apple sauce is very good if the whole apple is cooked, skin, core (unless wormy), and the seeds, then strain through a colander or sieve. Raisins added to apple sauce makes a very delicate dish.

Vegetables

asparagus	onions
beets	okra
beet tops	parsley
celery	greens of all kinds
cabbage (uncooked)	watercress
cauliflower	parsnip
carrots	pumpkin
cucumbers	rutabagas
turnips	sweet potatoes
tomatoes	squash
dandelions	Swiss chard
Irish potatoes (unpeeled)	sprouts from all
lettuce	beans, legumes, or grains
kale	spinach

Legumes

soybeans	garbanzos
green beans	chick peas

dried beans of any kind
split peas
lentils
lima beans

wax beans
navy beans
string beans
peas

Raw Diet

I believe in eating everything in its raw and natural state as far as possible, of the foods that can be digested. I just read an article by a man who thinks we should never cook anything, but eat it raw as people did in the beginning of time. But this fact is generally over-looked: Foods are not as they were in the beginning.

In the beginning, fruits, grains, and nuts grew all the year around, and there was no need to can, cook, and bake, as there is today. The wheat, rye, barley, oats, beans, and nuts were never hard and dry as they are now. There were fresh fruits and grains the year around, and they were eaten in their milky or grape-sugar state, in which they needed scarcely any digestion, like our green corn. We like to eat it when the milk comes out of the corn. It is then in the grape-sugar state, and can be easily digested. It requires very little cooking. After it matures and gets dry, it has turned into a starchy state, and no man has a digestive fluid with which to digest raw starch. Therefore we need to grind and bake it. If properly baked, it turns the starch back into grape-sugar, to a great extent.

Much impurity is produced in the system by too much protein. Now we know how to prepare our food, and what foods to eat to balance the amount of protein with other foods, to avoid overtaxing the system with too much protein. The corn, wheat, peas, and beans in their milky state, before they are full-grown, contain three or four per cent protein, but are high in minerals and life-giving properties. When they mature, the wheat has from eight to fourteen per cent protein; the dried corn a little less; while the beans have from twenty to thirty per cent more. All beans, lentils, and corn may be picked, and canned in the milky state. Being thus very low in protein, all can eat freely of them. Peas, beans, lentils, and grains can be sprouted (see Table of Contents how to sprout), which turns the protein into peptogen to a great extent, and the starches and sugars into dextrose and grape sugar. They are then very easy to digest. Also, the sprouts have a very good flavor, and are high in life-giving properties. Leafy vegetables, as spinach, lettuce, celery, and cabbage, are good taken in their natural state.

Fresh, cleanly prepared raw vegetable juices are excellent to supply the body with natural minerals, salt, and vitamins. It is necessary that they be properly macerated so that the life elements are released into the liquid.

Time Required for Digestion

Rice, boiled ....1 hr.	Bread, corn, baked 3¼ hrs.
Barley, boiled ....2 hrs.	Apples, hard and sour,
Milk, boiled ....2 hrs.	raw ....3 hrs.
Milk (raw) ....2½ hrs.	Apples, sweet and mellow,
Egg (soft boiled) ....3 hrs.	raw ....2 hrs.
Egg (hard boiled) ..3½ hrs.	Parsnips, boiled ....2½ hrs.
Egg (fried) ....3½ hrs.	Carrot, boiled ....3¼ hrs.
Egg (raw) ....2 hrs.	Beets, boiled ....3¾ hrs.
Butter ....3½ hrs.	Turnips, boiled ......3½ hrs.
Green corn and beans,	Potatoes, Irish
boiled ....3¾ hrs.	(baked) ....2½ hrs.
Vegetable hash,	Potatoes, Irish
warmed ....2½ hrs.	(boiled) ....3½ hrs.
Bread, whole wheat,	Cabbage, raw ....2½ hrs.
baked ....3½ hrs.	Cabbage, boiled ....4½ hrs.

Healthful Cookery

Food must be prepared properly to be well digested and thoroughly assimilated. Our physical well-being depends on this. Cooking does not receive the proper attention, due to its importance to health. A thorough knowledge of healthful cooking is as essential as well as good food.

Successful cooking depends largely upon the quality of the material used, which should be the best. Measurements must be accurate. The best food is often spoiled in preparation. When food is not prepared in a wholesome, appetizing manner, it cannot make good blood to build up wasting tissues. For health's sake it must be prepared in a simple form, and free from grease.

Ninety per cent of all human ills originate in the stomach, and are caused from overeating, wrong combinations of food, and unnatural foods.

Food properly cooked is always well digested.

Starch is converted into dextrin by dry heat at a temperature of 320° F.

All food should be prepared in one of the following ways: Boiled, steamed, broiled, baked, stewed, braising, roasting, or simmered. Do not use fried foods, except when you wish to occasionally warm something in a frying pan, but then it does not need to be fried hard. Fried foods are indigestible, and are poisonous to the system.

Cooking of Vegetables

The best way to cook vegetables is to bake them. Boiling is good if just enough water is used to cook them in and none thrown away. Waterless cooking, casserole baking, and low pressure steam cooking are also good.

When cooking vegetables in water, put them to cook in boiling water, using just enough water to cook them done; if there is any left, save it and add to your soups or broths. The vegetables must boil continuously after starting, otherwise they will be water soaked. It is not necessary for them to boil hard, just boil moderately.

Add salt in moderation just before they are entirely done; if salted when put to cook, it has a tendency to toughen them. Do not overcook vegetables, cook only until tender; overcooking destroys the life-giving properties. Do not add fats to vegetables when cooking; add your seasoning just before they are done, and serve at once.

Never peel or remove the eyes of Irish potatoes before cooking; the life of the potato is in the eyes and peeling. Do not peel any vegetable that can be used without peeling. Carrots, parsnips, salsify, rutabagas, and others may be scraped thinly, so as not to lose the minerals which are found just under their skins.

Green vegetables are very desirable during the winter months; if you think them expensive remember that they are far cheaper than the cost of sickness, and when they are properly prepared are real medicine.

Canned vegetables, if you get a good brand, are not as good as the fresh vegetables properly prepared, but they are good, and better than fresh vegetables poorly prepared.

For protein with your vegetables serve, Vegetose, Meatose, or To-Meta, or any nuts you like best. Nuts require thorough mastication, and they should be chewed to a creamy consistency so as to get the good of them, therefore, the meat substitutes which contain nuts are better for most people, as the nuts used in them have been ground.

Vegetables can be seasoned with soy mayonnaise, leaving out the lemon. Dilute it with cold water to the consistency of cream, or you can use as is. Rich soybean milk or one of the nut milks are good when added to hot vegetables; heat only a few minutes after milk has been added, and serve at once.

Good soybean milk can be purchased now, thus you can always have it on hand.

Eat all the non-starchy vegetables raw if they agree with you, such as, carrots, cabbage, cucumbers, radishes, and parsley.

VEGETABLES

Baked Potatoes

Select smooth, medium-sized potatoes, wash, and prick with a fork all over to let the moisture escape. Bake in a hot oven for forty to sixty minutes. Serve as soon as done, with soybean butter.

Mashed Potatoes

Boil potatoes with the skins on, or steam them until done. Remove skins, mash, season with salt and rich soybean milk, put in moderate to hot oven for one-half hour and serve at once.

Boiled Cabbage

Select a head of cabbage that has as many of the outside green leaves on as are fit to use. Slice in eighths, put in cooking pan and cover with sliced onion, pour boiling water over and cook for about twenty minutes, or until tender. Salt when about half done.

Carrots and Peas

Equal parts of carrots and peas can be cooked together until tender; season with rich soybean milk or soybean butter. Salt to taste.

String Beans

Wash, string and break beans about one-half inch long, or slice lengthwise. Cover bottom of pan with a little vegetable fat and put beans in pan. Salt and cover pan with tight lid until the beans are a bright green, stirring often so they will not stick, then, barely cover with boiling water, and cook until tender. Just before serving stir in soybean butter to taste.

Mixed Greens

Use as many kinds of greens as you wish, having them all as near the same tenderness as possible. Wash and chop. Rub kettle they are to be cooked in with a little garlic, add enough fat to just cover bottom of kettle well, put the greens in and cover tightly and cook about ten minutes. Salt and serve at once.

Eggplant

3 cups (diced about ½ inch size) raw, eggplant unpeeled	2 and ½ cups of tomatoes
	3 tablespoonfuls vegetable fat
½ cup chopped onions	Salt
½ cup green peppers	Flavor to suit with garlic

Put onions and peppers in hot fat and brown slightly, add eggplant and garlic and cook a few minutes, add 2 and ½ cups of tomatoes and put in oven and bake about 30 minutes in a moderate to hot oven. If you prefer—peel very thinly.

Beets

Use young beets. Cut the tops up fine and cook in hot water for fifteen minutes, add diced beets, dice about 1-8 inch square, add to the tops and cook until tender; salt and just before serving add a little soybean butter.

Okra

Select even-sized tender pods of okra, cook in just enough water to keep from burning until tender, salt and season with soybean butter just before serving.

Spinach

Wash until thoroughly clean, put in a tightly covered kettle and cook until tender, from five to ten minutes, salt when partly done.

Time Table for Cooking

Apples, sour	Medium hot oven,	30 min.
Apples, sweet	Medium hot oven,	45 min.
Asparagus	boiled	20 min.
Beets	boiled	until tender
Carrots	boiled	until tender
Cauliflower	boiled	until tender
Cookies	moderate oven	8 to 15 min.
Corn, green	boiled	5 to 8 min.
Cereals	1 hr. direct boiling,	2-4 hrs. in double boiler
Dried beans	boiled	'til tender, then bake
Eggplant, baked	hot oven	30 min.
Eggs, soft	put in boiling water,	turn fire off, 7-8 min.
Eggs, hard	boiled	30 min.
Gems and Muffins	quick oven, 375°F.	25 min.
Onions, boiled	boiled	until tender
Parsnips	boiled	45-60 min.
Peas	boiled	35-50 min.
Potatoes, boiled	boiled	35-45 min.
Potatoes, baked	hot oven	45-60 min.
Rice	boiled	20-30 min.
Rolled oats	direct boiling 45 min., double boiler 1 hr.	

Whole grain rolls and biscuits	quick oven	20-25 min.
Salsify	boiled	2 hrs.
Squash	boiled	until thoroughly done
String Beans	boiled	until tender
Sweet Potatoes	baked, hot oven	25 min.
Tomatoes	boiled	10 to 15 min.
Turnips	boiled	until tender

The Nutritional Value of the Soybean

"The soybean is going to revolutionize the food of humanity more than the potato did two hundred years ago, when it was a curiosity—and today is a staple food. It differs from the potato in the respect that it has been used for thousands of years as one of the principal foods of the Chinese.

"The Chinese nation exists today because of the use of the soybean as a food. China has survived five thousand years, its people have endured not only one, but hundreds of severe economic depressions, floods, earthquakes, famines and wars.

"Their recovery from these calamities is due largely to the use of the soybean, as it is a food which perfectly takes the place of disease producing meat, milk, and eggs. It contains all the life-sustaining properties of meat, milk, and eggs, and is far more economical and easier produced than any of these.

"If Americans were suddenly deprived of meat, milk and eggs and no more thought was given to planning our diet, than most of us do, the result would be a condition of malnutrition due to a shortage of protein in our food.

"The Chinese under similar circumstances have gone on living normal lives, simply by eating soybeans in some form. The Buddhist priests in the Orient are forbidden meat by their religion; in place of it they eat Tofu, a soybean curd and other soybean foods. The Chinese coolies, whose strength and endurance is traditional for carrying heavy burdens, rickshaws, etc., live chiefly on soybeans and rice. Chinese babies are dependent on the soybean for food, dairy products being rare in the Orient. Those babies which must be fed artificially are given milk made from soybeans. It is a scientific fact that physical development on a soybean diet is perfectly normal. History proves the value of soybeans as a food.

"Food chemists have conclusively proven that soybeans cannot only be substituted for more expensive foods but are more wholesome than those articles of diet. Today soybeans are one of the most economical sources of nourishment.

"Not only are soybeans suitable for all kinds of baked products, but soya flour or soybeans can also be used in breakfast foods, diabetic and infant foods, in pancake and self-rising flours, macoroni, doughnuts, pretzels, soy sauce, paté de foie gras, potted meats, meat loaf, and sandwich spreads, mayonnaise, soups, confectionary, beverages, coffee substitutes, beer, milk, cheese, ice cream, dog food, besides numerous industrial products. It is understood, of course, that food products containing soya flour should be properly labeled.

"Soya flour is considerably richer in protein than are the flours made from such other legumes as the navy bean, pea, lentil, lima bean, etc., and about four times as rich in this constituent as are the cereal flours. Soya flour protein is of especially good quality. Soya flour contains less than two per cent starch, whereas, starch is the main constituent in other cereal flour, containing as they do about thirty times as much.

"Soya flour is especially rich in the vitamines and in minerals. The amount of calcium is twenty times greater than in potatoes, twelve times that found in wheat flour, five times than that in eggs, about two times that amount present in liquid milk, and one-fourth as much as in dried milk. Milk has always been regarded as the calcium-food par excellence.

"One pound of soya flour is equivalent to two pounds of meat in protein content. To the extent that people might consume one-half pound of soya bread per day instead of ordinary bread, the extra amount of protein in the soya bread is sufficient to replace a quantity of protein in over one-fourth of the daily intake of meat on the average. Meat protein costs five times that of soya protein." *Taken from an address delivered by Dr. J. A. LeClerc, before the annual meeting of the America Soybean Association.* Sept. 15, 1936.

Proteins are muscle-builders and absolutely indispensable. There is a high quality protein content in soybeans, which makes them such a successful substitute for meat, milk, and eggs. They contain double the amount of protein found in beefsteak. They are the only natural food in the vegetable kingdom which contain higher protein nutritive value than meat, milk, and eggs.

Extensive experiments have shown that one can eat at least three times more soybean protein than meat protein or other beans higher in protein.

The soybean has life-giving properties which meat and other proteins do not have.

Uses of the Soybean for Industrial Purposes

Soybeans are used for the manufacture of artificial petroleum, automobile steering wheel rims, cable insulator, candles, casein, celluloid, core oil, crude and refined oil, emulsifier, electric distributor parts, illuminant (for lamps), hospital soap, hard and soft soaps, horn buttons, glue, hard curd soap, frying oil, glycerine, enamels, floating soap, foundry sand-cores, linoleum, lard, lubricant, laundry oil cloth, paints, photographic films, paper, plastic material, potassium soap, printer's ink, rubber substitute, silk-scouring soap, sea-water soap, shampoo mixture, silver soap, soy vinegar, toilet soap, varnish, textile dressing, transparent soap, waterproof cement, etc.

A knowledge of the value of the soybean here in America is one of the greatest things that was ever launched in the food line in the history of the nation, and at this time of great poverty, want, and disease, it is the most important thing that could be given the people.

Any one with a piece of ground may raise his own soybeans. They will not only greatly improve the soil and make virgin soil out of worn out soil, but at the same time they will supply the family with most delicious and nourishing food. Soybeans should be planted at different intervals throughout the summer in order to have shelled soybeans all summer. The green soybeans can be shelled just like any other bean or pea. Some varieties do not shell easily, but these can be easily removed from the shell by first boiling for just a few minutes.

Soybean milk can be made from soybeans at home for less than two cents a quart. The Yellow Mammoth, Dixie, Illinois, and Tokio soybeans are among the best varieties for soybean milk, but there are other varieties which are better for green shelled beans. W. J. Morse, Senior Agronomist, of the U. S. Agriculture Experimental Station, Washington, D. C. can give most valuable information along this line, as he has made, and is still making, extensive experiments with soybeans, and is thoroughly acquainted with that subject.

For stomach ulcers, duodenum ulcers, cancer and diabetes, as well as liver, kidney and bladder troubles, soybean milk is not only a good food, but a real medicine. It is easily digested, it does not curd, is highly alkaline, and is rich in mineral matter.

The soybean is one of the greatest and most complete foods that we have. In the Orient, it has been used for some time for stock feed, and to improve the soil. But only recently has much effort been made to use it for human consumption. At the present time, there are many people in various sections of the United States who are experimenting with it to some extent with considerable success.

The objection to the soybean is that it does not have a flavor as pleasant as some of the other beans. However, the flavor can be overcome by preparing the beans in a different way for human consumption.

I have experimented with soybeans for fifteen years and have produced a fine, acceptable soybean milk as well as many other soybean products.

I can make a soybean bread, buns, pie, pones, roast, cottage cheese, soybean cheese—which is very similar to Philadelphia Cream Cheese, also American Yellow Cheese. Also soybean coffee, ice cream, without any cane sugar in any product. My soybean milk is simply delicious, very palatable, and children like it as well as adults.

I use soybeans in more than fifty dishes. Soybean milk properly made is a wonderful food for the sick.

Soybean milk does not form hard curds in the stomach and putrify as cow's or goat's milk, and can be used in the same ways they are used. Beans and peas cook quicker when they are boiled in soybean milk, than when they are boiled in water. It will sour and clabber like cow's milk, and after souring, can be beaten up into most delicious buttermilk. The beauty of it is that it is highly alkaline, and is well adapted for the human system, for both adults and children.

Many pay a big price for goat's milk, while soybean milk is infinitely better for human consumption. It does not have the contamination of the animal in it, nor the liability to disease and putrefaction.

The following is an analysis of human, cows, goats, soybean and nut milk as given by the United States Department of Agriculture, Bureau of Chemistry and Soils, Washington.

Milk	Water	Ash	Protein	Fat	Carbohydrates
HUMAN	89.95%	0.25%	1.30%	2.50%	6.00%
Cows	87.30	0.80	3.20	3.50	5.20
Goats	87.00	0.50	4.00	4.50	4.00
Soybean	87.03	0.52	2.40	3.15	6.90
Nut	87.00	2.03	5.60	5.50	7.23

To the soybean milk used for the above analysis, I had added a little emulsified soybean oil, and a little malt.

Soybean Cheese

5 lbs. raw peanut butter
1 qt. tomato puree
5 qts. soybean milk

(587)

Take five pounds of raw peanut butter, add one quart of tomato puree, or if you prefer a strong tomato flavor, use two quarts. Stir in gradually five quarts of soybean milk, and put in a warm place until it develops lactic acid, or until it gets about as sour as cottage cheese. After it has developed lactic acid enough and is as sour as you like, put it in cans (either No. 2 or No. 3), place in a large vessel, wash boiler or kettle, and cover with boiling water. Let this cook for four of five hours. If you have a steam pressure cooker, cook under five pounds pressure for two or three hours. The cheese is then ready for serving.

Soybean Cream Cheese

Use unsweetened soybean milk. Let stand until it thickens (not sour) put on the stove and boil a minute or two until the water separates from the whey. Put in a cheese cloth and wring dry. Run through the mill used in making the milk until it is a smooth paste. Add a little rich soybean milk to soften and make a creamy consistency. Salt to taste. Kloss' Mayonnaise may also be added with advantage.

Nut Cheese No. 1

1 lb. raw peanut butter
1½ pts. water, or soybean milk
½ lb. soybean butter
Salt to taste

Pour the water in the peanut butter very slowly, stirring to a paste, gradually adding water until the entire amount has been used. If soybean milk is used instead of water, a better product is obtained. Let stand until it sours to suit the taste, thus developing lactic acid like the lactic acid in buttermilk. Beat in the soybean butter. Put in cans, seal, and place in a vessel to cook for four or more hours as directed for cooking soybean cheese.

If you have a pressure cooker, the canned cheese should be cooked under five or six pounds of pressure for four hours.

Nut Cheese No. 2

    1 lb. raw peanut butter
    4 tablespoonfuls ground oatmeal flour
    1½ pts. water
    Salt to taste

Prepare in the same manner as directed for Nut Cheese No. 1.

Some of the Nut Cheese which I make is much like the yellow American Cheese and others are similar to cream cheese. They are very agreeable to the taste, are high in food value and emulsified nut oils, are much easier to digest, and contain none of the harmful bacteria of ordinary cheeses found on the market. These nut cheeses may be put up in cans to keep them pure and sanitary. They are prepared in a way that develops lactic acid such as is found in Yogurt buttermilk and cottage cheese.

Those who cannot eat ordinary cheese made with rennet can eat freely of nut cheese, and there is no exposure to disease as is the case with other cheeses.

Nut cheese is more economical, and may be used in any way that the cheeses on the market are used. More food value is obtained for the money.

Malted Nut Cream

    1 lb. raw peanut butter
    ¼ lbs. malt honey
    2 oz. Diastase malt powder

Mix the ingredients together and put up in cans. It will keep indefinitely. No cooking is required.

I prefer the malted nut cream to the malted nuts which are sold on the market at a high price.

Malted Nuts

1 cup raw peanut meal or raw peanut
butter (peanut meal is preferable)
½ cup malt honey
Few grains of salt

Mix well. Place in a slow oven until thoroughly dried out, but do not brown. Then run through a mill, but do not set mill too tight as it must remain in a powder form, and not be as a butter. If iron pans are to be used, lay heavy brown paper in the bottom of them so the nuts do not come in contact with the iron. If the oven is too hot, the nuts will turn too brown. Or, the nuts may be dried in the sun and put in the oven for a while, or just long enough to cook them.

Nut Milk

1 cup raw peanut butter
½ cup milk sweetening
1 cup boiling water
Few grains of salt

Mix the peanut butter and the milk sweetening thoroughly together. Use a heaping teaspoonful of this mixture to a cup of boiling water. Thoroughly mix, adding salt.

This may be used as any other milk.

Kokofat

This is the pure fat extracted from the cocoanut, and is one of the richest fats on the market. It takes one-fourth less kokofat than any other fat in cooking. For instance; if you need one pound of butter or Crisco in cooking or baking, you only need three-quarters of a pound of Kokofat to get the same results.

You can melt it, add some dandelion butter coloring, salt to taste, harden again, and use in place of cow's butter. It can be used for baking and cooking in any way that you would use butter. Makes very nice pie crust. Is sweet, has no foreign taste and keeps a long time without getting rancid.

Cocoanut Oil and Nut Butter

The ordinary cocoanut oil will melt between 70° and 80° F. When it is below 70° F. it is hard and quite white. When it is hard, melt it and add some salt and common "Dandelion" butter coloring to give it the shade of ordinary cow's butter.

When the weather is hot, we put it in the ice box or some cool place and are able to spread it on bread like butter. In the winter, we keep it in the cupboard or any place where it does not melt or get so hard it will not cut.

Cocoanut Oil Butter

> 1 lb cocoanut oil
> ½ lb. peanut oil
> Butter coloring
> Salt to taste

A fine butter is made by mixing these ingredients with an egg beater or an electric beater, beating until they are cold. It is a wholesome butter with a delicious flavor.

To Blanch Peanuts

Buy shelled nuts and heat slightly. Do not heat too much, only until a very light golden brown. Just heat enough so they are slightly dextrinized. Rub between the hands, or place on a table and lightly press with a rolling pin to loosen the skins sufficiently to enable one to blow them away.

Peanut Butter

1 lb. blanched, raw peanuts
1 lb. cocoanut oil
Butter coloring
Salt to taste

Boil peanuts until they are done, but not enough to make them fall to pieces. Do not use too much water. Run the peanuts and cocoanut oil through a peanut butter mill, salt, add a very little dandelion butter coloring. This is a very excellent and wholesome butter. Peanut butter made this way can be diluted with water and used like cream, or spread on bread.

Mock Almond Butter

Take one pound blanched peanuts, cover with water, boil until they just begin to get tender, but not mushy. Drain off the water and dry the peanuts thoroughly. This can be done in the sun, or in a very slow oven if they are stirred frequently, *but the nuts must not be browned at all.* Grind them fine. This makes an excellent butter which can be used in many ways. Add water until it is of the consistency of milk or cream to eat with vegetables or fruit.

This same butter may be reduced with water, beaten in cocoanut oil with butter coloring added, and salted to taste, making a palatable and nourishing butter which is easy to digest.

Canned Soybeans

Soak the beans overnight in water. In the morning pour the water off, put them in a warm place, and let them sprout about a half inch. Parboil for four or five minutes, pour the water off; then put them in any kind of a vessel and let boil until they are tender. A little tomato and onion added makes a very palatable and wholesome dish.

They are much better if cooked in a steam pressure cooker for about forty minutes or more. Some beans require more and some less cooking, depending on the variety.

Soybeans and Rice

Boil the sprouted soybeans until tender. Boil rice separately. Mix approximately equal parts, add tomato sauce and some cubes of nut-meat. Mix these all together and place in the oven.

If the flavor of the soybeans is too strong, they may first be parboiled in strong salt water for a few minutes.

Baked Beans with Tomato Sauce

Use any kind of beans, soak them overnight in cold water, and the next morning mix them with the tomato sauce, or other seasoning if you prefer, and bake in a stone jar about four hours in a hot oven. One who cannot eat beans prepared in the ordinary way can eat them baked in this fashion.

These beans after soaking overnight, may also be put in cans about three-quarters full, and fill the can to the top with water, salting the water before pouring it in the can. Or use half tomato sauce and half water. Seal and cook in steam pressure cooker, using ten pounds pressure for about an hour and a half. Some beans require a little less and some a little more cooking. Test them out for yourself. Old beans require longer cooking than new ones, but all beans should be thoroughly soft and tender. Prepared properly, they will not produce gas and will digest more easily.

Another way to prepare beans is to cook them until almost dry, then put them in a pan or some kind of a dish, add some soybean milk, put in the oven and bake thoroughly. This adds to the flavor and digestibility of the beans, and makes them more alkaline.

The marrowfat bean is very fine and cooks easily. The lima bean is alkaline and therefore one can eat it more freely than the navy bean, and some of the others.

Soybeans are, no doubt, the best of all beans, but the flavor is not as pleasant. This can be overcome by using various seasonings, such as tomato sauce, a little onion, and celery.

Vegetable Roast

8 ounces strong cereal coffee
1 pound washed gluten
5 ounces of raw peanut meal
Salt to taste

Run this mixture through an Enterprise mill two or three times. Put it in cans, seal, and cook in steam pressure cooker for about four hours under five pounds of pressure; or if in an open kettle, for six hours. This can also be put in a stone crock, placing the crock in a dish of water and baked four hours in a moderate oven. The placing of the crock in the dish of water is to prevent the meat from burning.

This product will be found to be an excellent product when cut in cubes, to combine with any kind of a vegetable stew that the housewife may wish to prepare.

Vegetarian Roast No. 1

2 tablespoonfuls ground onions
2 cups raw peanut butter
½ cup boiled kidney beans
3 cups water
Ground celery seed to suit taste

Mix the ingredients, put in cans, seal, and cook for four hours under five pounds pressure. This can be placed in a crock and baked in the oven as described in directions for Vegetable Roast.

Vegetarian Roast can be used diced in roasts, stews, and soups. It is good sliced and browned for sandwiches.

Vegetarian Roast No. 2

1 pound raw peanut butter
1½ pints water added slowly, stirring continuously to make paste free from lumps.
Salt to taste.
Boil from one to four hours

Can be boiled in a double boiler or in the oven by placing the dish containing the roast in a dish of water to prevent it from burning on bottom and sides. May also be cooked in sealed cans.

This should be of such consistency that when it is cold it can be sliced and eaten. Children and people with delicate digestions may eat this. This is good made up into sandwiches, also diced in roasts or in stews and soups.

Original Meat

1 pound of washed gluten
8 ounces strong cereal coffee
5 ounces of raw peanut meal
Salt to taste

Run this mixture through an Enterprize mill two or three times. Put in cans and cook for four hours under 5 pounds pressure, or 6 hours in an open kettle.

Vegetarian Meat

1 pound raw peanut butter.
1½ pints of water added slowly stirring

continuously to make a paste free from
lumps

Salt to taste

Boil from one to four hours

Can be boiled in a double boiler or in the oven by putting dish containing it in a dish of water to prevent it from burning on bottom and sides or put in cans, and seal and cook under five pounds steam pressure for four hours.

Tometo

Work it just like the Vegetarian meat, except take one-half water and half tomato juice; or you can take all tomato juice if you like.

Tomato Vegetarian Roast

Work like the Vegetarian Roast No. 2, except take one-half water and half tomato juice. If a strong flavor of the tomato is desired, use all tomato juice and no water.

Vegetable Salmon

1 lb. raw peanut butter

1 medium sized carrot (grind very fine)

1 No. 2 can of tomatoes, put through a fine
sieve

1 pt. water

Mix ingredients thoroughly, salt to taste. It is then ready to be put in cans, if desired, and cook under five pounds steam pressure for fours hours. If cooked in an ordinary kettle, well covered with water, it will require a little longer boiling, one and a half to two hours longer. The mixture can also be baked in the oven. First, boil it a few minutes in an open saucepan, stirring constantly until it thickens, and bake in a slow oven for one hour. It is then ready to serve. This is a very wholesome and palatable dish.

Vegetable Protein

Take five pounds of strong gluten flour, which is ordinarily called bread flour. (It can be obtained at large mills, bakeries, or wholesale grocers.) Add two quarts of water, and make into a fairly stiff dough, about the consistency of bread dough. Let stand for one hour after mixing. Then put in a large pan and cover with water Wash out the starch by working it with both hands. When the water becomes white with starch, pour it off, and put on fresh water. Repeat this until the water is clear; then all the starch will be washed out.

If it is desired to have it very tender, cover this gluten with water and let stand a day or two under water. If the weather is cool it should stand about two days, but in warm weather, a day will be sufficient time. Do not let it stand too long, however, for the gluten will dissolve.

Then cut the gluten mass in small pieces, dropping, as it is cut, into a pan of boiling water, containing enough water so that the gluten will float. Stir with a pancake turner on the bottom so it will not burn. Let cook for half an hour.

Remove from the water what is desired for immediate use and add a little soybean sauce, or Behrend's Horta Extract. This gives it a meaty flavor.

Always keep the gluten covered with water, both before it is cooked and afterwards.

It can be warmed in a frying pan with a little Mazola or corn oil, seasoning with finely cut oinions, if desired. Too much frying makes it tough, however.

This vegetable protein can be used in stews, pot pies, vegetable roasts, or any place where lean beefsteak is used. It is excellent in vegetable soup.

The flour used is not like the ordinary white flour, for it has more food value and more vitamins.

Pillsbury's Best, Gold Medal, and other bread flours that are used by the bakers are high in gluten.

Nut Loaf

2 cups brown rice, cooked	2 tablespoonfuls soy sauce
1 cup nuts, chopped	2 tablespoonfuls onions
½ cup whole wheat bread crumbs, toasted	2 tablespoonfuls celery
Soy milk to moisten	Salt to taste

Chop onions and celery fine, mix all ingredients together thoroughly, add more soy milk if too dry and bake in moderate oven ¾ hour.

Nut Roast

2 cups sprouted lentils
2 cups washed gluten

Mix together and run through an Enterprise grinder two or three times. Season with a little tomato, Vegex or sage. Salt to taste. Cook four hours in sealed tins under five pounds pressure. If cooked in an open vessel or double boiler, six hours cooking is required.

To cook in the oven, make the material into a loaf and cover with water—not too much. Place this dish into another containing water and bake. (This is done to prevent burning.) When done pour the liquid off the loaf and use this for a gravy. It may be thickened with corn meal and seasoned with Vegex or Vegetable Extract.

Malt Honey

Take one pound of wheat or cornmeal. Add eight quarts of water. Let it come to a boil and boil it until it thickens so that the starch is cooked. Cool to between 140° F. and 170° F. Then add two ounces of barley malt, either in powder or syrup form. Stir. Let stand until the starch is changed into dextrose or malt honey. When the water is clear, pour or siphon it off, being careful not to get any mash from the bottom, otherwise the malt honey will not be clear. Now boil it down to the consistency of syrup.

Old Fashioned Granola

Take whole wheat flour and enough water to make a stiff dough. Roll it out about a quarter or half an inch thick. Put in oven and bake until it is partly dextrinized, nearly a golden brown. Take a hammer and break it up, and grind through a Quaker City Mill made by the A. W. Straub Company of Philadelphia. After grinding, put in a baking pan and reheat to slightly dextrinize it.

Kloss' Granola

2 cups whole wheat flour
1 cup soybean mash (or 1 cup soybean flour)
Soybean milk

Prepare this in the same way as given in the recipe for old fashioned granola, using a sufficient quantity of soybean milk to make a stiff dough.

Granola No. 1

1 cup whole wheat flour
1 cup cornmeal
1 cup cotton seed meal

Mix and prepare in the same way as given in the recipe for old fashioned granola.

These granola recipes can be baked into loaves of bread, raised with yeast, and when a day or two old, can be broken up while the bread is still a little moist and run through a mill, then put in a baking pan and reheated.

Boiled Rice

1 cup natural brown rice
4 cups water
Salt to taste

After washing the rice, place it into the boiling salted water, stirring until it rolls up in the rapidly boiling water. Let it boil in this way until it swells, then set into the outer boiler (of double boiler) and cook more slowly. Do not stir after it begins to swell. It will require one hour or more to thoroughly cook brown rice. The kernels should be very tender.

Baked Rice

½ to ¾ cup natural brown rice
2 cups soybean milk
½ teaspoon salt

Wash and drain the rice. Pour the hot milk into a baking dish and add the rice. Cover and bake in a slow oven two to three hours without stirring, or until the milk is thickened and creamy with rice. If the milk boils out under the cover, the oven is too hot.

This makes a very delicious dish, and does not require any additions. However, if a dressing is desired, milk sweetening, the recipe for which is given in this book, may be diluted with a little water or soybean milk and poured over the rice. Fig marmalade, the recipe of which is also given in this book, may be diluted and served with it.

An excellent rice pudding can be made by adding one-half cup malt honey and one cup of raisins just before placing the rice in the oven to bake.

Breakfast Wheat

1 cup natural whole grain wheat
3 cups water
Salt to taste

Place in a double boiler and cook until the kernels burst. Raisins, stoned dates, or chopped figs may be stirred into the wheat just before serving. These give a natural sweetness, and are far better for the system than adding sugar.

This may also be cooked in a steam pressure cooker until the kernels are done, or in a crock in the oven, having the crock setting in a pan of water to keep the wheat from burning. This requires about four hours.

Dixie Kernel No. 1

1 cup cornmeal
1 cup oatmeal
1 cup whole wheat flour
1 cup finely ground bran
1 teaspoonful salt

Mix these ingredients and add enough water to make a stiff dough. Roll out to about one-half inch thickness. Bake in a moderate oven until slightly browned. When a day old, grind up while still a little moist.

Add one cup of water to a cup of malt honey, mixing thoroughly. Sprinkle this over the ground cereal product. Do not let the mixture get too moist. Now spread out to partly dry, and then place in an oven to dextrinize, making a slight golden brown.

This is a very delicate breakfast food and is tasty.

Old Fashioned Dixie Kernel

Take various kinds of broken crackers, such as bran, whole wheat, oatmeal, graham and white, and grind them together.

Take equal parts each of malt honey and water, stirring well together, and sprinkle over the ground crackers, mixing them up thoroughly to slightly moisten them. Place in the oven, stirring frequently to prevent burning, and slightly dextrinize to a golden brown.

This makes a very delightful breakfast food.

BEVERAGES

Soybean Coffee

Place the quantity of soybeans you desire in a dripping pan and heat in a hot oven, stirring frequently to prevent burning.

Watch them closely and thoroughly stir them as they have a tendency to burn, and will get much darker inside than on the outside while roasting. The outside hull seems to brown less rapidly than the inner portion, so you will find it necessary to take a few out occasionally, breaking them open with a hammer, to see just how they are roasting. To get a good flavored coffee, it is necessary to have an even roast. If part of the beans are not roasted quite enough, and some of them a little too much, it spoils the flavor of the coffee. After they are roasted, grind them through a mill quite coarse. Get some coffee and compare the color so you will know how brown to make it. Half bran and half soybeans may also be used for a good coffee.

Cereal Coffee

Cereal coffee is a product that is used very much nowadays, and can be made very easily at home.

Take the quantity of rye you desire and place in a dripping pan. Stir with a wooden paddle, until it becomes as brown as coffee. Grind rather coarse in any little hand mill. It is now ready for use.

Sometimes when roasting the whole grain, it is well when it gets nearly done to just take a little out with a spoon, lay it on a solid board and break up with a hammer in order to determine the brownness of it.

It is a good thing to have a little coffee, which was purchased in a store, in a little glass container so the brownness of it can be easily compared with the home-made coffee.

Cereal Coffee No. 2

Wheat bran is used in this recipe. Mix equal parts water and malt honey. Moisten the bran—a pound or whatever quantity you desire, with the water and malt honey mixture, let it get quite dry, or altogether dry before roasting. You may use Karo syrup in place of malt honey.

It may be placed in the sun or where it is airy to dry, so it does not sour before it gets dry.

When dry place in a dripping pan, in a hot oven, stirring frequently, until it is as brown as coffee. The flavor of this kind of coffee is very pleasing.

Half bran and half rye may also be used. The rye, however, must be ground, before mixing with the bran. This makes a fine-flavored coffee.

The bran for this coffee may be purchased from a feed store. It is much cheaper than bran put in packages and sold at the grocery stores. The ordinary bran run in large mills is just as clean as the flour from which the bran is taken, not touched by human hands. It runs out of the spout into a bag, and is perfectly clean and safe to use. Instead of paying ten cents to fifteen cents per pound for it, it will cost you only two cents or less per pound.

Bran Water

To two cups of bran, add one quart of water, let it stand overnight. In the morning strain through a fine sieve or cheese cloth.

To be used in any kind of soup stock, stew, or any breads in place of ordinary water.

Bran Broth

Cook one and a half cups of the bran water (as given above) for about five minutes. Add one-half cup of soybean milk. More or less of the bran water and soybean milk may be taken, depending, of course, upon the amount required to suit the need, but this is a good proportion to use. Season with Vegetable Extract or Vegex, and parsley.

Oatmeal Water

To one quart of water, add one cup of oatmeal, soak overnight. In the morning, strain through a fine sieve or cheese cloth.

This is to be used in soup stocks, stew, or breads in place of water. It increases the vitamins and makes soups creamy.

Soybean Broth

Soak two cups of wheat bran in one quart of unsweetened milk. (Soak one cup of oatmeal in one quart of soybean milk, strain overnight.) Stir up several times in the morning and strain. Pour one pint of boiling unsweetened soy milk on four heaping tablespoonfuls chickweed, let stand for half hour and strain. Mix the three ingredients together, adding one quart unsweetened soy milk. Add diced celery and onions for flavoring. Simmer together to thirty minutes, adding three tablespoonfuls Kloss' mayonnaise. A few minutes before it is finished, add one cup of very finely cut parsley. This broth contains all the ingredients the body requires.

Oatmeal Broth

Prepare oatmeal water as given in the recipe above, and cook five minutes. To every three-fourths cup of oatmeal water, add one-fourth cup soybean milk. Season with Vegetable Extract, or Vegex.

A very excellent drink can also be made by taking one part each, bran water, oatmeal water, heat together, adding soybean milk, and seasoning to taste. A little parsley or onion or celery lends a pleasing flavor.

Herb Broth

2 cups wheat bran
1 cup oatmeal
4 tablespoons chickweed water

Soak 2 cups wheat bran in one quart of water, also one cup oatmeal in a quart of water overnight. Stir up several times, then strain. Pour one pint of boiling water on the chickweed, let steep one-half hour, strain: Mix the three ingredients together, add one quart soybean milk. Parsley finely cut may be added for flavoring, or season with celery or oinons as preferred. Let simmer for a few minutes and serve. A little Kloss's mayonnaise may also be added.

This broth contains all the ingredients the body requires.

Soybean Buttermilk

Buttermilk is an excellent article of diet for everyday use, but is especially beneficial in malnutrition, tuberculosis, toxic conditions, and intestinal infections. Soybean buttermilk has the advantage of producing an alkaline effect and is more nourishing than ordinary buttermilk. It is rich in minerals and very palatable. More nourishing than yogurt buttermilk used under various names.

Use unsweetened soybean milk. It may be made of the whole milk, or let stand and skim. Let stand until sour as desired, or just clabbered and not sour, beat up with an egg-beater, and salt to taste.

Potassium Broth

2 cupfuls bran
1 cup oatmeal
4 quarts water

Soak overnight, beat up with egg beater and strain through a fine sieve.

Wash throughly 4 medium-sized potatoes and slice thin, also 2 large carrots, 2 medium sized onions (if onions are not liked, leave out), 2 large stalks celery with the green leaves, cut fine, ½ bunch of parsley cut up, 2 good sized vegetable oysters. Cook these in the bran or oatmeal water.

Let simmer in covered kettle until vegetables are done, mash up vegetables and strain again through fine sieve.

Herb Drinks or Teas

Coffee, tea, chocolate and cocoa are harmful to the system, but all of the teas named below are very fine to drink to take the place of harmful drinks. The herb teas are rich in medical and chemical properties. Some are very healing to the stomach and a good tonic, others prevent fermentation and gas in the stomach and bowels, also prevent griping. Some are very excellent to overcome nausea and vomiting and all of them have a splendid beneficial effect on the system. There are some that are nice to take in the evening before retiring to induce sleep. All of them are soothing and quieting to the system.

In order to select the one best suited to your need, look in the Table of Contents for the description of each of the herbs given. Some are most wonderful medicine for children and others are fine for pregnant women to prevent nausea and vomiting. Others are good for those with diarrhea, bowel and colon trouble. They are not expensive.

peppermint	fennel	hyssop
spearmint	strawberry leaves	rue
alfalfa	hop blossoms	chickweed
horsemint	sassafras	catnip
green celery leaves	yellow dock	wintergreen
mint	meadowsweet	camomile
sarsaparilla root	juniper berries	birch bark
chicory	red raspberry leaves	(small twigs)
calamus rt.	sage	
dandelion	wild cherry bark	
red clover blossoms	(the small twigs)	

Herb Tea

Use one heaping teaspoon of the herbs granulated, or if powdered use one-half teaspoon, to the cup of boiling water. Place the herbs in a pan, and pour the boiling water over them, allowing it to steep one half hour. Cover. This steeping draws the mineral elements out of the herbs which elements are very beneficial to the system.

These teas are less expensive than coffee, tea, etc., and they are healthful, beneficial and not harmful.

Soybean Cheese

5 lbs. raw peanut butter
1 quart tomato puree

5 quarts soybean milk
Salt to taste

Thoroughly mix the raw peanut butter with the tomato puree (you may use two quarts tomato puree if you prefer a strong tomato flavor). Stir in gradually five quarts soybean milk, put in a warm place until it develops lactic acid, or until it gets about as sour as sour cottage cheese. After it has developed lactic acid enough and is as sour as you like, put it in tin cans (either No. 2 or No. 3), seal them and place in a large vessel, wash boiler or kettle, and cover with boiling water. Let this cook for four or five hours, keeping covered with boiling water. If you have a steam pressure cooker, cook it under five pounds pressure for four hours. The cheese is then ready to be opened and served.

Soybean Cottage Cheese

Make in the same way as ordinary cottage cheese. Allow the milk to sour or clabber, then heat to body temperature until it separates from the whey. Drain in a very fine sieve, or through cheese cloth. When it has drained dry, add a little rich soybean milk to soften and flavor, as you would add cream to ordinary cottage cheese. The addition of a little Kloss' mayonnaise improves the flavor, makes a richer product, salt to taste. Some add a little honey, this makes it a tasty spread for children, and is a splendid nerve builder. Use unsweetened soybean milk.

Soybeans and Rice

Boil the sprouted soybeans until tender. Boil unpolished rice separately. Mix approximately equal parts, add tomato sauce and some cubes of nut meat. Mix all together, and place in the oven. Bake slowly, leaving uncovered the last few minutes to brown the top.

If the flavor of the soybeans is too strong, they may be parboiled in strong salt water for a few minutes, before mixing with the rice. Be sure to wash them thoroughly after parboiling.

To Sprout Soybeans, Lentils, or Grains

Cover well one pint or any amount you desire of soybeans (or others) with water and let stand overnight. Pour off water. Keep them moist. Rewash two or three times daily, keeping them moist, and in a dark place, for approximately three days until well-sprouted. Allow to stand until the sprouts are about one-half inch long. Lentils are prepared in the same manner, but do not take as long as soybeans. Soybeans may be allowed to sprout until they are an inch long, and then only the sprouts are eaten. The sprouts would need only ten or fifteen minutes cooking.

The sprouting of any bean or pea turns the protein into peptogen, to a great extent, and the starch into dextrose or maltose. The sprouts are very high in vitamins, more so than spinach, lettuce, or celery.

Cook sprouted beans or peas, as any bean or pea, only they do not require cooking as long. Salt to taste.

Soy Patties

2 cups soybean pulp
2 cups natural brown rice (cooked)
2 tablespoonfuls vegetable fat

Flavor with garlic or sage
1 onion chopped fine
1 tablespoonful soy sauce
½ teaspoonful salt

Mix ingredients thoroughly together, make into patties, roll in whole wheat bread crumbs and bake in greased pan until brown, or warm in a frying pan, but do not fry.

Gluten Patties

2 cups ground gluten
2 cups crumbled zwiebach, or cooked brown rice
1 onion finely chopped
½ cup soy sauce
½ teaspoonful salt

Flavor with garlic, vegex, or sage.

Mix thoroughly, make into patties, and brown in oven or frying pan.

Soybean Loaf

2 cups soybeans, cooked and ground
2 cups bean pulp
1 cup tomato juice
1 cup finely chopped nuts
1⅓ whole wheat zwiebach crumbs, toasted
1 onion chopped fine
2 tablespoons soy sauce
Salt to taste

Mix ingredients thoroughly together, add sage, celery seed, thyme, or some flavoring you like, put in greased baking dish and bake one hour in moderate oven.

Soybean Cottage Cheese Loaf

3 cups soybean cottage cheese
¾ cup raw peanut butter
1 cup whole wheat bread crumbs (toasted)
¼ cup peanut oil
6 tablespoonfuls lemon juice
6 tablespoonfuls soy sauce
1 tablespoonful chopped garlic
1 heaping teaspoon sage
pinch cayenne pepper
½ cup celery
Parsley
1 cup onion
½ cup green pepper
Salt to taste

Chop the celery, parsley, onion, and pepper fine; mix with the lemon juice, soy sauce, peanut butter, and cottage cheese, add the other ingredients, mix thoroughly, and bake in a moderate oven.

Soybean Milk

Take one pound soybeans, soak them overnight, well covered with water. In the morning wash them thoroughly, cover with fresh water and bring to a boil. If the water is changed again a couple of times and brought to a boil it helps to remove the soybean taste after the milk is made. Then drain, and grind. Put in a sugar sack, or cheese cloth that is not coarse, tie the top securely. Put the sack of ground soybeans in a large dish or pail. Pour two quarts of water over them; warm water is preferable as the milk has fat in it. Knead the sack of ground beans well, washing and squeezing the milk out—pour off in a large pan or pail. Pour on two more quarts of water—knead and squeeze out well again. Pour the second two quarts of milk with the first two quarts in large flat-bottomed dish, and boil twenty minutes or more—stirring constantly with a pancake turner from the bottom of the pan until it boils, when it is boiling it will not stick to the bottom of pan.

Sweeten with malt honey, honey, or malt sugar. Do not make it too sweet. Salt to taste. *Do not cook in aluminum.*

Soybean Milk No. 2

Take one pound soy meal (do not have it ground too fine), three quarts of cold water. Mix and boil 25 minutes, strain, sweeten and salt to taste. It is best to use a flat bottomed pan, and stir with a pancake turner, as it burns very easily. If you desire it richer add some soybean cream.

These soybean milks may be used in the same way as cow's milk. When using for cooking do not sweeten. This milk is highly alkaline. It must be handled in the same way as cow's milk. When cooled, keep in ice box or cool place, as it will sour in about the same length of time as cow's milk. You may add the sweetening to the milk as it is used—it keeps sweet longer before the sweetening is added.

This soybean milk makes a more nourishing and healthful chocolate milk than dairy milk.

The best grinder to use for grinding the wet soybeans is Enterprise Grinder No. 69, manufactured by the Enterprise Manufacturing Company, Philadelphia, Pennsylvania.

How to Curd Milk

After making the soybean milk, while the milk is boiling hot, add enough citric acid so it will curd at once. It takes three or four tablespoonfuls of the citric acid to the quart of boiling milk. Stir briskly and let set. The curds form within a few seconds, and it doesn't take long until the milk is curded. Skim the curd off the clear water and place in a double cheesecloth, squeezing out all the water, making the cheese as dry as possible.

If a smooth cheese is desired, use less citric acid. If a granular cheese is liked, use more citric acid.

Soybean Jelly

4 cups soybean milk (unsweetened)
2 rounded tablespoonfuls agar-agar (flaky)
4 tablespoonfuls malt sugar

Soak the agar-agar in the soybean milk one hour. Put in a saucepan, bring to a boil and simmer slowly until the agar-agar is entirely dissolved, add the sweetening and cool.

Fresh fruit, or fruit juice may be added for flavoring, if desired. Put on ice.

Soybean Butter

½ pt. water
2 tablespoonfuls soybean flour

Mix together, and put in a heavy iron frying pan, boil five minutes, or until thickened. Strain into a mixing bowl. Pour in one pint of soybean oil, very slowly, as in making mayonnaise, beating constantly. (You may use any good vegetable oil.)

Soybean Cream

1 pt. rich soybean milk
½ pt. soybean oil (any vegetable oil)

Place this in a mixing bowl, and pour the oil in a very small stream, beating constantly, until it is the desired thickness; if you desire a thick cream use more oil, if a thin cream, use less.

If you do not have any soybean milk, use a heaping tablespoonful of soybean flour, and one-half pint of water. Place in a frying pan, stirring with a pancake turner, let it boil until thickened, five minutes or a little more, then strain, and proceed as above, beating in oil until you have the desired thickness.

Soybean Ice Cream

2 qts. rich soybean milk
2 lbs. malt sugar
½ pt. soybean butter, or soybean
    mayonnaise
1 tbsp. agar-agar

Soak the agar-agar in cold water until it swells, drain and put in soybean milk, add the malt sugar, and butter or mayonnaise. Put on stove and let boil for five minutes. Strain through a fine or cheesecloth. Add any crushed fruit or fruit juice you desire, or vanilla. Put in a freezer and freeze as any other ice cream. Ice cream made in this way can be melted and fed to invalids and infants. Ice cream should not be eaten with meals.

The Yolk of an Egg

You may use the following in any recipe where it is desired to use the yolk of an egg; it looks very much like egg yolk, tastes like it, and has very much the same properties.

Take one heaping tablespoonful soybean flour, mix with a half cup of water, put in a frying pan and boil until it thickens, stirring constantly so it does not stick. Strain into a mixing bowl, and beat in Soya bean oil until it becomes thick enough to be cut with a knife. Use this wherever a yolk of egg is desired. Season with a pinch of salt, and use dandelion butter coloring for a little added color.

Pancakes

1 cup cornmeal
1 cup soybean mash
1 cup soybean milk
½ cup malt sugar
½ cup soybean butter
Salt to taste

To the cornmeal and soybean mash add the soybean milk and beat up as ordinary pancake batter. Add the malt sugar, salt, and beat in the soybean butter.

If the batter is used when very cold, the pancakes can be made nicely without yeast or baking powder. If the pancakes are for breakfast, it is well to soak the cornmeal in the soybean milk the night before.

Some like it made with yeast: for this purpose, take one cake of Fleischmann's yeast, dissolved in the milk, and proceed as above, letting it rise about an hour before baking.

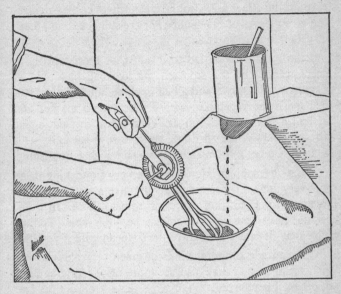

A UNIQUE ARRANGEMENT FOR POURING OIL IN MAKING MAYONNAISE OR SOYBEAN BUTTER AND CREAM.

SOUPS

Vegetable Soup

Take about one cup each of the following vegetables: carrots, cabbage, celery, one-half cup onions, potatoes, (do not peel the potatoes, but scrub with a wire brush, so the eyes will remain in the potatoes as they are the life-giving part). Add one gallon of water. After it has come to a boil, add one cup of brown rice, and simmer this slowly from one to two hours, or more. Salt to taste.

When soup is done, take off the fire and add one quart soybean milk, more or less to suit the taste. Use the green leaves of the celery and also the green leaves of the cabbage. The green leaves of the cauliflower are still better and these are generally thrown away.

If the soup is to be fed to invalids, or those who have ulcers, cancer of the stomach, or to small children, let it simmer at least two and a half or three hours slowly, and then mash the vegetables with a wire potato masher and let boil a few minutes longer. Then strain through a fine wire strainer. When all done, add the soybean milk. This is a most wonderful alkaline dish and highly nourishing.

When the soup gets cold, it is a very nourishing drink and very high in vitamins and life-giving properties, far superior to sauerkraut juice or tomato juice. In some certain cases tomato juice might be preferable. Tomato juice may be added instead of the soybean milk if you like.

One can add different kinds of green vegetables to suit his own taste, and may also use more of one kind and less of others if pereferred.

Vegetable Soup No. 2

2 large carrots (do not peel)
4 turnips
4 onions
parsley (use generously)
green leaves of cabbage (chopped)
medium bunch of celery (using leaves)
1 cup lima beans
1 cup green peas, or you may use a cup of puree made from the dried split peas and lima beans.

If you do not like onion, use soy sauce for
    flavoring, to suit your taste.

Cut the vegetables in small pieces, and do not boil hard,
let them simmer until cooked soft. Add a little salt when
finished.

Potato and Onion Soup

6 medium-sized potatoes (with peeling) sliced fine
3 good-sized onions (cut fine)
5 tablespoonfuls parsley (chopped)
2 quarts water

Let simmer for one hour, then add one heaping tablespoonful each of soybean flour, and oatmeal flour, mixed
thoroughly with a little cold water, then add to the soup
and let boil five minutes and serve.

Soybean butter can be used in place of the soybean and
oatmeal flours, using a heaping tablespoonful, to be added
to the soup just before serving. Use salt moderately.

Fruit Soup

(My parents used a great deal of fruit soup when I was
a child.)

2 cups raisins
2 cups prunes
2 lemons
1 cup grape juice (unsweetened)
4 quarts cold water

Use malt sugar or honey to sweeten to taste.

Add raisins and prunes to the water and let them simmer
until done (it would be good to first soak them overnight
in the water, then they will need very little cooking) add the
grape juice and lemon sliced very thin, and the sweetening
to taste. This can be served hot or cold as you desire.

(617)

Do not serve this soup with a vegetable meal; use the whole wheat zwiebach, whole wheat crackers, or any of the whole grain products, soybean gems, and nut products, or nuts; used in this way it makes a fine luncheon or fruit meal.

Cream of Tomato Soup

6 cups very rich soybean milk
6 cups rich tomato juice
6 rounding tablespoonfuls soybean flour (make into a thin paste with cold water)

You may also use a milk made from any nuts in place of soybean milk, milk made from raw peanut buter is excellent, and also almond milk.

Heat the tomato juice, add the soybean flour paste, stirring constantly; do not let it boil, just simmer; in five minutes stir in the thickened tomato juice into the hot milk, let heat a few minutes, add a pinch of salt and serve.

Tomato Soup

3 cups rich tomato juice
3 cups cold water
3 heaping tablespoonfuls soybean flour

Mix the tomato juice and water, and bring to a boil. Make a thin paste of the soybean flour mixed with cold water, stir this into the hot tomato juice, and let simmer five minutes. A heaping tablespoonful of soybean butter may be added to this (dilute the buter in a little cold water and put through a fine sieve before adding to the soup) let the soup get real hot, add a pinch of salt and serve.

All nut milks may be used in place of soybean milk. Flavor with a little soy sauce if desired, to taste.

Soups can be made from any combinations of vegetables one likes, celery, carrots, potatoes, parsley, onions, okra are very good. Dried beans such as navy, lima, marrowfat beans, green split peas, soaked overnight in water and cooked very slowly until throughly done, then put through a fine sieve or colander to remove any of the outside covering of the bean that may not have cooked up soft. If the sifted pulp is too thick, thin out with soy or nut milk, flavor with onion, garlic, or parsley, which should be cut very fine and added to the sifted pulp and heated about ten minutes before serving. Soy sauce, Savita, or Vegex is good for flavoring. Use salt moderately. Never use black or white pepper, read the description of cayenne (red pepper), in this book.

The soybean is king of the beans. It is a fine alkaline food, and there are many varieties of the soybean. For cooking purposes get the easy cook variety, as this one cooks much quicker than other varieties. It is best to cook soybeans under a low steam pressure, five pounds pressure for forty or sixty minutes for most varieties. They should be cooked until tender, not mushy. Always soak the beans overnight before cooking. It is best to cook all beans under a low steam pressure.

A good soy soup is made just as you make any other bean soup. They can be procured in cans, which makes it easier for the average home to use them more freely. They are a wonderful food.

Much is said about vegetable juices, and they are good, but everyone cannot take raw vegetables juices. Make your own vegetable juices by using any vegetable or vegetables you wish. The dark leafy vegetables are very good. Cut the leaves fine, put them in cold water, bring to a boil and boil gently until the juice is extracted, squeeze out all the juice by putting them in a bag (quite fine). Then you have a real vegetable juice; use hot or cold. Flavor with soy sauce, onion juice, or any vegetable flavoring you like.

Tomato Soup

1 quart water
1 tablespoonful 3-minute oats
1 quart tomatoes
1 tablespoonful cocoa fat
Salt to taste

Cook the three-minute oats in boiling water ten minutes; put the tomatoes through flour sieve, add to water and cocoa fat, boil five minutes. Salt and add a little of Kloss's mayonnaise before serving.

Cream of Tomato Soup

1 quart rich soybean milk
1 pint tomato juice
Salt to taste

Boil the milk for two or three minutes. Take it off the stove and let cool down a little. Add the pint of tomato juice and a little Kloss's mayonnaise and salt. Serve hot.

Do not boil the soup after the tomatoes are added. It can be reheated, but do not boil.

More tomato juice may be added if a strong tomato flavor is desired.

Oatmeal water made by soaking four parts of water to one part of oatmeal overnight and then strained is an excellent addition to any soup stock. It increases the vitamins and makes the soup creamy.

Cream of Corn Corn Soup

1 pt. fresh, or canned corn
3 pints rich soybean milk

Salt to taste

Heat the milk, put the corn through a sieve, add to hot milk, salt to taste and serve.

Cream Celery Soup

1 cup diced celery
1 pt. soybean milk
½ teaspoonful salt
½ pt. water
2 tablespoonfuls soybean butter

Cook the celery in the milk and water and when nearly done, add salt. Simmer until celery is soft. Add soybean butter just before serving.

Cream of Lentil Soup

1 qt. water
3 cups cooked lentils (sprouted preferable)
1 pt. rich soybean milk
Parsley

Put the lentils through a sieve, add the soybean milk, and one quart of water; salt to taste. Season with onion, and a little vegetable extract. Just before serving, add finely cut parsley, and 2 tablespoonfuls soybean butter.

Lentil Soup

2 cups cooked lentils
¼ cup chopped carrots (cooked)
¼ cup chopped green onions
1 cup tomato juice
2 cups lentil juice
½ cup finely cut parsley

Mix all the ingredients, heat to the boiling point, add one tablespoonful soybean butter, salt to taste, and serve.

Vegetable Oyster Soup

3 cups vegetable oysters (cut in small rings)
2 cups water
2 cups rich soy milk
1 tablespoonful soybean butter

Cook the vegetable oyster rings in the water until tender, add the soybean milk, and butter, salt to taste and serve.

Egplant Soup

3 cups diced eggplant (¼ inch square)
3 cups water
2 cups soybean milk

Cook the eggplant in the water until tender, then add the soybean milk, salt to taste, and add one tablespoonful soybean butter while very hot, just before serving.

Cream of Spinach Soup

1 cup spinach pulp
2 cups rich soy milk
1 cup mashed potatoes
(as given in this book)
2 cups potato water

Mix the spinach pulp and soybean milk, add the mashed potatoes and potato water, salt to taste, bring to a boil, add one tablespoonful soybean butter and serve.

Potato Soup

3 cups mashed potatoes
2 tablespoonfuls chopped onions
1 pt. rich soybean milk
1 quart water
Parsley or watercress for seasoning

Make the mashed potatoes by recipe in this book. Mix ingredients together, bring to a boil, add one tablespoonful soybean butter, and serve.

Split Pea Soup

Use green or yellow split peas. Rub the cooked peas through a sieve. To the pea puree add rich soybean milk until it reaches the desired consistency. Some gluten meat diced small will add greatly to this soup. Season with onions, garlic, parsley, or soybean sauce. Vegetable extract may also be used.

GRAVIES
Oatmeal Gravy

1 qt. boiling water
4 oz. oatmeal flour or three-minute oats
1 tablespoon mineral oil
Vegex or vegetable extract (to taste)
Salt

Season with bayleaf, onion, or desired flavoring.

Into one quart of boiling water stir gradually the four ounces of oatmeal flour, or three-minute oats. Boil until thickened. If three-minute oats are used, a little longer boiling is necessary than when oatmeal flour is used. Add about one tablespoonful mineral oil, or corn oil, or any other good oil. The gravy may be seasoned with a little onion, bay leaf, or other seasoning desired. Add a little (1 teaspoon) Vegex or vegetable extract which will give it a meaty flavor.

This makes a very wholesome and well-flavored gravy.

Soybean Gravy

Into one quart boiling soybean milk, add oatmeal flour

or three-minute oats to make the desired consistency, or thickness. Oatmeal works quickest.

Let simmer until thickened, stirring with a pancake turner so it will not burn on the bottom. Add a little soy sauce or vegetable extract to lend a meaty flavor.

This may be made with water instead of milk, and enriched with a little Kloss's butter, and a little fine cut onion to add to the flavor.

French Toast

Slice soybean bread about one-half inch thick and let dry in the sun or a moderately warm oven. When thoroughly dry, increase the heat in the oven enough to brown it golden clear through. This browning turns the starch into dextrose or grape sugar, making it practically like the juice in ripe fruit.

Now immerse the toast in soybean milk, being careful not to leave it too long. Lift out with a pancake turner, and spread a thin coating of Kloss's mayonnaise on each slice. Have your frying pan hot with a little oil in it, place the toast in with the side down that has the mayonnaise on it. Now, spread the top side with mayonnaise, leaving until the under side is browned, then turn it over until the top is browned.

Serve with diluted malt honey, honey, or maple syrup. French toast can be served with any meal, but is especially nice for breakfast. French toast, with a cup of hot soybean milk, is nice for a light supper.

This toast makes a wholesome and easily digested dish, containing all the necessary food elements.

Zwieback

Bread baked in the ordinary way is never entirely dextrinized, or the starch turned into grape sugar, therefore, zwiebach or twice-baked bread is very wholesome and easy to digest.

To make zwiebach, slice the bread about three-quarters of an inch thick, and let it dry out in the sun, or a slow oven, until it is entirely dry. Increase the temperature of the oven and brown the bread to a golden brown. It must be carefully watched, as it burns easily.

Canned Wheat

Soak two cups of the whole grain of the wheat as it comes from the field, in one quart of water, overnight. In the morning wash the wheat thoroughly, add one quart of water and boil in an open kettle, until thoroughly swelled.

Fill your cans with the wheat, within an inch of the top, add salt water, and seal. Cook one hour under five pounds steam pressure. If you do not have a steam cooker, boil on the stove, covering the cans with water, for one and a half hours.

Breakfast Wheat

1 cup natural whole grain wheat
3 cups water
A few grains of salt

Place in a double boiler and cook until the kernels burst. Raisins, stoned dates, or chopped figs may be stirred into the wheat just before serving. These give a natural sweetness and are far better for the system than adding sugar to cereals.

This can also be cooked in a steam pressure cooker until the kernels are done, about one hour, or in a crock in the oven; set the crock in a pan of water to keep the wheat from burning. This would require about one hour.

SALADS

Salads are refreshing and life-giving if made of any combination of vegetables which are fresh and crisp.

Do not combine fruits and vegetables in the same salad as it is not a healthful combination. Have your vegetable salads with your vegetable meals, or make a good nourishing vegetable salad and eat with nuts or some good meat substitute for luncheon. Another time have a fruit salad with nuts or some good meat substitute for luncheon or with a fruit meal.

Do not use mayonnaise that has vinegar, mustard, black or white pepper, or cane sugar in it. Make your own mayonnaise if you wish to use mayonnaise. (See recipe for soy oil mayonnaise.)

Vegetable Salad No. 1

1 cup finely diced or grated carrots
1 cup finely diced celery
1 cup cabbage chopped fine
1 green pepper cut in thin rings or fine slices
1 cup finely cut parsley

Mix the carrots, celery and cabbage together and put as large a serving as you wish of these on lettuce leaves, arranging the rings or slices of green pepper around the mixed vegetables and garnish with whole sprigs of parsley. Ground nuts sprinked over this makes a very nourishing salad or you can use the nuts whole; ground nuts are the best as very few people will chew the whole nuts enough to thoroughly emulsify them, thus they do not get the good of the nuts. Soy mayonnaise is very nice with this salad, and also a few olives arranged around or over it.

Vegetable Salad No. 2

Green peppers
Cucumbers
Celery

Green Onions (spring)
Parsley
Radishes

Watercress

Use equal parts of these vegetables, chop or dice the green onions and celery, and green peppers, mince the parsley and watercress, mix and place a serving on lettuce leaves. If the cucumbers are nice, with a thin fresh skin, do not peel, but wash well and cut in thin round slices, or lengthwise and arrange with radishes around and over the other vegetables.

Potato Salad

Potato
Onion (green preferred)
Parsley

Celery
Cucumbers

Prepare the potatoes by boiling with the skins on, and drying them out when done so they are dry and mealy. Cool the potatoes and skin them, making your salad for use immediately if you wish the best flavor.

Have the onions, celery, and ripe olives chopped quite fine, mince the parsley, and mix with your diced cucumbers and potatoes. Leave the skin on the cucumber if it is a nice thin skin. Salt moderately, add finely ground nuts or halves of walnuts, and a pinch of cayenne. Mix with soy oil mayonnaise, and garnish with radishes and parsley. Never use stale potatoes in making potato salad; it is much better to have them fresh cooked.

Fruit Salads

In making fruit salads be careful of your combinations. Citrus fruits do not combine well with other fruits, such as, dates, figs. Avocados may be used with citrus fruits. Combine these as you wish (avocados) using figs and dates as a garnish. When using avocados drop some lemon juice over them. Any kind of nuts may be used with a fruit salad, or finely ground nuts sprinkled over the salad makes it more nourishing.

Good Combinations for Fruit Salads

1. Ripe bananas, fresh cocoanut, shredded or ground, cherries and pineapple (Dried cocoanut may be used.)
2. Apples, raisins, walnuts
3. Bananas, apples, and pineapple
4. Ripe strawberries and ripe bananas
5. Red raspberries and bananas
6. Black raspberries and bananas
7. Ripe pears, strawberries, and bananas

Fresh cocoanut is a good combination with a fresh fruit.

All berries and fruits must be vine-ripened and tree-ripened to be really valuable for food. Be careful that bananas are fully ripened; they must not show any green on the ends and must be sprinkled with black spots generously over the entire skin, before they are really ripe, and valuable for food.

Fruit salads look nice served on fresh crisp lettuce leaves, but do not eat the lettuce if you serve them this way. Soy oil mayonnaise diluted to the consistency of cream is delicious with fruit salads.

Soy Oil Mayonnaise

1 heaping tablespoonful fine ground soy flour
½ pint cold water
½ pint soy oil

1 tablespoonful lemon juice (More or less to taste)
Pinch of salt

The addition of paprika or cayenne is healthful; read description of each in this book.

Color with a vegetable butter coloring.

Mix the soy flour into the cold water, boil for five minutes. Cook in a smooth flat-bottomed dish, using a pancake turner for stirring to keep free from the bottom of the dish, as it burns very quickly. Strain through a fine sieve into a medium size mixing bowl. While beating rapidly and continuously, pour in the soy oil in a very fine stream. If the oil is poured in fast, the mayonnaise will separate after standing a while. (If this should happen, pour the oil off, and beat again.) It will be very simple after you have made it a few times. Then add the salt, coloring, paprika and cayenne, and beat just enough to mix well. It needs only a small pinch of cayenne to make it taste snappy. Using more or less soy oil may make it any consistency you wish. Peanut oil may be used in place of soy oil. And a fine oatmeal flour can be used in place of soy flour, but I prefer the soy oil and soy flour.

A clove of garlic cut and rubbed on the bowl in which the mayonnaise is made greatly adds to the flavor.
Add soy oil buter here.

Kloss's Mayonnaise

1 egg
½ pint mazola or corn oil

Beak the egg into a mixing bowl with a round bottom and beat with an egg beater. Add the oil very slowly, beating continously until the oil is all beaten in. Salt to taste just before you finish beating.

This mayonnaise can be used anywhere that dairy cream is used. It makes a very fine dressing for cole slaw or any kind of greens.

Lemon juice and a little cayenne pepper may be added if a snappy mayonnaise is desired. To add the cayenne pepper, put a little in a cup and pour boiling water on it, then add this to your mayonnaise slowly until it has the desired flavor.

Red pepper or cayenne is a wonderful medicine, and does not injure the product. Cayenne pepper should not be classed with black and white pepper, or mustard and vinegar, which are found in the mayonnaise on the market and are highly injurious to the digestive tract, and stomach. Look in the Table of Contents for red pepper.

A little of the cayenne may be sprinkled directly into the mayonnaise, beating until it is throughly mixed.

Mayonnaise

Dilute one-half cup raw peanut butter (or mock almond butter as described in this book), with one cup of water. Then beat in one cup of oil, either corn, olive, or cotton seed oil. Add about 1 tablespoon lemon juice. Salt to taste.

This can also be boiled for two or three minutes, and then beaten thoroughly.

Sooth-o-Lax

1 lb. malt honey
1 lb. mineral oil

Add the oil to the malt honey very slowly, beating constantly, as when making mayonnaise. When finished it may be diluted with water and used as a dressing over fruits, puddings, vegetable jell-o, or oatmeal jelly.

Milk Sweetening

1 cup malt honey
1 cup corn oil, or olive oil

Pour the corn or olive oil into the malt honey, beating constantly, pour slowly. In this way the fat is emulsified and easily digested.

Fruit Salad

½ cup wheat flakes
½ cup diced or chopped raw apples
½ cup chopped raisins

It is best to soak the raisins overnight before using. More or less of any ingredient may be used to suit the convenience and taste. Mix ingredients together and serve. This makes a salad that anyone can live on.

Some like it very much with the Sooth-o-lax dressing, used as is, or diluted with a little water.

Wholesome Desserts

Fruit pies may be considered healthful when the crust is made of whole wheat flour and well baked; it has a rich nutty flavor, and requires a little less shortening than when made of white flour. The rich starchy pie fillings and custards are among the most objectionable of all desserts.

Brown Betty

1 tbsp. lemon juice
1 cup whole wheat zwie-
   bach crumbs
1½ cups seedless raisins
¼ tsp. salt
1 qt. chopped apples
1 scant cup brown sugar

Spread half the raisins over the bottom of a pudding dish, cover raisins with half the chopped apples, sprinkle over the apples half the sugar and half the crumbs, sprinkle over this the remainder of the raisins. Sprinkle on the rest of the sugar and crumbs, add salt and lemon juice to one half cup of water and pour this over top of pudding, set pudding in a pan of water, cover and bake an hour. Remove from the pan of water, and bake without the cover long enough to brown the top slightly. Serve with vanilla sauce.

Vannila Sauce

To the required amount of soybean cream you may add malt sugar and vanilla. This makes a delicious sauce, to be used in the place of starchy sauces, and whipping cream.

Vegetable Gelatin

To prepare agar-agar for dessert, soak one tablespoon of agar in one pint of warm water thirty minutes, drain and simmer twenty minutes in another pint of warm water, and boil until dissolved. To this amount, after straining, which will reduced by boiling, add a pint of any desired fresh fruit or fruit juice. Bananas, peaches, or any other fresh fruit may be sliced in the bottom of each mold to give variety. Before serving, decorate with crushed nut meats. For dressing, use the vanilla sauce, or soybean cream.

Orange Jelly

1 cup malt sugar	¾ cup orange juice
1 tsp. grated orange rind	¾ cup water
1 tbsp. vegetable gelatin	3 tbsp. lemon juice

Mix the orange juice, rind, lemon juice, pinch of salt and sugar, add the water; when boiled gelatin is ready, add the other ingredients, mold, and serve with soybean cream.

Strawberry Jelly

1 tbsp. agar	1¾ cups crushed straw-
2 tbsp. lemon juice	berries

1 cup malt sugar   Few grains salt
1 cup boiling water for agar

Prepare as for orange jelly; when cool decorate with strawberry halves, and serve with crushed nuts or soybean cream.

Baked Apples

Wash the apples and remove the cores without cutting open, fill the place from which cores were removed with raisins or dates, and bake in a flat baking dish with a little water in bottom. Nut meats may also be used with raisins, which add to the flavor. Serve with a nut cream.

Stuffed Dates

Remove the stones with a sharp knife, cutting lengthwise, and replace with pecan meats or others if preferred. If you wish to remove the skins, scald them, draining well. As a rule they should always be scalded to remove dirt.

Rice Pudding

1 cup soy cream   1 cup cooked natural rice
Pinch of salt   1 cup drained pineapple

Mix together, chill and serve. Other fruits may be used in place of pineapple.

Cream Tapioca

⅓ cup malt sugar   ½ cup tapioca (minute)
½ cup soy cream   2½ cups soybean milk

Soak the tapioca in soybean milk fifteen minutes, add the sugar, salt, and bring to a boil, stirring constantly. Place in a double boiler, and cook until tapioca is transparent. Add vanilla, chill and serve with soy cream.

(633)

- BREADS

Principles of Bread Making

Breads are divided into classes: fermented and unfermented. Fermented bread is made light by a ferment, yeast usually being employed. Unfermented bread is made light by the introduction of air into the dough or batter. This method will be spoken of later.

Yeast or Fermented Bread

Fermented bread is generally made by mixing flour, water, salt and yeast to a dough. A small amount of malt extract, malt honey, or honey may be added, if desired, as it increases the food value and hastens fermentation. This is the straight dough method. This dough is kneaded until it is elastic to the touch and does not stick to the board, the object being to incorporate air and to distribute the yeast uniformly. The dough is then covered and allowed to rise until it has doubled its bulk, and does not respond to the touch when tapped sharply, but gradually and stubbornly begins to sink. At this stage, the dough is "ripe," and ready to be worked down. It will require all the way from two to three and a half hours to rise, depending on the grade and consistency of the flour used, and the temperature of the room in which it is set, and the amount of yeast used. This process is best accomplished at a temperature ranging from 80° F. to 90° F. The bread is again worked down well, turned over in the bowl, and left to rise until about three-fourths its original bulk. Then it is turned out on a board, worked together enough to work out the air, and cut up in the size pieces desired for a loaf. For an ordinary loaf it takes a pound and three or four ounces of the dough to make a pound loaf after it is baked. Mould the pieces until the air has been worked out and leave it on the board a few minutes so it will rise just a little. You will find that this improves the texture of the bread. Then form into loaves and knead it just enough to work out the air. Do not knead too much. With a little experience you will become a master at bread making.

Sponge Bread

Bread is also made by setting a "sponge" at the beginning by making a batter of the water, the yeast, and part of the flour, and letting it rise until it is light, then adding the remaining ingredients and working all into a dough. This is called the sponge method. Bun and cracker dough is usually set with a sponge, as they require a very fine and light texture, which is best obtained by this method. Ordinary white and entire wheat breads are often made by the same process. A sponge is light enough when it appears frothy and full of bubbles. The time required will vary with the quantity and quality of yeast used, and with the temperature of the room in which it is set to rise.

Yeast

The most convenient yeast is compressed yeast which is always reliable and can be obtained in most grocery stores.

In Bible times they used to keep a little of their dough in an earthen vessel from one time to another. This sour dough was used for yeast in bread making. My mother used this kind of yeast. Sometimes in the early days we would go to a brewery and for two pennies we would get nearly a two-quart pail full of yeast. This yeast was just the same as the Fleischmann's yeast today, only it was in liquid form.

Bread Raising

A proper place for bread to rise when you make your own bread is of great importance in order to have good bread and have it good every time. I have at different times just taken an ordinary, clean drygoods box and put some shelves in it, and made a door through which I could put my big bread pan. Then I made a place below the lower shelf where I could set a lighted lamp with a little dish of water above it to keep this box an even temperature. You can put in a large dish of hot water, or heat some soapstones or bricks wrapped in a piece of paper or cloth for the purpose of maintaining an even temperature. There must be considerable space between these soapstones and the first shelf upon which your bread is set. In such a compartment the sponge can be raised as well as the bread after it is put in pans. In this way you can have good bread every time, because a proper place for raising the bread is very important.

However, I have found a common oats sprouter, made of galvanized iron, very convenient. This may be easily obtained, as they are sold everywhere, also by Sears, Roebuck and Company and Montgomery Ward and Company. This has a hot water tank over a lamp which can be regulated to get an even temperature to raise bread. This is a very valuable device to have in any household and it will pay for itself in a short time. You can use this to make malt, and you can use it in sprouting different grains and legumes for table use. It is very valuable and indispensable for success. Of course, anyone handy with a saw and hammer can make a wooden box, as previously described, to serve the purpose.

Often people have bread standing around on the table somewhere and it gets too cold while it is rising. I never advise that bread be set to rise all night, unless the proper yeast cannot be secured, and where a slow and long process of rising is made necessary on account of the yeast.

Put enough yeast in the bread to cause it to rise in two or three hours. The first time the bread should rise high enough just before it falls so that when it is touched it will go down. Should it happen that it rises so much that it falls, it is necessary that it be kneaded and allowed to rise again before it is put in the pans. After it is in the pans, it should rise half its size before it is put in the oven. If the bread rises too much while in the pan it will be coarse and full of holes. Should it accidentally rise too high, mold it over and let it rise again.

Whole wheat flour bread must not be permitted to rise as light in the pans as white flour bread. Care in this respect will preserve in the bread that sweet, nutty, wheat flavor which is so characteristic of bread made from the entire grain, but which will be lacking if the loaves rise too light in the pans.

Make it a business to have good bread, and do not give up until you do. Be determined, and say like many others have said, "I can make anything that anyone else can."

Some years ago I held a food demonstration in one of the Southern States. A Southern woman who attended one of these demonstrations had never made a loaf of bread in her life. All she had ever learned to make was soda and baking powder biscuits. She learned to make some very fine bread in only a single lesson. I furnished the flour, so I knew it was entire whole wheat flour. The first batch she made did not turn out very well, for the sole reason that the oven was not hot enough. The second batch was very fine. After one learns how, it is very easy to make good bread.

If you will only be determined to have good bread, with a little experimenting you will succeed. I know a twelve-year-old girl who bakes delicious bread.

The Oven

It is very important that one have a good oven in order to make good bread. I have many times found ovens in which the side of the bread nearest the fire box would burn, and sometimes it would burn on top, and sometimes it would burn on the bottom. This can be remedied to some extent in most of the ovens. If the bread does not bake evenly on the top, side, the bottom, there is something wrong with the oven. If it burns too quickly on the side where the fire is, you can take the grate out of the firebox, spread a layer of fire clay next to the oven, or put asbestos paper behind the grate. If it burns on top, you can put ashes on the top, and if it burns on the bottom, you can lay a piece of asbestos or a piece of tin on the bottom of the oven. Often if a piece of wire fencing with small mesh is placed on the bottom, a little bit of air space being left between the pan and the bottom of the oven prevents the burning of the bread on the bottom. If it does not bake enough on the bottom, it is evident that there is soot and ashes there and the stove needs cleaning out.

For whole wheat bread the oven heat should be 450° F., gradually being reduced from 350° to 300° F. It is well to have an oven thermometer, which you can find for sale in any bakers' supply house, and at both Sears, Roebuck and Company and Montgomery Ward and Company. The price is around $1.50 to $2.50. If you have no thermometer, the oven should be hot enough so the bread will begin to brown in fifteen minutes.

Be sure your oven is hot enough. If it is not, your bread will not be good. After the bread is thoroughly heated, reduce the oven temperature, for after the bread is partly dry if the same temperature were kept, it would burn it on the outside. Therefore, the temperature should be gradually reduced from 450 to about 350 degrees, then at last to about 300 or less. Bake your bread thoroughly, allowing at least an hour to one and one-quarter or one-half hours in the oven.

Old Fashioned Clay Oven

Anciently, and even to this day, before the iron stove came into existence, people baked bread in various ways. Sometimes they baked on the hearth of a fireplace, sometimes between two hot stones, and then they made ovens from clay, and sometimes they baked it in hot ashes, and toasted ears of corn upon the coals. They made ovens of clay and straw something like the Egyptians made brick.

My parents had one of these ovens. It was made like this: We built a platform about two and a half feet high of two-inch thick lumber—the one we had was about five feet wide and six or seven feet long—these boards were heavily covered with clay mixed with cut straw, then one layer of brick laid over them so it left a very smooth and nice surface on top. Then an arch from wooden slats was built over that. The arch was about two feet in height in the center. The back was closed except for a short chimney, and this was covered with a small piece of tin to hold the heat after the fire was taken out of the oven. The arch was covered with two or three layers of clay mixed with cut straw, and a door was left in front through which the oven was fired, and also for putting in and taking out of the bread. After the oven was all finished a slow fire would be started in it which would dry out the clay. After the clay was dried about so far, the fire would be increased, and it would burn this clay into brick in much the same way as bricks are made.

Then when we wanted to get the oven ready for bread making, a fire was made in this oven. When the bread was ready to go into the oven, all the coals and fire was raked out and the oven cleaned off. Many times the bread was put right on the brick, but we usually put it in pans and baked it the same as the people are doing nowadays in other ovens. This oven baked lovely bread with a beautiful crust. We generally arranged the fire so we could leave the bread in the oven from an hour to an hour and a half.

It would be great blessing if every home had an oven of this kind and people made their own bread today.

The finest bread may be made in this kind of an oven, because it bakes just right. The oven should be hot enough so that in fifteen minutes the bread will begin to brown. Then allow the heat to gradually diminish, as it naturally would in the clay oven, as the fire was all taken out of this oven. The ovens can also be made so there is a little fireplace on the front which opens into the oven, with a chimney on the opposite side. Then you can fire while you are baking.

Use of Steam in the Oven

It is much easier to get a good crust on bread without burning it if there is steam in the oven. This may be accomplished by placing a small pan of water in the oven. Some of the big bakers which have chain ovens bake bread under 900 degrees heat in 20 to 25 minutes with considerable steam in the oven to keep the bread from burning.

Importance of Bread

Bread is the most important health food. "There is more religion in a loaf of good bread than many think." (*Ministry of Healing,* page 302). Properly baked bread made from the right material, whole grain flours, has been the staff of life from the earliest history of Bible times, and has always been one of the principle foods that God gave to man; but it has indeed been made the staff of death by the modern inventions of milling baking.

God never intended that the wheat and other grains should be seperated in different parts, put out as a wonderful invention, and then sold for a big price. It is indeed an invention to destroy both soul and body. Untold harm is done by the baked stuff which is found on the market today.

From the earliest time a great deal of unleavened bread was used—more than leavened bread. The bread that Abraham's wife baked for the strangers, which were angels, was unleavened bread, for it took her just a short time to make this bread. In the sacrificial offering no leavened bread was ever used. Leaven was looked upon as a symbol of sin (Luke 12:1). If leaven or yeast of any kind is used in bread, it needs to be thoroughly baked so that the yeast germ is entirely destroyed.

Lately yeast has been much advertised to be eaten raw as a stomach remedy, but yeast should never be eaten unless it is first cooked. Yeast is highly nourishing and a wholesome product when it is cooked until the yeast germ is destroyed. The analysis of yeast is just the same as the analysis of Vegex, which is sold for such a high price on the market.

In recent times the fad has arisen claiming that no one should eat bread after he is thirty-five or forty years old. This advice is correct for most of the bread that is sold on the market, for it should not be eaten by anyone at any time. However, one can live on whole wheat bread, whole rye bread, whole barley bread, with vegetables or fruit added.

Oats also make a very excellent bread. Very delicious bread can be made by taking part whole wheat flour, whole corn flour, whole oats flour, and whole soybean flour. Add a little malt honey or karo syrup. This will make a bread that anyone could live and work on by eating just a little fruit with it. (Look in Table of Contents under "Bread Recipes" for recipe.)

All the grains before they are ripe, when they are in the milky state, can be eaten raw, as they are then in the grape sugar state and are like the sugar that is found in thoroughly ripe fruit. After the grain ripens it turns to starch, and the human system has no fluid to digest raw starch properly to make good blood. Animals have different fluids than man and can digest raw starch.

The baking process is very similar to the ripening of the fruit on the tree. The sun and the air gradually change the fruit from starch to grape sugar. When bread is put in the oven, it goes through the same process. The prolonged baking gradually changes the starch to a large extent into grape sugar, thus making it fit for digestion; or in other words, puts it in a form so the digestive fluids can properly act upon it and make good blood.

The baking process is instituted by God Himself to prepare the grains and starchy foods so they can be eaten by man and properly nourish him and make good blood.

Most of the baked stuff on the market is baked just enough to stand up, but not enough to kill the yeast germ, nor is it baked enough so that the starch is changed so it can be easily digested.

Fruit is the opposite of grains. Before it is ripe, fruit is in the starchy state and unfit to eat, but after it ripens in the sun it turns to grape sugar, is ready for assimilation and requires very little digestion.

Zwieback

No bread is entirely dextrinized, or turned into grape sugar; therefore zwieback or twice-backed bread, in which this process is completed is very wholesome and very easy to digest. A good way to make zwieback is to slice the bread about one-half inch thick, and let it dry out in the sun, or in a slow oven, until it is entirely dry.

I have kept zwiebach an entire year in fine shape in a common barrel lined with heavy brown paper. During this time there was a long period of wet weather, and it seemed as if the zwiebach had gathered a little moisture, but there was not a trace of mold; I put it outdoors on paper in the sun and let it dry out thoroughly again, and after it had been heated in the oven, it was just as good as when it was freshly made. I did this for experimental purposes.

Zwiebach should be made an important part of our diet, and if rightly handled, will save a great deal of time and expense. I have at times, when I was not in a position to bake my own bread, had some bakery make twenty-five, fifty, and even a hundred up to four hundred loaves of good, whole wheat bread, after my own recipe, for myself and neighbors. The bread can be sliced evenly and dried out in an oven, or better out-of -doors in the sun, until it is perfectly dry. Then heat the oven and brown slightly on both sides. Use for breakfast or lunch time. To make an excellent lunch, serve it with fruits, or fruit juices, soybean milk or malted nut cream. Use it any way you like, but make it a practice to have a large supply of zwiebach on hand.

Combination of Grains and Legumes
in Breads

In Bible times they used to combine different grains and legumes and make them into bread. "Take thou also unto thee wheat, and barley, and beans, and lentils, and millet and fitches, and put them in one vessel, and make thee bread thereof. . . ." (Eze. 4:9)

A number of seeds have been used in bread since Abraham's time and are still used by the Germans and others, such as caraway, gimmel, annis, rue, fennel, and dill. All of these have medicinal properties. They all are good for indigestion, and prevent fermentation. For gas and colic, rue was quite frequently used, even by the priests in Christ's time. It has a wonderfully quiet, soothing effect upon tired and weary brains.

People would do well today if they would use more of these things instead of the abundant luxuries which destroy both soul and body.

Bread Baking in Bible Times

In early Bible times when ovens were rare, sometimes a number of women would bake their bread in one oven, as in Leviticus 26:26, where ten women baked bread in one oven. All along down from ancient times until late years, bread, legumes and fruit seemed the main diet. Anciently bread, raisins and figs were used a great deal. Abigail carried two hundred loaves of bread, one hundred clusters of raisins, and two hundred cakes of figs with some other things to David. (1 Samuel 25:18)

Bread Recipes

There are many good bread recipes that can be found in almost any cookbook. Leave out the harmful ingredients and use only those which are wholesome.

Where these recipes advise grease or oils of any kind, use a little raw peanut butter, which is very rich in oil, and for the sweetening use malt sugar or Karo syrup which enriches the bread, gives it a very excellent flavor, and keeps it moist.

Whole Wheat Bread

3 cups warm water
1 cake compressed yeast
2 tablespoonfuls Karo Syrup
7 cups whole wheat flour
1 tablespoonful salt

Dissolve the yeast in a little lukewarm water, add the liquid, and mix all the ingredients to a medium soft dough. Turn out on a board slightly floured, and knead until elastic to the touch; then return to a bowl, cover, and let stand in warm room to rise until, when tapped sharply, it begins to sink. This takes about two hours. Work down well, turn over in the bowl, and let rise again one-half its size; then mold into loaves and put into pans for baking. Let rise until half again its original bulk, then bake in a good oven. Bake at least one hour or longer. These coarse breads must be watched closer during the rising than those made from white flour, as they get light in much less time. When taking bread from the oven, sponge it off with a cloth which has been dampened in cold water. Set it in a draft if possible, turn over so that it will cool off quickly, and the crust will be brittle and tender. If desired, it may be sponged off with a cloth saturated in oil.

Soybean or nut milk, however, may be used in place of water to improve bread.

Rye Bread

1 cake compressed yeast
3 cups lukewarm water

5 cups rye flour
1 cup sifted white flour
1 tablespoonful salt

The white flour should be flour strong in gluten. It should be the same as that used when making washed gluten for nut foods.

Dissolve the yeast in lukewarm water. Add two and one-half cups rye flour, or enough to make a sponge. Beat well. Cover and set aside in a warm place, free from draft, to rise for about two hours.

When light, add the white flour, the rest of the rye flour, or enough to make a soft dough, and the salt. Turn on a board and knead, or pound it five minutes. Place in bowl, cover, and let rise until it doubles in bulk. This takes about two hours.

Turn on board and shape into long loaves. Place in shallow pans, cover, and let rise again until light—about one hour. With a sharp knife cut lightly three strokes diagonally across the top, and place in oven. Bake in slower oven than when making white bread. Caraway seed may be used if desired.

Note.—By adding one-half cup of sour dough, left from a previous baking, an acid flavor is obtained which is considered by many a great improvement. This should be added to the sponge. My mother made nearly all her bread from sour dough, saved from previous baking, both rye and whole wheat. As nearly as I can remember now, she would save about a pint of dough from her baking and keep that until the next baking. It would be sour enough to start the yeast germs. Then she would work the bread the same as directed.

Rye bread can be worked much the same as whole wheat bread. Rye flour does not contain as much gluten as wheat, and therefore it does not rise as light as whole wheat flour without the addition of wheat flour strong in gluten. I have made a splendid rye bread with ninety pounds of rye flour and ten pounds of strong white gluten flour. Seventy-five pounds of whole rye flour and twenty-five pounds of whole wheat flour, strong in gluten, will make a splendid rye loaf.

Whole Wheat Raisin Bread

1 cake compressed yeast
1 cup lukewarm water
1 teaspoon salt
1 cup raw peanut butter
4 tablespoons mineral oil
6 cups whole wheat flour
¾ cup malt honey, malt sugar or Karo syrup
1 cup raisins

Dissolve the yeast in one cup lukewarm water. Add two cups of flour, also the ¾ cup of malt honey, and beat until smooth. Cover and set aside to rise in a warm place, free from draft, until light, which will take about one and one half hours.

When well risen, add raisins well floured, the rest of the flour, or enough to make a moderately soft dough, and the remainder of the ingredients. The raw peanut better should be dissolved in a cup of lukewarm water. If the dough is too soft, add a little more flour, and the next time use less water.

Knead lightly. Place in well-greased bowl, cover, and let rise again until double in bulk—about one and one-half hours. Mold into loaves, fill well greased pans half full, cover, and let rise until light—about one hour. Bake for from one hour to one and one-quarter hours.

Steamed Graham Bread

3½ cups of Graham flour
2 cups cornmeal
3 cups nut milk
1 cup malt honey or Karo syrup
1 teaspoon salt

Mix the nut milk, salt, and malt honey together; then mix the cornmeal and flour, and stir into the liquid. Put into basins, or empty cans under five pounds steam pressure, and steam for two and one-half or three hours. Then you can put it in the oven and brown it a little for fifteen minutes.

Soybean Bread No. 1

2 lbs. whole wheat flour
1 lb. soybean mash or ½ lb. soybean flour
1 cake compressed yeast
1 pint luke-warm water
½ cup malt sugar or Karo syrup
Salt to taste

Take two pounds fine whole wheat flour and one pound soybean mash, after the milk is taken out; or in place of the mash, ½ pound soybean flour may be used. If this does not make it stiff enough, add a little more flour.

Dissolve one cake of compressed yeast in a little luke-warm water, and add one pint of water. Also, a half cup of malt sugar should be added, and salt to taste. Mix this with the flour and mash to make a fairly stiff dough, about the consistency of regular bread dough.

Let it rise to about double its size in a warm place. Then knead it down and lap it over toward the inner side. Turn it over and let it rise again to about half again its size. Then knead it down, mold into loaves, put in pans, letting it rise to about double its size. Bake in a hot oven, about 450 degrees. It should begin to brown about fifteen minutes after placing in the oven. Bake the bread thoroughly; this gives it a good flavor, and makes it easy to digest.

Soybean Bread No. 2

3 lbs. Whole Wheat flour—finely ground.
1 lb. Soybean Meal (out of which the milk has been washed)

Mix this together and work it as in Bread No. 1
About 2 or 3 tablespoonfuls of malt honey added to the water will add very much to the flavor and value of the bread, giving it a deep nutty flavor. As the malt extract is high in diastase, which aids in the digestion of starch, to use malt extract would make the bread still better.

This bread, made into zwieback, thoroughly dried out until it is a light golden brown, diabetics can eat, because the starch has been changed into grape sugar. The zwieback is excellent for anyone to eat.

Health Gems or Crackers

Gems for those suffering with Bright's disease, diabetes, liver or kidney troubles may be made as follows:

Take whole wheat flour and put it in a pan on the stove. Stir it frequently with a wooden paddle until it is very slightly golden brown or what we call dextrinized.

Take two cups of the whole wheat flour, one cup of soybean flour, one cup of boiled spinach, or half a cup of powdered spinach, and add peanut milk, made from raw peanut butter. To make the peanut milk, mix raw peanut butter into a cream with water to the consistency of thin cream or cow's milk.

Beat the batter just thick enough so it will drop from a spoon, and salt to taste. If you wish to make a cracker, more flour will need to be added, roll it out to any thickness you want, and cut it to any size you desire. This makes a most wonderful product, either as a cracker or a gem. Carrots may be used in place of spinach. Two tablespoonfuls of malt honey or Karo syrup.

If products are not sweet enough, use more sweetening.

Soybean Buns or Cinnamon Rolls

4 cups whole wheat flour
1 cup soybean meal
½ cup soybean butter as given in this book
1 cup water or soybean milk
2 cakes compressed yeast

To the whole wheat flour and the soybean meal, add the half cup of soybean butter for shortening. Put in enough yeast so that the dough will rise in two or three hours. Mix down, turn over and let rise to half again its size. Now shape into the size of buns that you like and let rise to about half again their size. Bake from twenty to thirty minutes, according to the size of the buns.

Unleavened Bread

Unfermented or unleavened bread is made light by the introduction of air into the dough or batter. This is done by means of beating the batter breads, and kneading the dough breads.

Unleavened Gems

To make unleavened bread with any kind of meal, the whole thing in a nutshell is this:

Have your water and nut milk as cold as possible for gems or muffins, salted to taste. You can add a little soybean butter, a little malt honey or Karo syrup if you desire. Have your gem pans sizzling hot, and have your batter just stiff enough so that it will drop from the spoon. Place in the oven and bake. This will make a very palatable bread.

Cornmeal Gems

1 cup cornmeal
1 cup whole wheat flour
1 cup soybean milk
2 tablespoons oil
1 teaspoon salt

Take the milk, oil and salt and place in a bowl. Now beat the flour into this mixture. The ingredients should be cold as described above, and your iron gem pans sizzling hot. Bake in quick oven.

Oatmeal or Soybean Gems

1 cup cornmeal
1 cup whole wheat flour
1 cup oatmeal or soybean meal
1½ cups milk
3 tablespoons oil
1 teaspoon salt

Follow directions for making cornmeal gems.

Potato or Carrot Gems

2 cups whole wheat flour
1 cup mashed Irish potatoes, sweet potatoes, or mashed carrots
1 cup milk
3 tablespoons oil
Salt to taste

Follow directions for making cornmeal gems.

In place of the oil in the three foregoing recipes, soybean butter may be used instead, as it makes a better product, because the oil is emulsified and this renders it more easily digested.

Soybean Gems

½ lb. soybean mash (out of which soybean milk has been washed)

½ lb. dextrinized cornmeal (Put the meal in a large baking pan in the oven, and stir frequently with a pancake turner or a wooden paddle, until it gets a golden brown. Do not have the oven too hot as the meal should not be burned.) This turns the starch into dextrose and makes it palatable and easy of digestion.

½ cup soybean milk or water.

Mix the mash and the dextrinized cornmeal with the soybean milk. Salt to taste. Pour them in hot cast-iron gem pans and bake for 20 minutes in a hot oven.

This makes a very wholesome gem, one that diabetics can eat.

This mixture, made thin enough with more milk added, may be poured out in dots on a pan, as drop cookies and baked in a quick oven.

Pones

⅓ lb. cornmeal
⅓ lb. whole wheat flour
⅓ lb. oatmeal flour
1½ cups soybean milk or water
2 tablespoons malt honey or Karo syrup

Mix together all the ingredients. Have batter cold and pans hot, also oven hot. Bake thirty minutes, more or less, depending on the heat of the oven.

Beaten Biscuit

2 cups whole wheat flour
½ cup soybean butter
2 tablespoonfuls Karo syrup
⅔ cup soybean milk
Salt

Put your flour into a bowl, add the milk, then the soy bean butter and salt. Mix into a stiff dough as you would in making ordinary bread. Beat with a rolling pin or any heavy stick. This beating is done to make the biscuit tender and mellow.

Make into sticks or roll about one-half inch thick and cut in sizes to suit your taste. This can be rolled still thinner and made into a cracker if you like. Prick with a fork to keep it from blistering. Bake in a very hot oven to a light brown.

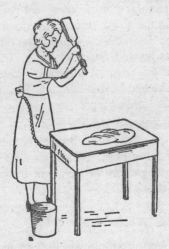

THIS WOMAN IS BEATING THE DOUGH FOR BEATEN BISCUITS

This woman is making beaten biscuits. The table is made with a six-inch board nailed to the legs, eighteen inches wide, and two feet long. Then I put a bottom on it, and filled it with cement, and made it smooth on top. It can also be made out of heavy planks. The club in her hand was made from a two by four, about three feet long. She has a piece of dough on the table beating it, she keeps folding it over and over, and repeating the folding and beating. After it has been well-beaten, about 10 or 15 minutes, make it into little biscuits, or cut it thin into little crackers or sticks, and when it is baked long enough to be thoroughly dextrinized it will be mellow enough to melt in your mouth. It makes one of the finest, most easily digested breads that can be made, without any shortening, baking powder, soda, or yeast. But a little shortening may be used, such as soybean butter, as given in this book, if you wish to use shortening. They are called old fashioned beaten biscuits. When I had a food factory, I made these old-fashioned beaten biscuits, and ran the dough through the dough brake about 20 or 30 times. It was then called a very fine article of food, by those who understood crackers. This would also make very fine pie crust. Always use whole wheat flour to make old fashioned beaten buiscuits. This makes a very fine bread for the Lord's supper.

In beating the dough, beat it until it is flattened out, then fold over and beat some more, continuing this way until the process has been repeated at least twenty times or more, depending upon the weight of the beater and the vigor put into beating it.

Whole Wheat Crisps

Take one pound of whole wheat flour and five ounces of raw peanut butter, made into a milk by dissolving in about half a pint of water. Stir the flour into the raw peanut butter milk, and salt to taste. Make the dough stiff enough so it can be rolled. This makes a lovely cracker.

It can be improved by adding to your milk about two big tablespoonfuls of malt honey or Karo syrup. This is a complete food and very palatable.

These crisps may also be made from raised dough. Make the dough as for bread. Take a scant pint and a half of water, and a half pound of malt honey or Karo syrup and about four ounces of raw peanut butter. Make the peanut butter into a milk, and set the sponge as for bread. Use for this amount about one cake of compressed yeast. When it has risen as for bread, knead it and work it into thin rolls. Prick them with a fork so they will not blister, cut into strips and bake in the oven until brown. This makes a very delicious cracker.

These recipes may be divided or multiplied, according to the size of the batch you desire to make.

PIES

Unleavened Pie Crust

1 cup whole wheat flour
1 cup zwieback bread crumbs
1 cup soybean flour or soybean mash
2 tablespoons Crisco or Kloss' mayonnaise
Water or soybean milk

Roll the zwieback bread crumbs with a rolling pin or run through a grinder. To the flour, crumbs and soybean flour or soybean mash, add the Crisco, cutting the shortening into the flour. Add the water or soybean milk, making a stiff dough so it can be rolled and placed in pie tins. After it has been placed in a tin, place another tin inside of the dough and bake to a light brown before putting in the filling. After placing the filling in the crust, bake in a moderate oven for about twenty minutes.

This crust may be used for any kind of a pie filling.

Raised Pie Crust

>   whole wheat flour
>   soybean flour or soybean mash
>   malt sugar
>   warm water
>   yeast cake

Dissolve the yeast cake in the warm water and add the melted Crisco and malt sugar. Now add the whole wheat flour and soybean flour or soybean mash. Mix the same as bread dough and let rise for an hour or more in a warm place. When it has risen, knead down and let rise ten or fifteen minutes before rolling out. Then roll out thin and put in pie tins, allowing it to rise about fifteen minutes.

Soybean Pumpkin Pie

>   1 cup dry mashed pumpkin
>   2 cups hot soybean milk
>   2 tablespoons fine zwiebach crumbs
>   ⅓ cup malt sugar, malt honey, or bee honey
>   ½ teaspoon, or less, of almond flavoring
>   A few grains of salt

Heat the milk. While the milk is heating, mix the zwiebach crumbs, sugar, salt, and stir them into the mashed pumpkin. Mix thoroughly and add the hot milk. Add seasoning. Pour into a crust and bake in a moderate oven until set.

The crust for this kind of pie should have a built-up edge.

Instead of vanilla and almond flavoring, nutmeg and cinnamon may be used.

Fig Marmalade Pie

1 cup figs
1 cup pitted dates
1 cup raisins
1 cup Sooth-O-Lax
3 cups soybean milk

Mix and run together through a food chopper. The holes in the plate of the mill should be quite fine so as to make the fruit fine as it is much easier to digest in this manner. Reduce the thickness of the fruit with soybean milk to the right consistency. Turn this filling into a raised pie crust, directions for which are given in the foregoing recipes, and bake for 15 to 20 minutes in a moderate oven. No top crust is needed for this pie.

About two teaspoons of agar-agar may be added to the cold milk, soaked for a short time, and then boiled before adding to the fruit. This will help to thicken the filling.

Vanilla may be added for seasoning, or, if desired, a teaspoonful of cocoa may be added, which gives the pie a very different flavor.

If the crust is about as thick as the filling, it makes a very nice pie. This makes a very healthful pie and one that would make an excellent school lunch for children. It is something they will like and which will nourish as well as satisfy them.

This pie filling may be prepared without the raisins. It may also be made with pitted dates alone, making a very sweet pie.

The old-fashioned turnovers may be made with this filling.

Grapes and Grape Juice

I have experimented with grape juice a great deal having gratifying results. The combining with a nut milk, about half and half, quickly furnishes the system with new blood of the purest kind. In anemia it is an excellent remedy.

Much of the grape juice found on the market is not good because it is adulterated. But there are good grape juices on the market that are pure and unadulterated, which is good medicine. The best way is to make your own, drinking it immediately after it has been squeezed, then you know it is pure and you lose nothing of the flavor or food value. If it stands any length of time after being squeezed it does lose something of the flavor and food value. The same rule applies to all fruit juices; drink at once after squeezing; if left standing, they undergo a change. You can also can your own fruit juices.

The very best way is to eat the grapes fresh from the vine when they are in season. A grape diet for a week or so is beneficial to the system. I have known people who thrived on eating the entire grape, skin, seeds, and all. But those who have weak digestion, and others with whom this would not agree, should not swallow the skin or seeds.

In cancer cases grape juice is particularly recommended. Or make a grape drink as follows: two-thirds grape juice, one-third water, adding a heaping teaspoonful of soybean flour. This is very nourishing.

Lemons

The medicinal value of the lemon is as follows: It is an antiseptic, or is an agent that will prevent sepsis or putrefaction. It is also anti-scorbutic, the term meaning a remedy which will prevent disease and assist in cleansing the system of impurities. The lemon is a wonderful stimulant to the liver and is a dissolvent of uric acid and other poisons, liquifies the bile, and is very good in cases of malaria. Sufferers from chronic rheumatism and gout will benefit by taking lemon juice, also those who have a tendency to bleed, uterine hemorrhages etc.; rickets and tuberculosis. In pregnancy it will help to build bone in the child. We find that the lemon contains certain elements which will go to build up a healthy system and keep that system healthy and well. As a food, we find, owing to its potassium content, it will nourish the brain and nerve cells. Its calcium builds up the bony structure and makes healthy teeth.

Its magnesium, in conjunction with calcium, has an important part to play in the formation of albumen in the blood. The lemon contains potassium 48.3, calcium 29.9, phosphorus 11.1, magnesium 4.4. Lemons are useful in treating asthma, biliousness, colds, coughs, sore throat, diptheria, la grippe, heart burn, liver complaint, scurvy, fevers, and rheumatism.

For diptheria, use pure lemon juice every hour or oftener if needed, either as a gargle or swab the throat with it and swallow some, until it cuts loose the false membrane in the throat.

For sore throat, dilute lemon juice with water and gargle frequently. Dilute one-half lemon juice, with one-half water, but it is still better to use it full strength.

A slice of lemon bound over a corn overnight will greatly relieve the pain.

A slice of lemon bound on a felon will not fail to bring the pus to the surface where it can be easily removed.

To relieve asthma, take a tablespoonful of lemon juice one hour before each meal.

For liver complaint, the juice of a lemon should be taken in a glass of hot water one hour before breakfast every morning.

To break up la grippe, take a large glass of hot water with the juice of a lemon added, while at the same time have the feet in a deep bucket or other vessel of hot water (Have the water deep enough so it comes almost to the knees.) with mustard added to it. Keep adding hot water as the patient can stand it for about 20-30 minutes, or until the patient is perspiring freely. Be sure there is no draft on the patient while this is being done. Patient should be near the bed so he can get in bed without moving around, thereby avoiding any danger of getting chilled. If it is convenient, a full hot tub bath would be good in place of the foot-bath. The lemon water should be taken every hour until the patient feels all symptoms of the cold gone.

A teaspoon of lemon juice in half glass of water relieves heartburn.

Lemon juice is an agreeable and refreshing beverage in fevers, where the bowels are not ulcerated.

For rheumatism, one or two ounces of lemon juice freely diluted, should be taken three times a day, one hour before meals, and at bed time. In cases of hemorrhage, lemon juice diluted and taken cold as possible will stop it.

Scurvy is treated by giving one to two ounces lemon juice diluted with water every two or four hours.

In excessive menstruation the juice of three or four lemons a day will help check it. Best to take the juice of one at a time in a glass of cold water.

The question may be asked: "How can one with an inflamed or ulcerated stomach partake of the juice? Would not a strong acid like that of the lemon act as an irritant?"

That would depend on how it was taken. If in quantity —yes: but to take it very weak at first (diluted with water), it will eventually cease to burn. The sufferer afflicted with ulcerated stomach has to use great perseverance to effect a cure, and it can be cured if care and patience is used.

The gastric juice in the stomach is four times as strong as lemon juice.

I wish that humanity would understand the real value of the lemon and learn to make a real medicine of it.

It should be especially remembered that it is a wonderful remedy for colds, la grippe, and all kinds of fevers.

ALWAYS TAKE WITHOUT SUGAR.

Lemon juice will sour sweet milk, suitable for cooking. Add a few drops, or a small teaspoonful to each cup of milk. The addition of one teaspoon lemon juice to a quart of very hot soybean milk, will make it curd—to make soybean cheese.

Lemon juice is excellent to take the place of vinegar; use just as you would vinegar.

The addition of a little lemon juice, and some of the grated lemon rind, adds greatly to the flavor of dried fruits, figs, prunes, peaches, etc. Add while stewing.

Household Uses

To bleach linen or muslin: Moisten with lemon juice and spread in the sun.

For the hands: After washing dishes, and to remove vegetable stains, rub the hands well with lemon juice; it will keep them white and soft; will also remove the odor of fish or onions.

To remove ink stains, iron rust, or fruit stains, rub the stain well with lemon juice, cover with salt, and put in the sun. Repeat if necessary.

Chapter XXXV

Oranges

The orange is one of nature's finest gifts to man. Orange juice contains predigested food in a most delicious and attractive form, ready for immediate absorption and utilization. The amount of food value contained in a single large orange is about equivalent to that found in a slice of bread. But orange juice differs from bread in that is needs no digestion, while bread, before it can be used for energizing and strengthening the body, must undergo digestion for several hours. A glass of orange juice is equivalent to a glass of milk. This is the reason oranges are so strengthening, and refreshing to invalids and feeble persons, as well as to those in health.

Orange juice is rich in salts, especially lime and alkaline salts, which counteract the tendency to acidosis. In such violent diseases as scurvy, beri-beri, neuritis, anemia, or any morbid condition in which the tissues are bathed in acid secretions, the alkaline mineral salts of fruits (fresh), will greatly benefit. The orange, lemon, and grapefruit are invaluable.

Orange juice has a general stimulating effect on the peristaltic activity of the colon. Orange juice should be taken one hour before breakfast.

In fevers, orange juice is perfectly suited to all requirements. Four to six quarts of liquids should be taken daily to relieve and quench the fever's fire, and eliminate poisons through the skin and kidneys, as fever is only nature's effort to rid the body of accumulated poisons. Fruit acid satisfies thirst, and the agreeable flavor of oranges, lemon juice, and other fruit juices make it possible for the patient to swallow the amount of liquid needed.

During the time of the severe epidemic of influenza, this country suffered following the World War, a doctor published in a paper that if the people would use quantities of orange juice, fever would be allayed and the patient would recover. He extolled the value of orange juice. It was found by practical experience that it would bring results. This caused the price of oranges to jump from $3 and $4 per case to between $18 and $25. This price jump caused the growers and shippers much alarm as they feared they would be prosecuted for raising prices, when in fact, they were not to blame, it was simply the increased demand. It so happened that it was just between seasons for oranges, and the supply was small in the States, so they offered all they had on hand to the government, and then the hospitals, but were not accepted as the officials of the food commission said that due to the small supply it would not be worth while, and it was better to let the individuals have the use of them, those that could afford them, as they would not go far in large institutions. But there was a great lesson in it for the people; if they would only use fruit juices in all fevers, what a blessing it would be to mankind.

Orange juice is indispensable in feeding bottle-fed babies. The use of orange juice will often prevent scurvy, pellagra, rickets, and infantile paralysis.

The acid of the orange and the sugar it contains aids digestion, and also stimulates and increases the activity of the gastric glands.

Oranges are capable of serving more useful purposes in the body than any of the other juicy fruits. The sweeter the orange the greater its food value.

As people become better educated in dietetics, oranges will be much more freely used and appreciated.

Orange Cleansing Diet

Drink from five to eight glasses of orange juice daily. Take during the time of the diet a high enema every night, herb enemas preferable, especially if there is any colon or intstinal trouble. It is also excellent to take slippery elm in connection with this, as slippery elm is very cleansing, nourishing, and healing to all the mucous surfaces in the body.

After taking the orange juice from five to ten days, eat a very plain, simple, and nourishing diet. This would improve anyone's health. If the person who wishes to take a cleansing diet is undernourished and weak, and feels that a little something else is necessary, eat apples, masticating them thoroughly. Also a few nuts might be eaten.

If troubled with skin diseases of any kind, boils, carbuncles, etc., a most wonderful treatment would be to take eight or ten oranges per day, and three or four glasses of sanicle tea per day. Take the tea after the orange juice has left the stomach, an hour or so. Take a high herb enema every evening for eight or ten days with white oak bark. This would bring results beyond all expectation.

CHAPTER XXXVI

POTATOES; GATHERING AND PRESERVING OF HERBS

We hear so much about mashed potatoes not being good to eat. It is true that the ordinary mashed potatoes which are eaten everywhere is a very unwholesome product. When potatoes are peeled, boiled, and then mashed with a large piece of butter, or other fat, they become unwholesome food. When potatoes are peeled, there is practically nothing left but starch. The alkaline part of the potato is cut away, when they are peeled, and the starch is acid forming.

I must not fail to mention that the eyes and the peeling of the Irish potato contains its life-giving properties. When the skin of the potato is not eaten, the best part of it is lost. Also, when the skin is baked too brown, the life-giving properties are destroyed.

A baked potato is the ideal way of cooking potatoes, but it must be properly baked. When properly baked the skin should be a little crisp, but not too dark brown, or black. Before putting potatoes in the oven to bake, after they have been thoroughly scrubbed, prick with a fork all over; this causes some of the moisture to evaporate, and helps to make them dry and mealy.

Another excellent way to prepare potatoes is to steam cook or pressure cook them. All vegetables may be excellently prepared in the steam pressure cooker under a low temperature, as the original food flavors are then preserved in an economical way. They can still be improved by placing them in an oven and allowing them to dry out for a few minutes. Many who have found it impossible to eat potatoes, prepared in other ways, are able to eat them prepared in this way.

Mashed Potatoes

Select the dry, mealy variety of potato, such as, Idaho, for instance. Wash them thoroughly and boil or steam until they are thoroughly done. Steaming is best. When done, peel the outer thin skin off, being careful not to remove the eyes. Mash, add rich soybean milk and salt to taste. Bake for twenty minutes in a hot oven.

Gathering and Preserving of Herbs

It must be understood that wide experience and knowledge of herbs is needed to successfully gather and preserve them. It is a study of a lifetime. Lack of knowledge in gathering and preserving herbs may render them of little or no medicinal value. Knowledge of soil is also necessary. Plants grown in virgin soil will contain far greater medicinal value than those grown on poor soil. The same plant grown in different localities will show a great difference in the amount of curative properties they will yield. There is a difference between cultivated plants and those growing in their natural wild state. For instance, the dandelion growing wild has rare medicinal properties, which are almost entirely lost when the plant is cultivated. Wild herbs are more effective for use in medicines than those grown in the garden.

Gather herbs only in dry weather, preferably when the plant is in full bloom, or the seeds getting ripe.

Barks.—The barks should be taken when the sap is rising in the spring. Shave off the outer rough part, then peel the inner part from the trunk of the tree. To dry, put in the sun for a short time (if desired), then complete the drying in the shade. Be sure they are thoroughly dry. If there is any moisture left in them when they are put away, they will mold.

Roots.—Dig up the roots either in the spring when the sap is rising, or in the late autumn, after the sap has gone down. Slice and dry the roots (in the shade), tie up in small bundles and put in the attic or some place where they are sure to be kept dry.

Flowers, seeds, and leaves should be gathered when they are in their prime, gathering only the perfect ones. These should also be dried in the shade. When thoroughly dry, put in heavy brown paper bags.

Do not preserve herbs in glass, as sometimes the glass sweats, and if any moisture comes in contact with the herbs they will become moldy.

When any barks, roots, or other herbs are thoroughly dried and kept dry, they will retain their medicinal value for years.

The bark, roots, flowers, seeds or leaves may all be dried for a short time in the sun, but always complete the drying process in the shade, as too much exposure to the sun tends to lessen the medicinal value. They may be dried entirely in the shade in an airy place. The only thing gained by putting them in the sun for a short time is hastening the drying process.

PERSONAL OBSERVATIONS

Here are a number of conditions that I have seen with my own eyes. One person who was very fleshy had almost three inches thick of pure fat. The colon in some parts was three or four times its natural size, but in some parts it had shrunk to the size of a finger and in other places until it was almost impossible for anything to pass through. The small intestines had shrunk in some places to the size of a lead pencil, with a heavy hard growth on the outside. Only a very small portion of the intestine was of natural size. The spleen was very much enlarged, and the stomach hung far down in the intestines. The kidneys were enlarged and very flabby, the lungs were much enlarged and almost black; and the liver was enlarged and hard.

In another case, the lungs and liver were very much enlarged and almost as hard as a rock. The colon and small intestines were also much enlarged although in some places they had shrunk so that almost nothing could pass through. The stomach was enlarged and flabby and hung far down out of its place. The kidneys were spongy; and the whole intestinal tract was out of its regular order.

In another case, the liver was very much enlarged. Over and around it were tumors, from the size of a small marble to that of a small potato. The heart was very much enlarged, very flabby, and in each lobe was a bunch of pure fat the size of a small potato. Both the colon and small intestines were very much enlarged, with pockets in various parts filled with hard fecal matter.

There was another case where the intestines had shrunk very much, with pockets in various parts of the colon; and the entire intestines were full of small growths. There were little hard growths under the skin over his entire body, from the top of his head to the soles of his feet.

Another case was one that was mere skin and bones. The liver was almost entirely eaten away, with just a little fibrous slush left; and the whole intestines were deformed. There was not a drop of blood in the whole system, and the body was full of pus and slime.

Some cases, where the X-ray revealed that the colon was full of deformities and that it and the stomach hung far down in the intestines, are alive and after treatment are getting along fairly well so that they are up and working.

One case had a colon shrunken in several places. In other places there were big pockets, and the rectum was full of hard growths. Through an operation the small places were cut out and the colon sewed together. The patient got well enough to be up and working, and to have normal bowel movements.

I could go on and tell of many more cases, but these suffice to illustrate what I say. All of these examples lived largely on foods that had been robbed of their life-giving properties, and ate mixtures that could not make good blood but cause only suffering. If you live as outlined in this book, it will prevent an untold amount of suffering and premature death.

One finds no such irregularity in the body of the animal creation. The animals eat their food as God has prepared it for them. Man has spoiled the food in its preparation, has robbed it of its life-giving properties. If man would eat the food as God has made it, his body would be symmetrical and beautiful and healthy.

"Lo, this only have I found, that God hath made man upright; but they have sought out many inventions." Ecclesiastes 7:29.

Man has made many inventions that are good and very useful, but many also which destroy both soul and body.

Who is she that goeth forth as the morning—fair as the moon, clear as the sun, and with banner floating above her? —The true healing art.

Whence art thou?—I come from nature.

What art thou?—Herbs, water, food, pure air, sunshine, exercise, and rest.

Where art thou going?—On the wings of the morning to the ends of the earth.

What is thy commission?—To go to every physician and nurse and whosoever will, to restore many families, prevent much suffering and premature death, and wipe the tears from many eyes.

Speed on thy flight, thou message of health and joy.

AUTHOR

———————

... If there is any uncertainty whatever as to the seriousness of a condition, one should seek competent medical assistance.

... The information in this book concerning any material or product may not be used in promoting the sale of such material or product.

PRAYER

Unanswered yet? Faith cannot be unanswered.
Her feet were firmly planted on the Rock;
Amid the wildest storms she stands undaunted,
Nor quails before the loudest thunder shock.
She knows Omnipotence has heard her prayer,
And cries, "It shall be done," sometime, somewhere.

Unanswered yet? Nay, do not say ungranted;
Perhaps your part is not yet wholly done.
The work began when your first prayer was uttered,
And God will finish what He has begun.
If you will keep the incense burning there,
His glory you shall see, sometime, somewhere.

—*Robert Browning.*

INDEX

ABSCESSES, herbs for treatment of, 339.

Aches, herbs for treatment of, 338.

Acidosis, how to correct, 385.

Adenoids, herbs for, 338.

Adulterated foods, 62; effects of, on the body, 62.

Ague, herbs for treatment of, 338.

Aloes, 197.

Alterative, water used as, 122.

Aluminum utensils, 89.

Angelica, 198.

Anemia, herbs for treatment of, 339.

Anise, 199.

Anodyne, water used as, 121.

Antispasmodic tincture, 274, 382.

Antispasmodic use of water, 121.

Apoplexy, herbs for treatment of, 339.

Appendicitis, causes, symptoms, and treatment of, 386.

Appetite, herbs used to improve, 338.

Apple tree bark, 200.

Arthritis, causes, symptoms, and treatment of, 536.

Asthma, causes, symptoms, and treatment of, 388; diet for, 389; herbs for, 339, 389.

Astringent, herbs used for, 338; water used as, 121.

BACKACHE, herbs for treatment of, 341, 356, 511.

Baking powder, 74.

Balm, 200.

Balomy, 200.

Basil sweet, 201.

Bathing, rules for, 124; sickroom, 150.

Baths: 124; ear, 131; electric light, 127; eye, 130; foot, 128, how to give Turkish, without a cabinet, 126; leg, 128; nose, 131; tub, 128; Turkish, 126.

Bay leaves, 203.

Bayberry, 201.

Bed, how to make a, 149.

Bed sores and chafing, causes and treatment of, 449; herbs for treatment of, 340.

Bed-wetting, causes and treatment of, 442; herbs for treatment of, 340.

Beech, 203.

Bethroot, 204.

Beverages: bran broth, 604; bran water, 604; cereal coffee, 602, 603; herb broth, 605; herb drinks or teas, 606; oatmeal broth, 605; oatmeal water, 604; potassium broth, 606; soybean broth, 604; soybean buttermilk, 605; soybean coffee, 602; soybean milk, 611.

Beverages, herbs used as, 342.

Biliousness, herbs for treatment of, 340, 341.

Bisort root, 204.

Bitterroot, 205.

Bittersweet, 205.

Black cohosh, 206.

Bladder trouble, causes, symptoms, and treatment of, 497, 563, 564; herbs for treatment of, 339.

Blanket pack, 137.

Bleeding, herbs for treatment of, 341.

Blood, impure; causes, symptoms, and treatment of, 501; herbs for cleansing, 340.

(673)

KIDNEYS and kidney stones, treatment of, 355, 507.
Kloss's granola, 599.
Kloss's mayonnaise, 629.
Kokofat, 590.
LA GRIPPE, causes, symptoms, and treatment of, 504; herbs for treating, 356.
Lame back, herbs for treatment of, 356.
Lavender, 252.
Laxative, foods good as, 79; herbal, 355, 380; water used as, 121.
Lemons, household uses of, 661; medicinal value of, 658.
Lentils, to sprout, 609.
Leprosy, causes, symptoms, and treatment of, 509; herbs for treatment of, 356.
Leucorrhea or whites, herbs for treatment of, 357.
Lily of the valley, 252.
Liniment, herbal, 218, 221, 379; how to make, 380.
Liquor habit, treatment for, 357, 512.
Liver, herbs for treatment of, 356.
Lobelia, 253.
Lobelia compound, 259.
Lockjaw, herbs for treatment of, 356.
Loss of speech, herbs for treatment of, 357.
Lumbago, causes and treatment of, 511; herbs for treatment of, 356.
Luncheon, 572.
Lung fever, causes, symptoms, and treatment of, 510; herbs for treatment of, 356.
Lungs, herbs used in treating, 356.
Lungwort, 281.
MAGNOLIA, 281.
Malt honey, 598.
Malted nut cream, 589.
Malted nuts, 590.
Mandrake, 282.
Marjoram, 282.
Marshmallow, 283.
Massage, 139: for constipation, 143; Swedish, 141; to abdo-

men, 140, 142; to arms, 140, 141; to back, 140, 142; to chest, 140, 141; to legs, 140, 142.
Masterwort, 283.
Mayonnaise, Kloss's, 629; nut, 630; soy oil, 628.
Measles, herbs for treatment of, 357; symptoms and treatment of, 517.
Meat-eating, 70.
Medicine, history of, 45.
Menstruation, 357, 358, 514.
Milk, cow's, 75; how to curd, 612; nut, 590; soybean, 605, 611.
Milk sweetening, 631.
Milkweed, 284.
Mineral salts, 76, 78; use of, 78.
Mineral water, 109.
Minerals, diseases caused by a deficiency of, 63; foods which supply, 77; found in body, 162.
Mint, 284.
Mistletoe, 284.
Mock almond butter, 592.
Motherwort, 285.
Mouth, causes and treatment of sore, 544.
Mucous membranes, herbs for treatment of, 358.
Mugwort, 285.
Mullein, 286.
Mumps, symptoms and treatment of, 516.
Muscles, strained, causes and treatment of, 542.
Mustard, 287.
Myrrh, 288.
NASAL TROUBLE, herbs for treatment of, 358.
Nausea, causes and treatment of, 522; herbs for treatment of, 358.
Nervousness, causes and treatment of, 419; herbs for relieving, 359.
Nettle, 288.
Neuralgia, causes, symptoms, and treatment of, 521; herbs for treatment of, 359.

(680)

(682)